Handbook of Sports Medicine and Science
Basketball

WITHDRAWN

088743
Aberdeen College Library

IOC Medical Commission
Sub-Commission on Publications
in the Sport Sciences

Howard G. Knuttgen PhD (Co-ordinator)
Boston, Massachusetts, USA

Harm Kuipers MD, PhD
Maastricht, The Netherlands

Per A.F.H. Renström MD, PhD
Stockholm, Sweden

Handbook of Sports Medicine and Science
Basketball

EDITED BY

DOUGLAS B. McKEAG

MD, MS
American United Life Professor of Preventive Health Medicine and
Chairman, Department of Family Medicine
Director, IU Center for Sports Medicine
Department of Family Medicine
Indiana University School of Medicine
Indianapolis, IN
USA

ABERDEEN COLLEGE
GORDON LIBRARY
WITHDRAWN

Blackwell
Science

© 2003 by Blackwell Science Ltd
a Blackwell Publishing company
Blackwell Science, Inc., 350 Main Street, Malden, Massachusetts 02148-5018, USA
Blackwell Publishing Ltd, 9600 Garsington Road, Oxford OX4 2DQ, UK
Blackwell Science Asia Pty Ltd, 550 Swanston Street, Carlton South, Victoria 3053, Australia
Blackwell Wissenschafts Verlag, Kurfürstendamm 57, 10707 Berlin, Germany

The right of the Author to be identified as the Author of this Work has been asserted in accordance with the Copyright, Designs and Patents Act 1988.

All rights reserved. No part of this publication may be reproduced, stored in a retrieval system, or transmitted, in any form or by any means, electronic, mechanical, photocopying, recording or otherwise, except as permitted by the UK Copyright, Designs and Patents Act 1988, without the prior permission of the publisher.

First published 2003

Library of Congress Cataloging-in-Publication Data

Basketball / edited by Douglas B. McKeag.
        p. cm. — (Handbook of sports medicine and science)
   ISBN 0-632-05912-5
   1. Basketball injuries.   2. Basketball—Physiological aspects.   I. McKeag, Douglas, 1945–   II. Series.
RC1220 .B33 B375 2003
617.1′027—dc21   2002152649

ISBN 0-632-05912-5

A catalogue record for this title is available from the British Library

Set in 8.75/12pt Stone by Graphicraft Limited, Hong Kong
Printed and bound in India by Replika Press Pvt. Ltd.

Commissioning Editor: Andrew Robinson
Production Editor: Nick Morgan
Production Controller: Kate Charman

For further information on Blackwell Publishing, visit our website:
http://www.blackwellpublishing.com

Contents

List of contributors

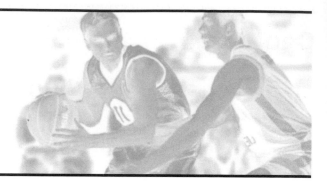

Eduardo Amy MD
Assistant Professor, Department of Physical Medicine, Rehabilitation and Sports Medicine, University of Puerto Rico, School of Medicine, PO Box 365067, San Juan, Puerto Rico 00936-5067

Enrique Amy DMD MDS
Director and Assistant Professor, Center for Sports Health and Exercise Sciences, Department of Physical Medicine, Rehabilitation and Sports Medicine, University of Puerto Rico, School of Medicine, PO Box 365067, San Juan, Puerto Rico 00936-5067

Leslie J. Bonci MPH RD
UPMC Center for Sports Medicine, 3200 S. Water Street, Pittsburgh, PA 15203, USA

Christopher M. Carr PhD
Methodist Sports Medicine Center, 201 Pennsylvania Parkway, Suite 200, Indianapolis, IN 46280, USA

Jill Cook PhD BAppSci (Phy)
Musculoskeletal Research Centre, School of Physiotherapy, La Trobe University, Victoria, 3086, Australia

Kevin B. Gebke MD
Assistant Professor of Clinical Family Medicine, and Fellowship Director, IU Center for Sports Medicine, Department of Family Medicine, Indiana University School of Medicine, 1110 W. Michigan Street, LO-200, Indianapolis, IN 46202-5102, USA

Jay R. Hoffman PhD
Department of Health and Exercise Science, The College of New Jersey, PO Box 7718, Ewing, NJ 08628-0718, USA

Karim Khan MD PhD
University of British Columbia, Department of Family Practice (Sports Medicine) & School of Human Kinetics, 211/2150 Western Parkway, Vancouver, BC V6T 1V6, Canada

Thomas J. Mackowiak ATC
Breslon Center, Z-22, Michigan State University, East Lansing, MI 48824, USA

Douglas B. McKeag MD MS
American United Life Professor of Preventive Health Medicine, and Chairman, Department of Family Medicine, Director, IU Center for Sports Medicine, Department of Family Medicine, Indiana University School of Medicine, 1110 W. Michigan Street, LO-200, Indianapolis, IN 46202-5102, USA

William F. Micheo MD
Department of Physical Medicine, Rehabilitation & Sports Medicine, University of Puerto Rico, School of Medicine, PO Box 365067, San Juan, Puerto Rico 00936-5067

Andrew L. Pipe MD
University of Ottawa Heart Institute, 40 Ruskin Street, Ottawa, ON K1Y 4W7, Canada

Margot Putukian MD
Center for Sports Medicine, Penn State University, Department of Orthopedics and Rehabilitation, Hershey Medical Center, 1850 East Park Avenue, University Park, PA 16802, USA

Forewords by the IOC

The birth date of basketball is usually identified as 21 December 1891, with the first game taking place in Springfield, Massachusetts, USA. Through the years, interest in the sport has appeared in practically every country in the world and participation spread internationally.

The sport of basketball was first included in the Olympic Games as a full medal sport for men in 1936 and for women in 1976. Certainly one of the most popular sports internationally, basketball presently attracts great attention from fans and media around the world. The admission of professional basketball players to Olympic competition in 1992 has further enhanced the popularity of the sport and the quality of play internationally.

The editor and contributing authors of this Handbook have covered in detail all of the basic science, the clinical aspects of injuries and other health concerns, and the practical information useful for the medical doctors and health personnel who care for basketball teams and players. The editor and authors are to be congratulated on this excellent contribution to sports medicine/sports science literature.

My sincere appreciation goes to the IOC Medical Commission Chairman, Prince Alexandre de Merode, and to the IOC Medical Commission's Sub-commission on Publications in the Sport Sciences for yet another high-quality publication.

Dr Jacques Rogge
IOC President

Basketball is one of the most demanding sports included in the Olympic programme as regards the many skills involved, the requirement for explosive muscle power, and the necessary combination of aerobic and anaerobic conditioning. Additionally, participation in the sport of basketball involves a unique constellation of injury risks and related health problems. Therefore, the health and medical care of every basketball team and each individual player requires an unusual assemblage of knowledge and skill on the part of every health professional involved.

This Handbook not only presents basic scientific and clinical information, but the editor and authors address every aspect of the health and medical care of the participating athlete. This includes injury prevention, the special needs of unique groups, the immediate care of injuries, injury treatment and athlete rehabilitation.

Professor Douglas McKeag and his international team of contributing authors have succeeded in producing this outstanding volume for the Handbooks of Sports Medicine and Science series.

Prince Alexandre de Merode
Chairman, IOC Medical Commission

Foreword by the FIBA

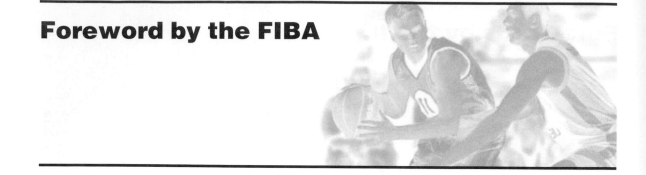

Among those who love the orange ball, the USA is widely regarded as the birthplace and the bastion of basketball. The sport, invented by James A. Naismith, has become a major Olympic event.

The last Men's World Championships organised in Indianapolis showed a universalisation of the quality of the athletes and the game being played. FIBA has 212 national affiliated federations and, one could consider, by including the huge number of Chinese, that the number of people practising the sport in the world is about 450 million.

The Handbook of Sports Medicine and Science on *Basketball*, which deals with players' health problems, is a wholly new and opportune book which will interest those responsible for the well-being of teams: doctors, surgeons, orthopaedists, trainers, chiropodists, psychologists and, one hopes, coaches. The authors have approached the preventive and curative aspect for all age groups. Professionalisation has grown enormously. In this aspect, the reader can find a collection offering solutions to technical pathology, a real sports medicine.

Citius, *Altius*, *Fortius* . . . Modern sport demands continuous self-improvement. To reinforce the intake and discharge of energy, specialists improve the fuel and the engine of the athlete. A well-balanced diet and muscle growth serve this purpose. The role of the doctor is to ensure that dangerous and prohibited 'supplementation'

methods are not used. The role of the doctor also consists of detecting, as much as possible, the risks induced by physical effort—preliminary medical examinations are a necessity at club and team level. Sudden death rarely strikes athletes and judges; however, it is our duty to evaluate this threat. The psychological aspect is also significant in the practice of basketball. The trainer is the provider of the right to participate. The dichotomic organisation of the game (five playing and five or seven watching them) has impacts on morale which interfere with motivation, performance and team spirit.

Naismith wanted a non-violent sport. Basketball does not have a reputation for being dangerous, but the injury rates are not declining: a phenomenon linked to the progression of athletic qualities and defensive toughness. A basketballer injures him/herself either alone or through contact, beneath the hoop most often. Sprained ankles are the most common accidents (around 30%), but new pathologies are appearing, in particular involving the arch of the foot—probably owing to repeated microtrauma, overuse by players or badly fitting shoes.

FIBA congratulates the IOC Medical Commission for publishing this indisputably useful Manual for the Basketball Family.

Jacques Huguet MD
President, FIBA Medical Council

Preface

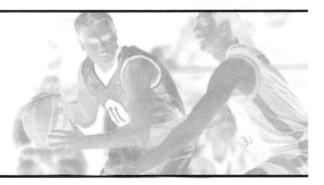

The perfect sport

I must have been around nine when it finally began to sink in. That is: why my brother smiled when he played, why my father smiled when he watched. At nine years old, it was just a game to me. I enjoyed playing it mainly because I enjoyed the socialization that took place with my friends. But to my father, it was like a beautiful choreographed dance. The slow motion that we so often see during televised games, he actually saw when he watched. He considered a successfully completed "pick-and-roll" play to be absolutely gorgeous. For the rest of my life as a high school and college basketball player it became apparent to me just what he was looking at—the perfect sport.

It is, by all measure, a contact sport, really more of a subtle collision sport in which no protective equipment is routinely worn. The player's expressions can be seen on a court much closer for spectators than most athletic contests. The muscle twitch that comes just before a quick move to elude a defender amply displays the biomechanical demands of a sport that requires an athlete to be able to run, jump, and exhibit upper and lower body strength, hand–eye coordination and most important, body control. This is also a sport that demands both aerobic endurance and anaerobic fitness—a sport that requires muscular proprioception and enhanced visual fields.

Basketball, when played right, is simply a beautiful thing to watch. This book, part of "The Olympic Handbook of Sports Medicine and Science" series attempts to present a sports-specific reference work for use by physicians, trainers and coaches for the care of their athletes. The demands of the sport create special problems for its players. Injuries and illnesses do occur. I have never seen a player yet who enjoys being injured or missing competition. The correct diagnosis and appropriate management in treatment of these injuries becomes of paramount importance to the athletes and teams they play for.

As editor of this volume, it was indeed an honor to work with the authors represented here. On the "world basketball scene", many of these names are familiar. Their work as reflected in this volume represents the most complete approach to the sport of basketball and its injuries yet published. I am proud to have edited this volume and want to take this opportunity to thank the authors for the excellence of their work. Thanks also to Howard G. Knuttgen who served as mentor in his role as overseer of the series and Julie Elliott and Nick Morgan, production editors at Blackwell.

My wish is that you find this book as interesting to use as I found it fun to put together. The entire world seems to have embraced this sport, it can only get better.

December 2002
Douglas B. McKeag, MD, MS
Indianapolis, Indiana

Dedication

This book is dedicated to my "basketball team",
  Di—point guard and play maker
  Kelly—shooting guard
  Heather—finesse forward
  Ian—power forward and re-bounder

Introduction

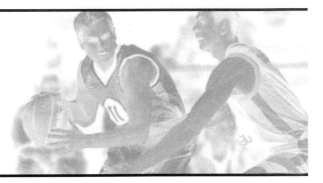

Basketball: how it began*

Basketball's origin is unique among world sports because it was actually invented.

Who: Dr James A. Naismith

When: December 21, 1891 at 11:30 a.m.

Where: The YMCA Training School located at the corner of State and Sherman in Springfield, Massachusetts

Why: *"The invention of Basketball was not an accident. It was developed to meet a need. Those boys simply would not play Drop the Handkerchief."*

Dr James A. Naismith

Dr Naismith was a young 30-year-old instructor at the Springfield YMCA Training School when he accepted a challenge from his boss, Dr Luther Gulick, to invent a winter game to be played indoors. Those "boys" referred to in his quote were a class of 18 rowdy future YMCA directors that two previous instructors had given up on.

Naismith had boasted that he could invent a sport. Now he had two weeks in which to accomplish this challenge before the first class. For 13 days he tried to adapt Rugby, Soccer, American Football and Lacrosse—all sports in which he excelled. This

---

* This history is written by Ian Naismith, grandson of Dr James A. Naismith. Ian is currently the Founder and Director of the Naismith International Basketball Foundation, headquartered in Chicago, Illinois. Phone: (312) 782-8470, Fax: (312) 782-8475.

failed because of possible injuries from physical contact.

The game started taking shape when he realized that the ball had to be passed or shot at some kind of goal without any running or walking which eliminated tackling. Next, he had to decide on a goal and decided on two 18-inch boxes at either side of the gym. Remembering a childhood game called "Duck on a Rock" where a rock had to be thrown in an arc at an opponent rock, he decided that he must elevate the boxes and put them on a horizontal plane so that the opposing team could not surround them.

Now, with the fundamentals in place, he worked late into the night and drafted the 13 "Original Rules" (see Fig. 1 on pages xii and xiii).

"The first game of Basketball was played in my bed the night before the first class."

Dr James A. Naismith

Dr Naismith woke up in the morning and hurried to the Secretary, Mrs Lyons. Mrs Lyons was asked to type the "Rules" while he went to the Janitor, Mr Stebbins, to locate boxes. Mr Stebbins told Dr Naismith that he did not have any 18-inch boxes, but that he had two peach baskets in the basement. Naismith and Stebbins nailed the peach baskets to the lower track railing of the gym—which happened to be exactly ten feet from the floor. The height of the basket today is still ten feet. Just think, we could all be playing "Box Ball"!

Then, at 11:30 a.m. on December 21, 1891, James pinned the two typed sheets of the "Original Rules" to the bulletin board. The first game of Basketball

Basket Ball.

The ball to be an ordinary Association   foot ball.

1. The ball may be thrown in any direction with one or both hands.

2.   The ball may be batted in any direction with one or both hands (never with the fist).

3.   A player cannot run with the ball, the player must throw it from the spot   on which he catches it, allowance to be made for a man who catches the ball when running at a good speed.

4.   The ball must be held in or between the hands, the arms or body must not be used for holding it.

5. No shouldering, holding, pushing, tripping or striking in any way the person of an opponent shall be allowed.   The first infringement of this rule by any person shall count as a foul, the second shall disqualify him until the next goal is made, or if there was evident intent to injure the person, for the whole of the game , no substitute allowed.

6.   A foul is striking at the ball with the fist, violation of rules 3 and 4, and such as described in rule 5.

7.   If either side makes three consecutive fouls it shall count a goal for the opponents (consecutive means without the opponents in the meantime making a foul).

8.   A goal shall be made when the ball is thrown or batted *into the basket* from the grounds and stays there, providing those defending the goal do not touch or disturbe the goal.   If the ball rests on the edge and the opponent   moves the basket it shall count as a

Fig. 1 The original 'Rules' of basketball, typed and corrected by James A. Naismith himself. Anyone with an appreciation of the sport will be interested in how basketball has evolved from its origins. Reprinted here with permission from his grandson Ian Naismith.

#2.

goal.

9.   When the ball goes out of bounds it shall be thrown into the field, and played by the person first touching it.   In case of a dispute the umpire shall throw it straight into the field. The thrower in is allowed five seconds, if he holds it longer it shall go to the opponent.   If any side presists in delaying the game, the umpire shall call a foul on them.

10. The umpire shall be judge of the men, and shall note the fouls, and notify the referee when three consecutive fouls have been made.   He shall have power to disqualify men according to Rule 5.

11.   The referee shall be judge of the ball and shall decide when the ball is in play, in bounds, and to which side it belongs, and shall keep the time.   He shall decide when a goal has been made, and keep account of the goals with any other duties that are usually performed by a referee.

12.   The time shall be two fifteen minutes halves, with five minutes rest between.

13.   The side making the most goals in that time shall be declared the winners.   In case of a draw the game may, by agreement of the captains, be continued until another goal is made.

*First draft of Basket Ball rules.
thing in the gym that the boys might
learn the rules - Dec. 1891 James Naismith
6-28-31.*

was played. There were nine men per side and the score was 1 to 0. Mr Stebbins stood on a ladder to retrieve the ball after a goal was made because nobody thought of cutting the bottom out of the baskets.

Basketball caught on like wild fire spreading across the country and overseas in a matter of months. Naismith credited the fact that the game was invented in the YMCA as a major factor. The students took the game back to their home towns and countries. Basketball was played in China in 1893 and the first women's game was played at the Springfield, Massachusetts YMCA in February 1892. Maude Sherman, James' future wife, played in the first women's game. Senda Bernenson introduced a modified version to the girls of Smith College in 1893.

The dribble was always in the game, according to James. When a player caught the ball, he had 15 seconds to shoot or pass. If he could do neither, they would drop the ball and catch it to restart the 15 seconds. Sometimes they would roll the ball on the floor and pick it up to restart the clock. This technique was called "Rollyball".

Dr Naismith invented the backboard not to bank the shots, but to protect the basketball from the fingers of the opposing fans that would deflect the ball from the goal.

If you were to see a basketball game played according to the 13 "Original Rules", the game would look much the same. Much has been added, but little taken away.

Dr Naismith was a lifetime member of the International Rules Committee and introduced the game to the Olympics in 1936, one of his proudest moments.

I often say that to understand Basketball, you have to understand Dr Naismith:

"I am sure that no man can derive more pleasure from money or power than I do from seeing a pair of basketball goals in some out of the way place deep in the Wisconsin woods an old barrel hoop nailed to a tree, or a weather-beaten shed on the Mexican border with a rusty iron hoop nailed to one end. These sights are constant reminders that I have in some measure accomplished the objective that was set years ago. Thousands of times, especially in the last few years, I have been asked whether I ever got anything out of basketball. To answer this question, I can only smile. It would be impossible for me to explain my feelings to the great masses of people who ask this question, as my pay has not been in dollars, but in satisfaction of giving something to the world that is a benefit to masses of people."

Dr James A. Naismith, 1939

Chapter 1
Epidemiology of basketball injuries

Jay R. Hoffman

Basketball is a sport that is generally not associated with a high risk for injury. This is likely a result from the primarily noncontact nature of the sport. When a player is on offense they often avoid contact by using their athletic skills (e.g., running, slashing and cutting movements) to free themselves for an uncontested shot. On defense the player is taught to use their athletic skills to defend the opposing player and prevent them from getting free. Although the rules of basketball discourage most forms of contact (e.g., illegal contact will result in a foul), close interactions occurring during picks and box-outs do allow some physical contact to occur. Nevertheless, the intensity at which the sport is played is increasing (see Chapter 2), and as a result contact is thought to be becoming a significant factor in the increase in the number of injuries reported (Zvijac & Thompson 1996).

Epidemiological studies on basketball injuries are quite limited. Often descriptions of basketball injuries are part of a larger study examining a multitude of sports without specific reference to any sport. The National Collegiate Athletic Association (NCAA) is perhaps the only organization that provides data on injuries for each specific sport through their injury surveillance system. No other major sports governing body provides similar information. Thus, data appear to be incomplete concerning injury patterns in professional or scholastic basketball athletes. In addition, the ability to compare injury patterns between countries may also be compromised by the relatively few studies published on injury patterns of basketball players outside of the

United States. Since playing styles may differ among countries the injury rates may be difficult to compare. This chapter will review the epidemiology of injuries in basketball. When possible, particular reference will be given to differences in injury patterns between different levels of play and between genders. In consideration of possible differences in the style that basketball is played today (i.e., higher intensity and a greater emphasis placed on strength and power development) compared to previous years (Hoffman & Maresh 2000), it was decided to focus this review on only studies published during the past decade.

Incidence of injury

Injury rate

The injury rate for basketball has been difficult to ascertain due to differences in the reporting methodology between studies. Some studies have reported injury rate as a function of the number of total injuries divided by the total number of participants, while others have computed injury rate as a function of 1000 athlete exposures. An athlete exposure has been defined as one athlete participating in one practice or contest where he or she is exposed to the possibility of injury (NCAA 1998). In addition, many examinations of basketball-related injuries have focused on the occurrence of a specific injury (i.e., anterior cruciate ligament injuries) and did not report the injury rate inclusive of all other injuries.

A recent study examined over 12 000 high school basketball players for 3 years (Powell & Barber-Foss 2000). These investigators reported an injury rate of 28.3% and 28.7% in both male and female athletes ($p > 0.05$), respectively. Other studies performed during this past decade on high school basketball players have reported injury rates ranging from 15% to 56% (DuRant et al. 1992; Gomez et al. 1996; Messina et al. 1999). Although several studies have been unable to demonstrate any significant difference in the risk for injury between males and females (Kingma & Jan ten Duis 1998; NCAA 1998), others have shown that females are injured at a frequency that is more than twice that of males in high school basketball (33% vs. 15%, respectively) (DuRant et al. 1992).

At the collegiate level the injury rate for male and female intercollegiate basketball players has been reported to be 5.7 and 5.6 injuries per 1000 athlete exposures, respectively (NCAA 1998). The data collected during this investigation were from the NCAA Injury Surveillance System (ISS). The ISS was developed to provide data on injury trends in NCAA sports and records injuries from a random sample of NCAA Division I, II and III institutions. In this system an injury was defined as an incident resulting from participation in either a practice or game that required medical attention by the team's trainer or physician. In addition, the athlete's participation in performance was restricted by one or more days beyond the day of injury. The ISS has been the most comprehensive report to date that has detailed injury patterns among intercollegiate athletes.

The injury rate during intramural basketball for college-age recreational basketball players (8.2 injuries per 1000 player-games) appears to be slightly higher than that seen for competitive intercollegiate players (Barrett 1993). The better physical condition of the intercollegiate athletes is likely a major factor attributing to the lower injury rate. In another study reporting on the injury rate in recreational basketball players in the United States, 6.2% of the participants were reported injured during community center basketball competition (Shambaugh et al. 1991). In comparison, a 5-year retrospective study on sports-related injuries in the Netherlands reported an even lower injury rate (2.3%) for basketball

(Kingma & Jan ten Duis 1998). The studies on recreational basketball have been unclear concerning gender-based differences in injury occurrence.

Injury rate comparing practice vs. games

Most injuries appear to occur during practice rather than games in organized competitve basketball. In college athletes, between 62% and 64% of the injuries reported in men's and women's basketball occur during practices (NCAA 1998). In high school basketball players, between 53% and 58% of the injuries reported occurred during practice for both males and females (Powell & Barber-Foss 2000). In contrast, other reports have suggested that basketball injuries occur more often during games (Yde & Nielsen 1990; Backx et al. 1991; Gutgesell 1991). For example, Gutgesell (1991) has reported that 90% of the injuries occurring during recreational basketball are seen during games, although this would be expected when one considers the limited number of practices common in recreational basketball.

When injury rates are expressed relative to hours or exposures to practice and games it appears that games do present a higher risk for injury than practice (Backx et al. 1991; NCAA 1998). In high school basketball players the injury rate during practice has been reported to be 1 per 1000 h, while the injury rate during games was reported to be 23 per 1000 h (Backx et al. 1991). Similarly, when expressed relative to 1000 athlete exposures collegiate male and female basketball players were injured during practice at a rate of 4.5 and 4.7 per 1000 athlete exposures, respectively (NCAA 1998). During games the injury rate for college basketball players increased to 10.2 and 9.3 per 1000 athlete exposures for men and women, respectively (NCAA 1998). These results are depicted in Fig. 1.1. The higher rate of injury seen during games is likely related to the greater levels of intensity, competitiveness and contact that occur in games compared to practices. Nevertheless, athletes that participate in competitive basketball (either at the scholastic or collegiate levels), in which practices are an integral and regular part of the program, may be injured more frequently during practices primarily because there are considerably more practices than games.

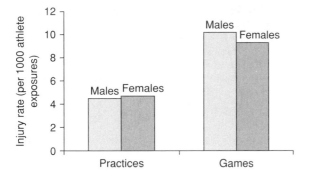

Fig. 1.1 Injury rate (per 1000 athlete exposures) Comparisons between men and women NCAA college basketball players during games and practices. (Data from NCAA 1998.)

Injury characteristics

Types of injury

Sprains appear to be the most common injury in both male and female basketball players at all levels of competition (Paris 1992; Gomez *et al.* 1996; Kingma & Jan ten Duis 1998; Messina *et al.* 1999; Powell & Barber-Foss 2000). Sprains have been reported to range between 32% and 56% of the total injuries reported. In gender comparisons women appear to suffer more sprains than men. In collegiate basketball players sprains account for 34% of the injuries in females and 32% of the injuries in male players (NCAA 1998). At the high school level sprains account for 56% of the injuries in the female basketball player and 47% in the male player (Messina *et al.* 1999). Strains, contusions, fractures and lacerations account for the majority of the other injuries common to both male and female basketball players. The range in the occurrence of these injuries can be seen in Table 1.1.

Injury location

The anatomical location of basketball-related injuries can be seen in Table 1.2. The results for the college athletes represent the three most common locations for injuries reported for NCAA basketball players. The lower extremity appears to be the area

Table 1.1 Common basketball injuries across level of play and gender. (Data from Gomez *et al.* 1996, Kingma & Jan ten Duis 1998, Messina *et al.* 1999, NCAA 1998, Powell & Barber-Foss 2000.)

	% Occurrence
Sprains	32–56
Strains	15–18
Contusions	6–20
Fractures	5–7
Lacerations	2–9

most frequently injured in either gender and across various levels of competition. Further examination of the lower extremity shows that the ankle is the most common area of injury followed by the knee. There does not appear to be any gender effect on the occurrence of ankle injuries. However, differences in the occurrence of knee injuries between males and females seen in Table 1.2 are consistent with a number of studies suggesting that females are at a greater risk for knee injuries than male athletes (Arendt & Dick 1995; Arendt *et al.* 1999; Gwinn *et al.* 2000). Above the lower extremity the wrist and hand are the most frequent sites of injury. For the remainder of this section discussion will focus on studies that have examined basketball-related injuries to specific anatomical locations.

Head

Injuries to the head do not appear to occur as frequently as those seen in both the upper extremity (shoulder, elbow, wrist, and hand) and lower extremity (hips, knee, ankle, and foot). The occurrence of mild traumatic brain injury (MTBI) in high school basketball players was examined for 3 years in 114 high schools as part of the National Athletic Trainers Association injury surveillance program (Powell & Barber-Foss 1999). A MTBI was identified and reported if the injury required the cessation of a player's participation for initial observation and evaluation of the injury signs and symptoms before returning to play. In addition, any facial fracture or dental injury was also recorded as an injury. Results revealed that MTBIs comprised 4.2% and 5.2% of

Table 1.2 Comparison of injuries by anatomical location in both men's and women's basketball (reported as percentage of total injuries).

| | High school | | | | College | | Recreational |
	Males		Females		Males	Females	Males and females
Reference:	a	b	a	b	c	c	d
Number of injuries:	1931	543	1748	436			525
Head							
Skull	–	3%	–	3%			3%
Face	10%	11%	7%	5%			5%
Upper extremity							
Shoulder	2%	4%	2%	3%			39%
Elbow							
Wrist/hand	11%	12%	10%	10%			
Spine/trunk							
Neck	11%	–	12%	–			2%
Back	–	6%	–	6%			
Ribs	–	<1%	–	1%			
Lower extremity							
Pelvis/hip/groin/thigh	14%	10%	16%	9%	6%		51%
Knee	11%	10%	16%	20%	10%	18%	
Ankle	39%	32%	37%	31%	25%	23%	
Foot	–	4%	–	5%	–	6%	

a, Powell & Barber-Foss (2000); b, Messina *et al.* (1999); c, NCAA (1998); d, Kingma & Jan ten Duis (1998).

the total injuries reported in males and females, respectively. The injury rate for MTBIs in male high school players was 0.11 per 1000 athlete exposures and 0.16 per 1000 athlete exposures in the female athlete. Most MTBIs appeared to occur during games for both male (63%) and female (68%) basketball players. An injury rate of 0.06 and 0.07 per 1000 practice exposures was seen in male and female basketball players, respectively, while the injury rates during games were 0.28 and 0.42 per 1000 game exposures in male and females, respectively. The MTBI occurred most often as a result of a collision between two players. These collisions were reported to occur more often in the open court rather than underneath the basket where more contact is generally seen.

The time lost from participation as a result of an MTBI in both male and female high school basketball players can be seen in Table 1.3. Most head

Table 1.3 Time lost from participation as a result of a mild traumatic brain injury (MTBI). (Data from Powell & Barber-Foss 1999.)

Time lost (days)	Males (%)	Females (%)
<8	88.2	83.1
8–21	9.8	13.8
>21	2.0	3.1

injuries resulted in less than 8 days lost from participation in either gender. During the course of the 3-year study only one male and two female players who sustained a MTBI were unable to participate for more than 21 days following their injury. The occurence of head injuries is quite low in basketball compared to other sports (i.e., football, wrestling and soccer) (Powell & Barber-Foss 1999). Most often head contact is the result of an inadvertent action,

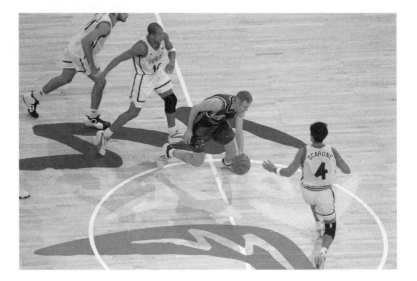

Fig. 1.2 Quick changes in direction can result in injuries to the knee. Photo © Getty Images/Jed Jacobsohn.

and not the result of a deliberate hit as seen in these other sports.

Upper extremity

As seen in Table 1.2 the hand and wrist are the most common upper extremity structures that are injured. The proximal interphalangeal (PIP) joint is the most frequently sprained and dislocated joint in the hand, with dorsal PIP joint dislocations being the most common subtype (Wilson & McGinty 1993; Zvijac & Thompson 1996). These generally occur as a result of hyperextension of the finger (Zvijac & Thompson 1996). Thumb metacarpal–phalangeal joint injuries are the next most frequent upper extremity injuries reported (Wilson & McGinty 1993; Zvijac & Thompson 1996); trapezial–metacarpal fractures and ulnar collateral ligament sprains are the most common injuries to this joint (Zvijac & Thompson 1996). The relative infrequency of upper body injuries when compared to the lower extremity in basketball is related to the nature of the sport. Generally, contact is only made during picks or box-outs in a nonaggressive manner. Typically these actions are performed to force the opponent to alter their direction or to get in a better position to grab a rebound. Rarely do these actions result in injuries that are commonly seen in more aggressive sports such as football or hockey.

Lower extremity

Studies examining the epidemiology of basketball injuries have been consistent in their findings that the majority of injuries sustained during basketball occur to the lower extremity (Zvijac & Thompson 1996; Kingma & Jan ten Duis 1998; NCAA 1998; Messina *et al.* 1999; Powell & Barber-Foss 2000) (Fig. 1.2). In recreational basketball players, injuries to the lower extremity account for 51% of the total injuries reported (Kingma & Jan ten Duis 1998). Injuries to the lower extremity in high school basketball players range between 56% and 69% of the total injuries recorded (Gomez *et al.* 1996; Messina *et al.* 1999; Powell & Barber-Foss 2000). Similar injury patterns are also observed for the college athlete (NCAA 1998). When examining gender differences it appears that females tend to have a greater percentage of lower extremity injuries than males. In the study of Powell and Barber-Foss (1999), 64% of the injuries observed in the male athletes were to the lower extremity, while in the female athlete 69% of the total injuries seen in that subject population was to the lower extremity. Likewise, Messina and colleagues (1999) reported that 56% of the injuries to male basketball players occurred in the lower extremities compared to 65% in the female players. These differences are likely related to the greater risk for knee injuries seen in the female athlete (Arendt

Table 1.4 Ankle structures most commonly injured during basketball. (Data from Sitler *et al.* 1994.)

	% Occurrence
Anterior talofibular ligament	66
Calcaneofibular ligament	17
Deltoids ligament	7
Posterior talofibular ligament	5
Syndesmosis joint	5

& Dick 1995; Arendt *et al.* 1999; Gwinn *et al.* 2000), and will be discussed in more detail later.

As seen in Table 1.2 ankle injuries are the most common injury seen in the basketball player, male or female. Sitler and colleagues (1994), in a 2-year study on a college intramural basketball program, showed that inversion sprains were the most predominant mechanism resulting in ankle injury, accounting for 87% of the total ankle injuries reported. Generally, these sprains (70% of all total ankle injuries) occurred as a result of contact with an opposing player (landing on the player's foot). The ankle structures most commonly injured can be seen in Table 1.4. The anterior talofibular ligament is the most common site of injury in the ankle, accounting for 66% of the total ligament injuries of the ankle.

Injuries to the knee are less common than ankle injuries in basketball. However, knee injuries are generally more devastating to the athlete because they are associated with a greater loss of playing time (Zvijac & Thompson 1996). Knee injuries have received a tremendous amount of attention over the last few years. This is a result of a clear difference in injury patterns between male and female athletes. With the increase in the number of female athletes participating in intercollegiate athletics since the 1970s (as a result of the passage of Title IX, which mandated equal sports participation for females), female athletes have been suffering knee injuries in a disproportionate number. In a 5-year study on NCAA College basketball players 12% of all injuries recorded for men were knee injuries, while injuries to the knee accounted for 19% of the total injuries in women (Arendt & Dick 1995). During this time period the knee injury rate for men was 0.7 injuries per 1000 athlete exposures, while for women it was 1.0 per 1000 athlete exposures. The knee structures that were injured can be seen in Table 1.5. The structure most frequently injured for the male athlete was the patella or patella tendon, while anterior cruciate ligament (ACL) and meniscus injuries were the most common in the female athlete.

The higher incidence of ACL injuries in female basketball players is a medical issue that has been seen in several studies in a number of different sports (Arendt & Dick 1995; Hutchinson & Ireland 1995; Arendt *et al.* 1999; Gwinn *et al.* 2000). Injuries to the ACL during basketball appear to occur with no apparent contact or collision with another player (77% of all cases including men and women) (Arendt & Dick 1995). The mechanism behind these noncontact injuries appears to be the same in both men and women. Planting and pivoting movements appear to be the primary mechanisms reported for noncontact ACL injuries. Table 1.6 shows the common mechanisms reported for ACL injuries during basketball. Injury occurs when the athlete lands in an uncontrolled fashion with their upper leg and hips adducted and internally rotated, their knee is extended or only slightly flexed and in a valgus position, and their tibia is externally rotated. Contact with the ground is made with the athlete not in

Table 1.5 Knee structures most commonly injured in the male and female basketball player. (Data from Sitler *et al.* 1994.)

Males		Females	
Injury	% Occurrence	Injury	% Occurrence
Patella or patella ligament	38	Anterior cruciate ligament	26
Collateral ligaments	31	Torn cartilage	26
Torn cartilage	20	Collateral ligaments	25
Anterior cruciate ligament	10	Patella or patella ligament	22
Posterior cruciate ligament	1	Posterior cruciate ligament	1

Table 1.6 Common mechanisms causing ACL injuries during basketball. (Data from Arendt *et al.* 1999.)

Mechanism	% Occurrence
Planting/pivoting	57.2
Hyperextension	12.3
Landing from a jump	12.2
Deceleration	12.2
Going up for a jump	4.1
Unsure	2.0

control or well balanced. The positioning of these anatomical structures upon landing is known as the point-of-no-return and is thought to be primarily responsible for the noncontact ACL injury common to the basketball player (Ireland 1999). The higher risk for ACL injuries seen in the female athlete compared to the male athlete has been attributed to both intrinsic factors (noncontrollable), extrinsic factors (controllable) or a combination of the two (Arendt & Dick 1995; Ireland 1999).

Intrinsic factors include lower limb alignment, intercondylar notch shape, joint laxity, ACL size, hormonal influences, and body weight (Bonci 1999; Heitz *et al.* 1999; Ireland 1999; Rozzi *et al.* 1999). Extrinsic factors include muscle strength and conditioning, skill level, playing experience, technique, shoes and field or court conditions (Bonci 1999; Ireland 1999; Gwinn *et al.* 2000). In addition, factors that may be considered a combination of both intrinsic and extrinsic factors such as neuromuscular activation patterns and muscle proprioception may also contribute to the risk for knee injury (Ireland 1999). A complete description of these factors is beyond the scope of this chapter. However, for further insight into the mechanisms that have been attributed to the increased incidence in ACL injury in the female athlete the reader should refer to the reviews of Bonci (1999) and Ireland (1999).

Injury severity

Time loss due to injuries

Most studies examining the epidemiology of basketball-related injuries have primarily reported on the incidence of injury and injury characteristics.

Table 1.7 Percentage of injuries resulting in seven or more days of time loss, or less than seven days of time loss in college basketball players. (Data from NCAA 1998.)

	Males	Females
<7 days	76%	70%
≥7 days	24%	30%

There have been far fewer reports on the severity of injuries. Powell and Barber-Foss (2000) have shown that most injuries occurring in male (75.5%) and female (72.1%) high school basketball players can be classified as minor. However, females were observed to have a higher proportion ($p < 0.05$) of major injuries (12.4%) in comparison to the male players (9.9%). The NCAA ISS has the most comprehensive report on time lost to injury. Table 1.7 shows the percentage of injuries that resulted in either seven or more days of time loss, or less than seven days of time loss, in both men and women collegiate basketball players. Injuries to either gender were normally associated with less than seven days of lost time from practice and games (≥70%). This proportion appears to be consistent over the duration of years (>10 years) that the NCAA has collected data. At the professional level the only report on time loss due to injury was observed in a study on meniscus injuries over a 6-year period in the NBA (Krinsky 1992). In this study there were a total of 38 meniscus injuries reported during this time. Fifty-eight percent of the injuries were to the lateral meniscus and resulted in an average (± SD) of 14.7 ± 9.6 practices missed and 15.0 ± 8.5 games missed. In comparison, injuries to the medial meniscus resulted in 18.4 ± 16.3 practices missed and 20.1 ± 18.9 games missed. The difference in the time lost between lateral and medial meniscus injuries was significant ($p < 0.05$).

Injury prediction

Structural measures as predictors of injury

Over the past 30 years there have been various studies that have examined a number of biomechanical and structural measures as potential markers for indicating increased risk for injury. The results of these studies, which primarily examined football players, have been inconclusive. In the past 10 years a couple of studies have examined the ability of different physical, biomechanical and structural features in the basketball player to predict injury risk (Shambaugh *et al.* 1991; Grubbs *et al.* 1997). The investigation by Shambaugh and colleagues (1991) followed 45 recreational basketball players during a season. They performed various measurements such as: bilateral anthropometrical differences (thigh girth, calf girth and the weight difference between right and left side of body), Q-angle, leg length inequality (short leg), range of motion of various lower extremity joints (e.g., ankle, subtalar, and midfoot), forefoot varus, and rearfoot valgus. During the study 15 injuries were recorded in 14 players. Based upon the injuries and the values obtained from their measurements the investigators developed a three-variable regression analysis using the variables weight difference, abnormal Q-angle left and abnormal Q-angle right. A formula was developed to provide an injury score:

Score = (weight imbalance × 0.36) +
(right abnormal Q-angle × 0.48) +
(left abnormal Q-angle × 0.86) − 7.04

For example, if a male athlete had a weight imbalance of 8.5 lb., a right Q-angle of 8.5° and a left Q-angle of 13° the formula would be calculated as such:

Score = (8.5 × 0.36) + (8.5 × 0.48) + (13 × 0.86) − 7.04
= 11.28

A positive score (anything above zero) would indicate that the athlete was at risk for injury. A negative score indicates that the athlete is at a reduced risk for injury.

This three-variable regression equation was shown to be successful in predicting injury with a 91.1% accuracy (Shambaugh *et al.* 1991). In a follow-up study of 11 NCAA Division III male basketball players reported within the same publication (Shambaugh *et al.* 1991), of the three players that tested with positive scores the player with the highest positive score was the only player to miss a game with an injury. Of the other two players with positive scores, one was hurt, but did not miss any games, while the

other was uninjured. This study demonstrated that structural asymmetry was able to discriminate injured from noninjured basketball players and that the use of such measures may be able to predict potential risk for injury. For players that are shown to be at a higher risk, manipulation, orthotics or special training can be incorporated to reduce the structural imbalance (Shambaugh *et al.* 1991).

A later study that examined the predictive validity of the above-mentioned equation was unable to duplicate those findings (Grubbs *et al.* 1997). In a study on both male and female high school basketball players Grubbs *et al.* (1997) showed a sensitivity of only 16.7% and a specificity of 66.1% for that predictive equation. There were several methodological differences between the studies that likely resulted in these conflicting results. In the initial study the regression equation was developed using male subjects only, while the second study utilized both male and female subjects. Differences between the genders on Q-angle (females reportedly have a larger Q-angle than males) could be a significant factor affecting the relationship between the structural variables and the incidence of injury. In addition, other differences in study design (i.e., definition of injury, age of the athletes, level of competition and length of the season) may make study to study comparisons difficult to perform.

The ability of structural or biomechanical variables to predict injury in basketball players is still inconclusive. However, structural symmetry may have a greater influence in overuse injuries secondary to repetitive microtrauma in sports such as running. In basketball most injuries are the result of a macrotrauma (i.e., landing on an opponent's foot, poor landing from a jump or a pivot shift) (Grubbs *et al.* 1997). Nevertheless, further research is still warranted to understand more clearly the relationship between structural factors and injury risk. If such a relationship can be established then effective intervention strategies can be employed.

Injury prevention

Shoes

As mentioned previously, ankle inversion injuries are the most common injury seen in basketball. It is thought that the ankle's susceptibility to injury is related to the position of both the ankle and foot (Johnson & Markolf 1983; Ottaviani et al. 1995). During plantar flexion it appears that changes in the orientation of the ligaments of the foot and ankle place the ankle in a position of vulnerability increasing the likelihood of injury (Johnson & Markolf 1983). In a neutral or plantar flexed position the peroneal muscles are responsible for supporting externally induced inversion activity. However if this rotational movement were not supported, injury to the anterior talofibular and calcanofibular ligaments would likely be seen (Ottaviani et al. 1995). The use of high-top basketball shoes are commonly used as an intervention to help prevent ankle sprains by providing additional support to the rotational movements occurring about the ankle joint (Shapiro et al. 1994; Ottaviani et al. 1995).

The ability of basketball shoe height to reduce incidence of ankle injury has been examined by several investigations (Garrick & Requa 1973; Barrett et al. 1993). In a study of 622 college intramural basketball players no difference in injury rate was observed between athletes wearing high-top sneakers compared to athletes in low-top sneakers (Barrett et al. 1993). One of the problems of that study was the low incidence of injury: 8.21 per 1000 player games. In addition, it is difficult to extrapolate the results of this study on intramural athletes to more competitive intercollegiate athletes, considering that the subjects in this study played 30-minute games and their season was only 2 months in duration. Games at the intercollegiate level are 40 min in duration, and the season typically lasts between 5 and 6 months. Fatigue within a game, or cumulative fatigue occurring during a season may impact on injury rate. In an earlier study of intramural basketball players by Garrick and Requa (1973), an injury rate between 30.4 and 33.4 injuries per 1000 player-games was reported. Players that wore high-top sneakers, or had their ankles supported by prophylactic taping, had a lower rate of ankle sprains than the athletes wearing low-top shoes.

Ankle stabilizers

Taping has been the traditional method used to prevent ankle injuries in athletes. As mentioned,

the study by Garrick and Requa (1973) showed a significant benefit of ankle taping as a prophylaxis against ankle injuries. However, concern has been addressed of the ability of taping to maintain its initial support with continued exercise. Reductions of up to 50% in support have been reported in football players during 2–3 h practice sessions (Furnich et al. 1981). This has led to the development of various ankle stabilizers (i.e., leather lace-up braces and semirigid orthoses made of thermoplastics and plastic polymers) that provide continued support during prolonged activity. The efficacy of ankle stabilizers was demonstrated in a study of 1601 college intramural basketball players over 2 years (Sitler et al. 1994). The use of a semirigid ankle stabilizer was shown to significantly reduce the incidence of ankle injury. In addition, subjects wearing the ankle stabilizer had a lower percentage of multiple ligament or grade II ankle injuries (18%) than did control subjects (37%). Although the results on reductions in the severity of injury were impressive, these differences did not reach statistical significance. This appeared to be related to the low statistical power of the injury severity data. Despite the positive results concerning ankle braces, athletes appear reluctant to endorse these products for fear that they may inhibit athletic performance (Burks et al. 1991; Paris 1992). Recent research has demonstrated that prolonged wearing (> 1 week) of ankle stabilizers does not appear to have any detrimental effects on performance (Pienkowski et al. 1995). Thus, it appears that some period of acclimation is needed while wearing the brace to maintain joint mobility and athletic performance, as well as gain acceptability by the athlete.

Strength and conditioning

The importance of strength and conditioning to the basketball athlete can be reviewed elsewhere (Hoffman & Maresh 2000) and in Chapter 2. Strength training appears to be able to reduce the incidence or severity of injury by increasing the strength of the tendon–muscle complex and increasing bone mineral density. In addition, an athlete who is in better condition will reduce his or her rate of fatigue, which will also reduce the stresses on the musculoskeletal system. However, there have not been any prospective studies performed to date on the effect that strength and conditioning has on the injury rate in basketball players. Future research should focus on this important avenue of research.

Conclusion

Differences in how injuries are reported have made it difficult to compare injury rates between different studies. The most comprehensive system to date is the NCAA ISS. From this data set it appears that the injury rate for male and female college basketball players are similar (5.6 and 5.7 injuries per 1000 athlete exposures, respectively). Most of these injuries appear to occur during practice. However, actual games present the highest risk for injury to the athlete. Ankle sprains are the most common injury seen in basketball, for either gender and across all levels of play. Women basketball players, however, do appear to be more susceptible to knee injuries (specifically ACL injuries) than male players.

Research still appears to be inconclusive concerning the ability of structural or biomechanical measures to predict risk for injury. Although the efficacy of ankle stabilizers has been demonstrated, it does appear that to reduce the risk for any decrement in performance and to enhance athlete acceptability a period of acclimation with the brace is needed. Finally, comprehensive studies on both scholastic and professional basketball players are warranted considering the paucity of data that exists at those levels.

References

Arendt, E. & Dick, R. (1995) Knee injury patterns among men and women in collegiate basketball and soccer. *Am J Sports Med* **23**, 694–701.

Arendt, E., Agel, J. & Dick, R. (1999) Anterior cruciate ligament injury patterns among collegiate men and women. *J Athletic Training* **24**, 86–92.

Backx, F.J., Beijer, H.J., Bol, E. & Erich, W.B. (1991) Injuries in high-risk persons and high-risk sports. A longitudinal study of 1818 school children. *Am J Sports Med* **19**, 124–130.

Barrett, J.R., Tanji, J.L., Drake, C., Fuller, D., Kawasaki, R.I. & Fenton, R.M. (1993) High- versus low-top shoes for the prevention of ankle sprains in basketball players. *Am J Sports Med* **21**, 582–585.

Bonci, C.M. (1999) Assessment and evaluation of predisposing factors to anterior cruciate ligament injury. *J Athletic Training* **34**, 155–164.

Burks, R.T., Bean, B.G., Marcus, R. & Barker, H.B. (1991) Analysis of athletic performance with prophylactic ankle devices. *Am J Sports Med* **19**, 104–106.

DuRant, R.H., Pendergrast, R.A., Seymore, C., Gaillard, G. & Donner, J. (1992) Findings from the preparticipation athletic examination and athletic injuries. *Am J Dis Children* **146**, 85–91.

Furnich, R.M., Ellison, A.E., Guerin, G.J. & Grace, P.D. (1981) The measured effect of taping on combined foot and ankle motion before and after exercise. *Am J Sports Med* **9**, 165–170.

Garrick, J.G. & Requa, R.K. (1973) Role of external support in the prevention of ankle sprains. *Med Sci Sports* **5**, 200–205.

Gomez, E., DeLee, J.C. & Farney, W.C. (1996) Incidence of injury in Texas girls' high school basketball. *Am J Sports Med* **24**, 684–687.

Grubbs, N., Nelson, R.T. & Bandy, W. (1997) Predictive validity of an injury score among high school basketball players. *Med Sci Sports Exercise* **29**, 1279–1285.

Gutgesell, M.E. (1991) Safety of a preadolescent basketball program. *Am J Dis Children* **145**, 1023–1025.

Gwinn, D.E., Wilckens, J.H., McDevitt, E.R., Ross, G. & Kao, T. (2000) The relative incidence of anterior cruciate ligament injury in men and women at the United States Naval Academy. *Am J Sports Med* **28**, 98–102.

Heitz, N.A., Eisenman, P.A., Beck, C.L. & Walker, J.A. (1999) Hormonal changes throughout the menstrual cycle and increased anterior cruciate ligament laxity in females. *J Athletic Training* **34**, 144–149.

Hoffman, J.R. & Maresh, C.M. (2000) Physiology of basketball. In: W.E. Garrett, D.T. Kirkendall, eds. *Exercise and Sport Science*. Philadelphia: Lippincott, Williams & Wilkins, 733–744.

Hutchinson, M.R. & Ireland, M.L. (1995) Knee injuries in female athletes. *Sports Med* **19**, 288–302.

Ireland, M.L. (1999) Anterior cruciate ligament injury in female athletes: Epidemiology. *J Athletic Training* **34**, 150–154.

Johnson, E.E. & Markolf, K.L. (1983) The contribution of the anterior talofibular ligament to ankle laxity. *J Bone Joint Surg* **65A**, 81–88.

Kingma, J. & Jan ten Duis, H. (1998) Sports members participation in assessment of incidence rate in five sports from records of hospital-based clinical treatment. *Perceptual Motor Skills* **86**, 675–686.

Krinsky, M.B., Abdenour, T.E., Starkey, C., Albo, R.A. & Chu, D.A. (1992) Incidence of meniscus injury in professional basketball players. *Am J Sports Med* **20**, 17–19.

Messina, D.F., Farney, W.C. & DeLee, J.C. (1999) The incidence of injury in Texas high school basketball. *Am J Sports Med* **27**, 294–299.

National Collegiate Athletic Association (1998) *NCAA Injury Surveillance System for All Sports*. National Collegiate Athletic Association, Overland Park, KA.

Ottaviani, R.A., Ashton-Miller, J.A., Kothari, S.U. & Wojtys, E.M. (1995) Basketball shoe height and the maximal muscular resistance to applied ankle inversion and eversion moments. *Am J Sports Med* **23**, 418–423.

Paris, D.L. (1992) The effects of Swede-O, New Cross, and McDavid ankle braces and adhesive ankle taping on speed, balance, agility, and vertical jump. *J Athletic Training* **27**, 253–256.

Pienkowski, D., McMorrow, M., Shapiro, R., Caborn, D.N. & Stayton, J. (1995) The effect of ankle stabilizers on athletic performance. *Am J Sports Med* **23**, 757–762.

Powell, J.W. & Barber-Foss, K.D. (1999) Traumatic brain injury in high school athletes. *J Am Med Assoc* **282**, 958–963.

Powell, J.W. & Barber-Foss, K.D. (2000) Sex-related injury patterns among selected high school sports. *Am J Sports Med* **28**, 385–391.

Rozzi, S.L., Lephart, S.M., Gear, W.S. & Fu, F.H. (1999) Knee joint laxity and neuromuscular characteristics of male and female soccer and basketball players. *Am J Sports Med* **27**, 312–319.

Shambaugh, J.P., Klein, A. & Herbert, J.H. (1991) Structural measures as predictors of injury in basketball players. *Med Sci Sports Exercise* **23**, 522–527.

Shapiro, M.S., Kabo, J.M., Mitchell, P.W., Loren, G. & Tsenter, M. (1994) Ankle sprain prophylaxis. An analysis of the stabilizing effects of braces and tape. *Am J Sports Med* **22**, 78–82.

Sitler, M., Ryan, J. & Wheeler, B. *et al.* (1994) The efficacy of a semirigid ankle stabilizer to reduce acute ankle injuries in basketball. *Am J Sports Med* **22**, 454–461.

Wilson, R.L. & McGinty, L.D. (1993) Common hand and wrist injuries in basketball players. *Clin Sports Med* **12**, 265–291.

Yde, J. & Nielsen, A.B. (1990) Sports injuries in adolescents' ball games: soccer, handball and basketball. *Br J Sports Med* **24**, 51–54.

Zvijac, J. & Thompson, W. (1996) Basketball. In: D.J. Caine, C.G. Caine, K.J. Lindner, eds. *Epidemiology of Sports Injuries*. Human Kinetics: Champaign, IL, 86–97.

Chapter 2
Physiology of basketball

Jay R. Hoffman

Basketball has achieved an impressive level of popularity in the world today with both males and females. It is a sport that originated in the United States, but individuals can be seen playing basketball in almost every country in the world. Basketball in the United States is considered by many to be at the level that most countries strive to reach. Although the style of play may vary between countries, the number of foreign athletes playing basketball in the United States, and the broadcast of National Basketball Association (NBA) basketball games throughout the world has encouraged many foreign teams to try and emulate the American style of play. Nevertheless, there are still large differences in the way that basketball can be played that will influence the physiological requirements of the athlete, and determine the direction of the athlete's training program.

One of the first differences that are seen in basketball, regardless of the style of play, is the duration of a basketball game. The length of a basketball game is dependent upon the league. Typical high school basketball games are played with four 8- or 10-minute quarters. Collegiate basketball games are played with two 20-minute halves, and professional basketball games (i.e., NBA) are played with four 12-minute quarters. European games (governed by the International Basketball Federation) are similar in duration to intercollegiate contests. However, the duration of basketball contests in other parts of the world among various leagues may be different.

The intensity of the game is intermittent in its nature. Depending upon the coach's strategy the game can generally be played at either a high intensity (i.e., fast transition from defense to offense) or at a low intensity (i.e., slow deliberate half court style) of play. However, depending upon the opponent or the circumstances in a game (e.g., point differential), the coach may decide to alter the team's style of play. In addition, the athleticism, basketball skills and physical condition of the players on a team may also influence the type of strategy employed by the coach. If a coach believes his or her team would be more successful in playing a style of basketball that emphasizes pressure defense and a fast transition from defense to offense, the physiological demand on those athletes would be quite different than a team that plays at a much slower intensity. These strategic differences in how the game of basketball is played would have a large impact on the physiological requirements of the basketball player, and would have important implications in the development of the athlete's training program.

Physiology of the game of basketball

Movement patterns

The game of basketball is played in a continuous movement. There is a smooth transition from offense to defense and all players perform similar movements (i.e., rebounding and shooting) on the basketball court during a game. These movements differ in their mode of activity (e.g., running, shuffling or jumping) and degree of intensity (from a jog to a sprint). In a study of an Australian National League basketball game, close to 1000 changes in movement were reported during a 48-minute basketball game (McInnes *et al.* 1995). This equated to a change in movement every 2 seconds, clearly illustrating the intermittent nature of basketball. Shuffle movements (performed at varying intensities) were seen in 34.6% of the activity patterns of a basketball game, while running at intensities ranging from a jog to a sprint were observed in 31.2% of all movements. Jumps comprised 4.6% of all movements while standing or walking was observed during 29.6% of the playing time. Movements characterized as high intensity were recorded once every 21 seconds of play. When considering both high intensity shuffles and jumps, the investigators reported that only 15% of the actual playing time was spent engaged in high intensity activity. Sixty-five percent of playing time was reported to be engaged in activities that were of greater intensity than walking. The results of this study suggest that the movements occurring during a basketball game are performed at an intensity that is primarily aerobic in nature. However, successful basketball performance also has been suggested to be dependent upon anaerobic performance (Hoffman & Maresh 2000). These contrasting results are likely related to the different styles of play seen between international and American (i.e., NCAA, NBA) basketball.

Physiological demands during competition

As previously mentioned the physiological demands imposed during a basketball game are quite dependent upon the style of play. Although there are limited data available on the physiological responses during a competitive game, several studies have examined the heart rate response during competition. These measures do provide some indication of the intensity of play. In a study on male professional basketball players, heart rates during competition averaged 169 ± 9 beats·min^{-1}, which corresponded to $89 \pm 9\%$ of the athlete's peak heart rate (McInnes *et al.* 1995). Seventy-five percent of the actual play occurred at a heart rate that was 85% of the athlete's peak heart rate, while 15% of the contest heart rate exceeded 95% of peak heart rate.

There appears to have been only one study that has reported on blood lactate concentrations during an actual basketball game (McInnes *et al.* 1995). During the game mean blood lactate concentration for the eight players examined was 6.8 ± 2.8 mmol·l^{-1}. The average maximal blood lactate concentration was 8.5 ± 3.1 mmol·l^{-1}, with the highest value recorded for one player reaching 13.2 mmol·l^{-1}. No significant differences in lactate concentrations were seen between quarters. In addition, significant correlations were seen between lactate concentration and both the time spent in high intensity activity ($r = 0.64$; $p < 0.05$) and the mean percentage of peak heart rate ($r = 0.45$; $p < 0.05$). Lactate concentrations during a basketball game are likely influenced by the intensity at which the game is played, and could vary considerably from game to game.

Physiological profile of the basketball player

The physiological profile of a sport provides a set of performance characteristics of the athlete that can be used to identify talent and develop sport-specific training programs. Although several sports have well established and well accepted standardized testing profiles (e.g., 40-yard sprint and maximal strength tests in football), basketball has yet to become associated with any standard testing regimen. Most physical performance testing performed on basketball players has been quite varied in its methodology, which has made it difficult to establish specific standards. In addition, a question concerning whether to characterize basketball as an aerobic or anaerobic sport has been a subject of debate, and may have caused confusion amongst coaches and conditioning professionals as to how to properly direct their conditioning programs. Latin *et al.* (1994) published the most comprehensive survey to date on the physical fitness and performance profile for Division I NCAA Men's College Basketball players. However, they did acknowledge a poor compliance rate (15.2% survey return), and a large inconsistency in variables reported. In this section the physiological profile of the basketball player will be examined by focusing in on specific fitness components and their relation to the sport.

Aerobic capacity

Both laboratory measures and field tests common to athletic conditioning programs (i.e., 1.5 mile run or 12 minute run) have been used to describe the aerobic capacity of basketball players. The maximal oxygen consumption ($\dot{V}o_{2max}$) of male basketball players has been reported to range from 42 to 59 mL·kg^{-1}·min^{-1} (Latin *et al.* 1994; Hoffman & Maresh 2000). Although no significant differences were noted in $\dot{V}o_{2max}$ between positions, guards tend to have a greater aerobic capacity than either forwards or centers at both the collegiate and professional level of basketball.

The values reported for aerobic capacity in male basketball are similar to values seen in sedentary individuals of comparable age and of athletes that participate in nonendurance events. This wide span of $\dot{V}o_{2max}$ values encompasses more than 25 years of studies performed on basketball players, and likely reflects differences in playing styles and changes in conditioning programs over the course of a generation. Although anaerobic metabolism has been suggested to be the primary energy source for playing basketball, there still appears to be an important aerobic component to basketball performance (Hoffman & Maresh 2000). Aerobic capacity may have more importance in the recovery processes (e.g., lactate clearance, cardiodeceleration patterns), rather than in providing a direct performance benefit. However, several indications suggest that there may be a limit to the benefits provided by a high aerobic capacity during recovery from an anaerobic activity (Hoffman *et al.* 1999a). It appears that a certain threshold of aerobic capacity is needed, and once this threshold is achieved further improvement in aerobic capacity may not provide any additional advantage. Interestingly, a high aerobic capacity has been reported to have a negative relationship with playing time in elite male college basketball players (Hoffman *et al.* 1996).

Maximal aerobic capacity levels in female basketball players have been reported to range between 39.5 ± 5.7 and 51.3 ± 4.9 mL·kg^{-1}·min^{-1} (Smith & Thomas 1991; Hoffman & Maresh 2000). Guards (54.3 ± 4.9 mL·kg^{-1}·min^{-1}) have been reported to have a significantly higher aerobic capacity than small forwards (47.0 ± 4.3 mL·kg^{-1}·min^{-1}) (Smith &

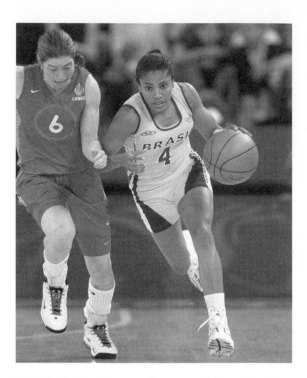

Fig. 2.1 Gender differences deserve careful consideration by physicians and coaches. Photo © Getty Images/ J. Squire.

Thomas 1991), but no other significant differences between position have been noted. However, in contrast to the relationship noted between aerobic capacity and basketball performance in males, in the female athlete aerobic power is reported to be not only related to basketball performance, but it also appears to be able to discriminate between higher and lesser skilled players (Riezebos *et al.* 1983). This gender difference in the relationship between aerobic capacity and basketball performance is likely related to differences in the style of play (Fig. 2.1).

Anaerobic power

It has been suggested by a number of investigators that success in basketball appears to be more dependent upon the athlete's anaerobic power and endurance rather than on aerobic power, *per se* (Hoffman & Maresh 2000). Although only 15% of the playing time in a basketball game has been described as high intensity (McInnes *et al.* 1995), it is these actions that can determine the outcome of a contest. The quick change of direction and explosive speed needed to free oneself for an open shot or defend, the ability to jump quickly and repetitively, and the speed needed to reach loose balls and run a fast break, are examples of high intensity activities common to basketball. These components of anaerobic ability (i.e., speed, vertical jump and agility) have also been demonstrated to be strong predictors of playing time in male college basketball players (Hoffman *et al.* 1996).

A wide range of tests has been used to assess anaerobic power and endurance in basketball players. Anaerobic power in basketball players have been determined from both laboratory (i.e., Wingate Anaerobic Power Test, vertical jumps with force plates) and field tests (i.e., vertical jump height, line drill). The number of testing modalities has made it quite difficult to generate normative data for anaerobic power performance in basketball players. The most frequent test employed appears to be the vertical jump. This is a relatively simple test to perform, and quite easy to interpret for both the player and coach. Latin *et al.* (1994) have reported that the mean vertical jump in NCAA Division I male basketball players was 71.4 ± 10.4 cm (range 25.4–105.4 cm). Vertical jump power (using the Lewis formula) in these athletes was 1669.9 ± 209.7 W (range 1073.1–2521.5 W). Significant differences were seen between positions. Guards and forwards jumped significantly higher (73.4 ± 9.6 cm and 71.4 ± 10.4 cm, respectively) than centers (66.8 ± 10.7 cm) (Latin *et al.* 1994). Vertical jump power, however, was reported to be significantly greater in both forwards (1749.3 ± 210.7 W) and centers (1784.6 ± 162.7 W) than in guards (1550.4 ± 161.7 W) (Latin *et al.* 1994).

There have been far fewer studies performed on anaerobic power output in female basketball players. In a review of several studies reporting on vertical jump heights on female basketball players, Hoffman and Maresh (2000) reported jump heights ranging from 26.3 ± 2.9 cm to 48.2 ± 8.5 cm. The vertical jump height of North American female basketball players (mean jump heights ranging from 44.7 to 48.2 cm) appear to be much greater than their European counterparts (mean jump heights ranging from 26.3 to 29.0 cm). In comparisons be-

tween positions the vertical jump height for guards (49.4 ± 6.2 cm) and forwards (49.4 ± 11.1 cm) tended ($p > 0.05$) to be higher than the jump height seen for centers (43.5 ± 4.5 cm) (Lamonte *et al.* 1999). When anaerobic power output was examined relative to body mass, both guards and forwards had significantly greater peak (23% and 15%, respectively) and mean (23% and 12%, respectively) power outputs than centers (Lamonte *et al.* 1999).

Strength

Strength in basketball players has primarily been reported as the 1RM strength (repetition maximum; see Kraemer & Häkkinen 2002) in the bench press, squat and power clean exercises. These dynamic constant resistance exercise tests are used to assess upper body strength, lower body strength and explosive strength, respectively. Lower body strength (1RM squat) has been shown to be a strong predictor for playing time in NCAA Division I male basketball players (Hoffman *et al.* 1996). Squat strength has been reported to average 152.2 ± 36.5 kg in NCAA Division I male college basketball players (Hoffman & Maresh 2000). In a position-by-position analysis collegiate forwards (161.9 ± 37.7 kg) were significantly stronger than centers (138.1 ± 32.1 kg) but similar to guards (151.1 ± 35.5 kg) (Latin *et al.* 1994). When lower body strength was expressed relative to body weight, centers were significantly weaker than both the guards and forwards. The importance of lower body strength for the basketball player is for "boxing-out" and positioning during a basketball game. In addition, the importance of leg strength for these athletes may also be related to its positive relationship to both speed and agility (Hoffman & Maresh 2000).

The power clean may be as good, or even a more appropriate, exercise than the squat for improving jumping height, speed and agility. The explosive action of the power clean, and its ability to integrate strength, explosive power, and neuromuscular coordination among several muscle groups suggests that this exercise has similarity to many of the actions common to basketball players. Thus, improving strength in this exercise may provide for a better transfer of strength to the basketball court. However, the power clean is not as common as the squat or bench press exercises for use as a strength test in basketball players. Limited data have reported maximal strength in the power clean to be 99.2 ± 15.2 kg (range 59.0–137.3 kg) in NCAA Division I male college basketball players (Latin *et al.* 1994). In comparison between positions, forwards (105.1 ± 16.9 kg) have been reported to be significantly stronger than guards (94.5 ± 13.0 kg) but not the centers (99.8 ± 13.7 kg) (Latin *et al.* 1994).

Strength in the bench press appears to be the most common strength testing measure reported in basketball players. Hoffman and Maresh (2000) reviewing studies examining strength measures in NCAA Division I college basketball players reported that maximal upper body strength (e.g. 1RM bench press) is 102.7 ± 18.9 kg for these athletes. However, upper body strength has been shown to be poorly correlated with playing time (r's from –0.04 to 0.14) in male college basketball players (Hoffman *et al.* 1996). It has been suggested that although the bench press may not be a determining factor for playing time, it is likely that certain positions such as power forward and center require more upper body strength than other positions. Still, no significant differences in upper body strength have been seen between guards (100.8 ± 17.6 kg), forwards (104.0 ± 21.5 kg) and centers (104.4 ± 17.0) at the collegiate level (Latin *et al.* 1994). Interestingly, guards were significantly stronger than both forwards and centers when strength was reported relative to body mass. Most of the published studies on strength in basketball players have been on collegiate basketball players. The only study to report on strength in NBA players occurred nearly 20 years previous. In that study maximal bench press strength was reported to be 86.8 ± 15.0 kg, 101.3 ± 20.8 kg, and 70.0 ± 0.0 kg in NBA guards, forwards and center, respectively (Parr *et al.* 1978). A large strength difference is apparent when comparing the results of the collegiate and professional basketball players. However, these differences most likely reflect the greater emphasis on strength training of basketball players in recent years.

Speed and agility

Speed and agility have been both reported to be a consistent predictor of playing time in NCAA Division I male basketball players (Hoffman *et al.* 1996). Speed has been generally determined by a timed 40- or 30-yard sprint. The 40-yard sprint may have greater popularity due to the familiarity with performance times associated with football players. However, the 30-yard sprint may be more specific for the basketball athlete because of the similarity between this distance and the length of the basketball court (Hoffman & Maresh 2000). Times (mean ± SD) for the 40- and 30-yard sprint in collegiate basketball players have been reported to be 4.81 ± 0.26 s and 3.79 ± 0.19 s, respectively (Latin *et al.* 1994). Guards were observed to be significantly faster than centers in both 40-yard (4.68 ± 0.20 s vs. 4.97 ± 0.21 s, respectively) and 30-yard (3.68 ± 0.14 s vs. 3.97 ± 0.21 s, respectively) sprints (Latin *et al.* 1994). The times for forwards were 4.84 ± 0.29 s and 3.83 ± 0.16 s in both the 40-yard and 30-yard sprints, respectively. These times were not significantly different than either guards or centers.

Agility is also considered an important component in basketball performance (Hoffman *et al.* 1996). This is not surprising considering the rapid changes in movement and direction during the game of basketball. However, there does not appear to be any widely accepted method of measuring agility in basketball players. Only 7% of the NCAA Division I schools which complied with a survey on testing of their basketball athletes reported agility performance scores (Latin *et al.* 1994). Although there are several tests that are available to measure agility, the *T*-test may be the most appropriate for the basketball player. This drill utilizes the basic movements performed in a game: forward sprint, side shuffle, and backwards run. No significant differences between positions in the *T*-test (mean ± SD; 8.95 ± 0.53 s) have been reported (Latin *et al.* 1994), however, this is more likely due to the small number of schools reporting this measure, considering that guards were 0.20 s and 0.54 s faster than forwards and centers, respectively.

Flexibility

Flexibility is the ability to move muscles through their full range of motion about a joint. However, flexibility is joint specific and inference from one joint to another cannot be done without specifically measuring the flexibility of that particular joint. The sit and reach test appears to be the most popular exercise used to measure flexibility in the basketball player. Several studies have reported sit and reach mean scores ranging from 1.4 cm to 4.9 cm in collegiate basketball players (Hunter *et al.* 1993). NBA players appear to have slightly better scores in the sit and reach test (mean scores ranges between positions 6.7 cm to 7.4 cm) (Parr *et al.* 1978). Being highly flexible does not appear to provide any performance advantage. The only benefit that flexibility likely has is on reducing the athlete's risk for injury. Recent evidence suggests that flexibility exercises performed prior to a power activity (e.g., vertical jump) may reduce power performance by causing changes in muscle–tendon length (Schilling & Stone 2000). Subsequently, force output and the rate of force development is decreased. Although the benefit of flexibility exercises is not being questioned, the timing of when these exercises are performed may have an impact on acute power performance.

Body mass and body composition

The body mass of Division I collegiate basketball players appears to be quite similar between teams (Latin *et al.* 1994). In a recent survey of NCAA Division I college basketball teams (Latin *et al.* 1994) the range in body mass (84.5–97.9 kg) reported is consistent with the body mass reported in collegiate basketball players over the past 25 years. Significant differences between each position have also been noted (Latin *et al.* 1994). Guards (82.9 ± 6.8 kg) are the lightest players, followed by forwards (95.1 ± 8.3 kg) and then centers (101.9 ± 9.7 kg).

In a review by Hoffman and Maresh (2000) on studies of basketball players over the past 25 years, it was reported that the body composition of both college and professional male basketball players had ranged from 8.3 to 13.5%. The body fat percentages in NCAA Division I collegiate basketball players were lower than those observed in NCAA Division II or III basketball players or in European players. Comparisons between positions have shown that guards have a significantly lower body fat percentage (8.4 ± 3.0%) than centers (11.2 ± 4.5%) but not forwards (9.7 ± 3.9%) (Latin *et al.* 1994). This may reflect the greater mass needed by centers to play the "low post" position, which involves considerable body contact during box-outs, picks and rebounding.

The body mass of female basketball players has been reported to range from 61.5 to 70.4 kg, while body composition is reported to range between 17.0 and 26.2% (Smith & Thomas 1991; Lamonte *et al.* 1999; Hoffman & Maresh 2000). Interestingly, Hoffman and Maresh (2000) report that recent studies show a trend towards a higher body mass and a lower percentage of body fat in female basketball players. This likely reflects the greater emphasis on resistance training programs over the last 10–15 years. Similar to male players there appears to be significant differences in body mass between positions. Guards are lighter ($p < 0.05$), and have the lower body fat percentages ($p < 0.05$), when compared to both forwards and centers (Smith & Thomas 1991; Lamonte *et al.* 1999). Centers also appear to be heavier ($p < 0.05$) than forwards (Lamonte *et al.* 1999), but no significant differences in body fat percentage was seen between those positions.

Effect of a season on the physiological profile of the basketball player

It appears that aerobic fitness can be maintained during a basketball season by participation in basketball practice and games only, without any supplemental training (Caterisano *et al.* 1997; Hoffman & Maresh 2000). However, this may be dependent upon the extent of playing time for each player. It has been shown that reserve players (defined as those athletes playing less than 10 min per game) may be unable to maintain their aerobic fitness (Caterisano *et al.* 1997). For those players it may be beneficial to consider supplemental training.

Anaerobic power has generally been shown to be maintained or increased during the basketball season. This is not surprising considering the highly anaerobic nature of practice and games. Hoffman and colleagues (Hoffman *et al.* 1991a) have reported significant improvements in both speed and vertical jump height during a competitive basketball season. Interestingly, by the end of the season vertical jump height returned to preseason levels. It is likely that the decrease in jump performance was related to an over-reaching phenomenon. It is thought that these fitness components (speed and vertical jump height) are sensitive to changes in training volume and may be potential markers for predicting fatigue in basketball players (Hoffman & Maresh 2000).

The ability to maintain upper and lower body strength during a basketball season has met with contrasting results. It appears that maintenance of strength may be influenced to a large extent by the resistance training experience of the athlete (Hoffman *et al.* 1991b). In basketball players with only 5 weeks of resistance training experience it appears that both upper and lower body strength can be maintained during the season, even when no in-season strength training program was incorporated (Hoffman *et al.* 1991a). It was apparent that the players did not achieve "full-fledged strength training adaptations" during the 5-week preseason training program, and that the strength gains made were the result of primarily neural contributions. However, that study was unable to determine whether strength gains could be maintained in basketball players that were more experienced in resistance training. A later study by the same investigators (Hoffman *et al.* 1991b), examined the effects of a 2-day·week^{-1} in-season resistance training program in experienced resistance-trained basketball players. The results of that study demonstrated that not only were strength levels able to be maintained in the experienced resistance-trained players, but that upper body strength could be increased during the season in basketball players with minimal (5 weeks) resistance training experience. However, the ability to improve or maintain strength during a basketball season may be related to the intensity of the in-season resistance training sessions. A later study by Caterisano and colleagues (1997) reported that basketball players were unable to maintain their strength during the season. Although the frequency of training was similar between the studies (2 day·week^{-1}), the intensity of training in the former study required players to perform a 5–8 RM depending upon the exercise, while the intensity level in the latter study was 10 repetitions at 70% of the player's 1 RM. Apparently, the intensity of the in-season resistance training program is an important variable for maintaining strength during a competitive basketball season.

Training the basketball player

Once the basketball season is completed the athletes are generally given some time to recover before beginning their preparation for the next season. The length of the recovery time is quite arbitrary and there are no specific investigations that have examined ideal recovery times following a season. Empirically, 2 weeks of passive rest has been used in collegiate basketball players before they begin their off-season training program. Whether this is a sufficient recovery time for professional athletes that compete in a season of greater duration is unknown. A recent study examining professional athletes that participate in the European League suggested that recovery was still not complete, even 4 weeks following a 9-month basketball season (Hoffman *et al.* 1999b).

The training program is based upon the principles of periodization. Typically, periodization is a planned variation of acute training variables (i.e., intensity and volume) which are manipulated to bring an athlete to maximal strength and power for a single competition. However, in contrast to a powerlifter or weightlifter, in whom training is focused on peaking for a particular competition that normally culminates the training program, the basketball player emphasizes peak performance throughout the season and needs to begin the season in peak condition. Furthermore, the basketball player needs to maintain this level of condition throughout the competitive year. In addition, the basketball player needs to train multiple components of fitness. Thus, the athlete will concurrently perform various modes of training (e.g., strength, anaerobic, endurance). The training program needs to be developed with the understanding that concurrent training may effect maximal performance gains. Therefore, to maximize the training effect, a proper manipulation of these various stimuli must be performed.

There are a number of recommendations and suggestions that can be found in the literature on conditioning for basketball. Examinations of off-season resistance training programs have shown significant increases (range 8–17%) in both upper and lower body strength (Hoffman *et al.* 1991b; Hunter *et al.* 1993), but the magnitude of these increases appears to be related to the resistance training experience of the athlete. An examination of male basketball players during their 4-year playing career at a Division I basketball program showed significant increases in 1RM bench press (24%) and 1RM squat strength (32%) over that time (Hunter *et al*. 1993). The greatest strength increases were observed in the year between the athletes' freshman and sophomore seasons.

Off-season conditioning programs do not appear to cause any changes in the aerobic capacity of college basketball players (Hunter *et al*. 1993). It appears that the aerobic component of the off-season training program is focused more on maintaining an aerobic base rather than in improving it and is consistent with what has been demonstrated with the relationship between aerobic capacity and basketball performance.

The ability of the basketball player to improve agility, speed and vertical jump height during an off-season training program is not very clear. During a college basketball player's career (spanning four seasons), significant improvements in vertical jump height (range from 8 to 12%) have been seen (Hunter *et al*. 1993). Similar to improvements in strength, the increase in jump height appeared to occur primarily between the athletes' first and second year of college. As the athletes' performance in these fitness components improved, it became more difficult to make further improvements even with the greater training experience. This may partly explain the results of Hoffman and colleagues (Hoffman *et al*. 1991b) showing no improvement in sprint time and a less than 1% improvement in both vertical jump height and *T*-test time after an off-season training program in experienced resistance-trained basketball players. In that same study, significant increases in 1RM bench press (17%) and 1RM squat (16%) were observed, suggesting that these athletes were closer to their full potential in speed, agility and vertical jump than they were to their strength potential.

Resistance training program

Strength appears to be an important component to the success of a basketball player. It also appears that of all the athletic components comprising the basketball player, strength has the greatest potential to be developed. This is likely related to a lack of exposure of many basketball players to a weight room. For most basketball players the large improvements seen in strength appear to occur with only minor improvements in athletic skills (i.e. agility, speed and vertical jump height). However, these minor improvements may have great practical significance in the success of the player.

The frequency of training is dependent on the resistance training experience of the athlete. A 3 day·week^{-1} off-season resistance training program is thought to be an effective frequency of training for basketball players, however, depending upon the resistance training experience of the athlete, a greater frequency of training may be more appropriate (Hoffman & Maresh 2000). Considering that team members with varying levels of resistance training experience will train together, it may be prudent and more manageable to use a training program that will benefit both experienced and novice lifters. Therefore, a 4 day·week^{-1} resistance training program for basketball players is recommended.

The resistance training program can be divided into three phases. The initial phase is the off-season, followed by the preseason and then the in-season (maintenance) phases. The off-season program is similar to what would be expected from a basic periodized training system. An example of a periodized off-season resistance training program for basketball can be seen in Table 2.1. The duration of this program is dependent upon the length of the off-season. The example provided in Table 2.1 is of a collegiate off-season resistance training program. The collegiate athlete generally plays a shorter season, and has a much longer off-season than professional athletes in both North America and Europe.

The first phase of the periodized training program is the hypertrophy or preparatory phase. This phase concentrates on developing muscle mass, and building basic strength for the more complicated exercises in the strength and strength/power phases. The intensity of training for this is low (8–10 RM), volume of training is high, and the rest periods are short (about 1 minute) between exercises.

In the second or strength phase, additional multijoint structural exercises (i.e. power clean and push press) are added, while several of the assistance

Table 2.1 Example of a periodized off-season resistance training program for college basketball players (adapted from Hoffman & Maresh 2000).

	Phase	Hypertrophy (7-week)	Strength (7-week)	Strength/power (4-week)
Days 1 and 3	Power clean	–	1,4 × 4–6 RM	1,4 × 3–5 RM
	Push press	–	1,4 × 4–6 RM	1,4 × 3–5 RM
	Bench press	1,4 × 8–10 RM	1,4 × 6–8 RM	1,4 × 4–6 RM
	Incline bench press	1,3 × 8–10 RM	1,3 × 6–8 RM	1,3 × 4–6 RM
	Incline dumbell flys	3 × 8–10 RM	–	–
	Shoulder press	1,3 × 8–10 RM	–	–
	Upright row	1,3 × 8–10 RM	–	–
	Lateral raise	3 × 8–10 RM	–	–
	Triceps pushdown	3 × 8–10 RM	3 × 8–10 RM	3 × 6–8 RM
	Triceps extension	3 × 8–10 RM	3 × 8–10 RM	–
	Abdominal exercise	3 sets	3 sets	3 sets
Days 2 and 4	Squat	1,4 × 8–10 RM	1,4 × 6–8 RM	1,4 × 4–6 RM
	Leg extension	3 × 8–10 RM	3 × 8–10 RM	3 × 6–8 RM
	Leg curl	3 × 8–10 RM	3 × 8–10 RM	3 × 6–8 RM
	Standing calf raise	3 × 8–10 RM	3 × 8–10 RM	3 × 6–8 RM
	Lat pulldown	1,3 × 8–10 RM	1,3 × 6–8 RM	1,3 × 6–8 RM
	Seated row	1,3 × 8–10 RM	1,3 × 6–8 RM	1,3 × 6–8 RM
	Biceps exercise I	3 × 8–10 RM	3 × 8–10 RM	3 × 6–8 RM
	Biceps exercise II	3 × 8–10 RM	3 × 8–10 RM	–
	Abdominal exercise	3 sets	3 sets	3 sets

RM, repetition maximum.

exercises used in the previous phase are eliminated. During this phase more sport-specific and explosive power exercises, which better simulate the movement of a basketball player, are used. The push press exercise simulates jumping for a rebound movement and shooting a jump shot. This exercise uses a slight countermovement before an explosive push upward. In addition, the lat pulldown, which is normally performed with the hands in a wide grip position, may be better performed with a closed pronated grip while lowering the bar to the chest. This technique may better simulate the "rebound-grab" movement performed on the basketball court. During this phase, the volume of training is lower but intensity is increased. Note that intensity remained slightly higher in the assistance exercises. The rest period between sets may be increased to 2–3 min to maximize strength gains.

The third or strength/power phase is much shorter in duration and precedes the preseason training. Intensity is even higher, while volume is lowered. The rest period between sets is similar to the previous macrocycle. Several assistance exercises can be

eliminated during this phase. At the conclusion of each phase of training there is a 1-week active recovery period in which the athlete does not perform any resistance training. However, he or she could be active in training other fitness components.

The preseason period is not easily defined. For instance, in a collegiate basketball player the preseason period (as it relates to the conditioning program) may be defined as the time when the athlete returns from summer break (end of August/beginning of September) until the start of official basketball practice (mid-October). In other leagues, in which the off-season training program is of shorter duration, a separate preseason period for a resistance program may not be considered. In such a situation the off-season program is followed immediately by the in-season training program. In the example of the college athlete, the resistance training program during the preseason period may be comprised of several different microcycles that may resemble the off-season training program. For example, a 6-week preseason resistance training program may be comprised of a 2-week hypertrophy phase, a 2-week

Table 2.2 In-season resistance training program (adapted from Hoffman & Maresh 2000).

1 Power clean	$1 \times 10, 3 \times 4-6$ RM
2 Push press	$1 \times 10, 3 \times 4-6$ RM
3 Squat	$1 \times 10, 3 \times 6-8$ RM
4 Bench press	$1 \times 10, 3 \times 6-8$ RM
5 Lat pulldown	$3 \times 8-10$ RM
6 Leg curl	$3 \times 8-10$ RM
7 Tricep pushdown	$3 \times 8-10$ RM
8 Bicep curl	$3 \times 8-10$ RM
9 Abdominal exercise	3 sets

RM, repetition maximum.

strength phase and a 2-week strength/power phase. During this time a greater emphasis on the conditioning program is devoted to anaerobic (e.g., intervals and sprint) and sport specific (e.g., agility, plyometrics) training.

During the season, the primary concern is to maintain the strength gains achieved during the off-season. For first year, or inexperienced resistance-trained players, there is some evidence that supports the benefit of an in-season resistance training program to increase strength during the season (Hoffman *et al.* 1991b). The in-season training program is generally referred to as a maintenance program. An example of an in-season resistance training program can be seen in Table 2.2.

Endurance program

It appears that once an aerobic base is reached (apparently a value between 42 and 59 mL·kg^{-1}·min^{-1} for male basketball players) any further increase in aerobic capacity may not provide any additional benefit to the basketball player (Hoffman *et al.* 1999a). Therefore, the goal of the endurance training program should be to maintain aerobic capacity levels within this range. To maintain an aerobic base during the off-season training program the basketball player should run at least 3 day·week^{-1} for 20–30 min each session. Alternative means of aerobic training (e.g., cycling) may also be a good training program variation for the athlete. The intensity for this exercise should be near 70–75% of age-predicted maximal heart rate. The coach or strength and conditioning specialist should be aware if the players will be required to participate

in "unsupervised" basketball scrimmages that may run for 2 h per day, 5–6 day·week^{-1}. If so, this may be a sufficient stimulus to maintain an aerobic base. If the goal of the off-season training program is to increase strength and body mass then too much emphasis on an aerobic program (including the daily basketball scrimmages) may reduce the ability of these athletes to maximize strength and body mass gains (Hoffman & Maresh 2000). However, if there is an athlete whose primary goal is to reduce body fat, then a greater emphasis should be directed at increasing the aerobic component of the athlete's off-season training program.

Anaerobic conditioning

Specifically conditioning the anaerobic energy system is generally not initiated until the preseason training program begins (upon return to campus) for the collegiate athlete. For other athletes this may occur during the last phase of the off-season training program. Up until this phase of training, the athlete's conditioning program has focused primarily on resistance training, maintaining an aerobic base, performing sport-specific drills (this may include both agility and speed development), and playing basketball (either scrimmages or in summer leagues). Anaerobic conditioning until this point was avoided to prevent any possible overtraining syndrome to occur during the season. The preseason (at the collegiate level) is approximately 6 weeks in duration. During this phase of training the goal is to condition the athlete in order to prepare him or her for official basketball practice, but not to reach peak conditioning. Once official basketball practice starts the team will begin practicing with the basketball coaching staff. During this period of time, before the competitive season begins, conditioning levels will peak. The conditioning program is designed in this order to reduce the chances of fatigue, or overreaching developing if the athlete "peaks" too soon (Hoffman & Maresh 2000).

An example of an anaerobic conditioning program can be seen in Table 2.3. The program is performed 4 day·week^{-1}, with a progression in both the intensity and volume of training. The work/rest ratio during the sprint training is manipulated to increase the intensity of exercise. The aim in reducing

Table 2.3 Example of a 6-week preseason anaerobic conditioning program (adapted from Hoffman & Maresh 2000).

	Exercise	Frequency	Work/rest ratio
Weeks 1–2			
Day 1	Intervals	3–4 laps	–
Day 2	400-m sprints	× 1	1 : 4
	100-m sprints	× 2	1 : 4
	30-m sprints	× 8	1 : 4
Day 3	Intervals	3–4 laps	–
Day 4	200-m sprints	× 4–5	1 : 4
Weeks 3–4			
Day 1	Intervals	4–5 laps	–
Day 2	400-m sprints	× 1	1 : 4
	100-m sprints	× 3–4	1 : 4
	30-m sprints	× 8–10	1 : 4
Day 3	Intervals	4–5 laps	–
Day 4	200-m sprints	× 5–6	1 : 4
Weeks 5–6			
Day 1	Intervals	5–6 laps	–
Day 2	400-m sprints	× 2	1 : 3
	100-m sprints	× 4–5	1 : 3
	30-m sprints	× 10–12	1 : 3
Day 3	Intervals	5–6 laps	–
Day 4	200-m sprints	× 6–7	1 : 3

the work/rest ratio is to improve the recovery time from high-intensity activity during a basketball game. Interval or fartlek training can also be used to simulate the energy demands experienced during competition. During interval training the athlete sprints the straight portions of a track (approximately 100 m) and jogs the turns (100 m). The required number of laps is performed continuously. Fartlek training is another method of anaerobic training that intersperses high-intensity sprints with lower-intensity running, and can be substituted for any of the anaerobic conditioning activities shown.

Speed, agility and basketball skills training

Speed and agility training is usually performed during the preseason conditioning program. However, some athletes looking to enhance their speed or agility may begin such training during the off-season conditioning program. Many different exercises are available for improving agility in basketball players. Ideally, an exercise should be selected that incorporates movements that are common to the game of basketball and can be performed on the court. To improve sprint speed many athletes will incorporate more explosive exercises in their resistance training program and perform drills to enhance running technique. Examples of both agility and running technique drills can be seen in Table 2.4.

Basketball-specific drills should be performed throughout the training program. It is imperative that the athlete continues to shoot and play basketball during the off-season conditioning program.

Table 2.4 Examples of agility and running-technique drills (adapted from Hoffman & Maresh 2000).

Agility drills	Description	Running technique drills
Side shuffle	Place two cones 5–7 m apart and side shuffle between cones for 10 s	15-m knee to chest
Quick feet	Using baseline of a basketball court, attempt to take short choppy steps over and under the baseline. The object is to stay as close to the line without touching, and be as quick as possible	15-m heels to butt run
Four-corner drill	Place cones in a square (can use foul line extended) 5–7 m each side. Player performs a backwards run from cone 1 to cone 2 with a tight transition around the cone the player side shuffles to cone 3. The player makes a tight transition around cone 3 and performs a karioki exercise (shuffle over—shuffle under) till cone 4, where the player then sprints to cone 1	Striders
T drill	Cones set in a T-formation. Player sprints from baseline to cone 1 (9 m), side shuffles to cone 2 (4.5 m), side shuffles to cone 3 (9 m), side shuffles back to cone 1 (4.5 m) and does a backward sprint back to baseline	Power skips
Jump rope		

As long as the athlete continues to play basketball during the off-season resistance training program there does not appear to be any adverse effect on the fine-motor skills needed for shooting a basketball. In addition, resistance training may enhance shooting skills by increasing the shooting range of the player, accelerating release time and accelerating the time to peak height during the vertical phase of the jump shot (Hoffman & Maresh 2000).

Plyometric training

Plyometrics is a term that is used to describe exercises that involve the muscle being stretched and then shortened to accelerate the body or limb. As such, plyometrics is often described as a stretch-shortening exercise, a description that may be more appropriate. Most plyometric exercises, although not all drills, require the athlete to rapidly accelerate and decelerate their body weight during a dynamic movement. Plyometric training is generally incorporated into an athlete's training program to improve power and increase vertical jump height. Plyometric drills are often combined with a traditional resistance training program with the premise that vertical jump performance may be enhanced to a significantly greater extent than if performing either resistance training or plyometric training alone (Hoffman & Maresh 2000). However, most of the studies demonstrating the effectiveness of plyometric training on jump performance have used primarily untrained or recreationally trained athletes, and not basketball players. Thus, it has been difficult to determine whether improved vertical jump ability is directly related to the utilization of plyometric training, or whether it is related to improved leg strength in this population group. Although the efficacy of plyometric training has been demonstrated, the ability of plyometric training to improve jumping ability in the experienced basketball player is still not well understood.

If plyometric exercises are to be incorporated into the athlete's training program it should be used primarily during the off-season and preseason training programs. During the season the number of plyometric sessions, although not necessarily eliminated, are substantially reduced. However, common sense should prevail when using plyometric drills during the season. For basketball players that play several games per week and are continuously scrimmaging during practice, the addition of plyometric exercises may pose more of a risk for injury than enhancing power performance.

Conclusion

Basketball is one of the most popular sports in the world today. This chapter has reviewed the physiological demands that comprise the game of basketball as well as the physical requirements needed by the athlete to succeed in this sport. Discussion also included the development of the optimal training program for the basketball player. A true challenge for the player or coach is to begin the season in near-peak condition, and maintain peak performance throughout the season. Recommendations for off-season, preseason and inseason conditioning programs were also provided.

References

Caterisano, A., Patrick, B.T., Edenfield, W.L. & Batson, M.J. (1997) The effects of a basketball season on aerobic and strength parameters among college men: Starters vs. reserves. *Journal of Strength and Conditioning Research* **11**, 21–24.

Hoffman, J.R. & Maresh, C.M. (2000) Physiology of Basketball. In: W.E. Garrett & D.T. Kirkendall, eds. *Exercise and Sport Science*, pp. 733–744. Philadelphia: Lippicott Williams & Wilkins.

Hoffman, J.R., Fry, A.C., Howard, R., Maresh, C.M. & Kraemer, W.J. (1991a) Strength, speed and endurance changes during the course of a division I basketball season. *Journal of Applied Sport Science Research* **5**, 144–149.

Hoffman, J.R., Maresh, C.M., Armstrong, L.E. & Kraemer, W.J. (1991b) Effects of off-season and in-season resistance training programs on a collegiate male basketball team. *Journal of Human Muscle Performance* **1**, 48–55.

Hoffman, J.R., Tennenbaum, G., Maresh, C.M. & Kraemer, W.J. (1996) Relationship between athletic performance tests and playing time in elite college basketball players. *Journal of Strength and Conditioning Research* **10**, 67–71.

Hoffman, J.R., Epstein, S., Einbinder, M. & Weinstein, I. (1999a) The influence of aerobic capacity on anaerobic performance and recovery indices in basketball players. *Journal of Strength and Conditioning Research* **13**, 407–411.

Hoffman, J.R., Epstein, S., Yarom, Y., Zigel, L. & Einbinder, M. (1999b) Hormonal and biochemical changes in elite basketball players during a 4-week training camp. *Journal of Strength and Conditioning Research* **13**, 280–285.

Hunter, G.R., Hilyer, J. & Forster, M.A. (1993) Changes in fitness during 4 years of intercollegiate basketball. *Journal of Strength and Conditioning Research* **7**, 26–29.

Kraemer, W.J. & Häkkinen, K. (eds) (2002) *Strength Training for Sport*. Blackwell Science, Oxford.

Lamonte, M.J., McKinney, J.T., Quinn, S.M., Bainbridge, C.N. & Eisenman, P.A. (1999) Comparison of physical and physiological variables for female college basketball players. *Journal of Strength and Conditioning Research* **13**, 264–270.

Latin, R.W., Berg, K. & Baechle, T. (1994) Physical and performance characteristics of NCAA division I male basketball players. *Journal of Strength and Conditioning Research* **8**, 214–218.

McInnes, S.E., Carlson, J.S., Jones, C.J. & McKenna, M.J. (1995) The physiological load imposed on basketball players during competition. *Journal of Sport Science* **13**, 387–397.

Parr, R.B., Hoover, R., Wilmore, J.H., Bachman, D. & Kerlan, R.K. (1978) Professional basketball players: Athletic profiles. *Physician and Sportsmedicine* **6**, 77–84.

Riezebos, M.L., Paterson, D.H., Hall, C.R. & Yuhasz, M.S. (1983) Relationship of selected variables to performance in women's basketball. *Canadian Journal of Applied Sport Science* **8**, 34–40.

Schilling, B.K. & Stone, M.H. (2000) Stretching: acute effects on strength and power performance. *National Strength and Conditioning Association Journal* **22**, 44–47.

Smith, H.K. & Thomas, S.G. (1991) Physiological characteristics of elite female basketball players. *Canadian Journal of Sport Science* **16**, 289–295.

Chapter 3
Nutrition guidelines for basketball

Leslie J. Bonci

Introduction

The game of basketball is a combination of intermittent and high intensity exercise, which places great physical demands on the body. The frequency of practices and games, coupled with off-court training and conditioning sessions can be exhausting. Basketball players often practice 6 days a week, often with twice a day practices and two to three games a week in season (Fig. 3.1).

The nutrition goals for basketball focus on maximizing speed, agility and power. Emphasis is placed on the necessary energy requirements before, during and post practice and competition for optimal performance and recovery.

One of the obstacles to eating appropriately and regularly is the hectic lifestyle and schedule of the basketball player. Games are often played in the evening, practices may occur during meal times, and the ability to eat well and often can be compromised. Athletes may be too tired to prepare a meal after an evening game or practice, and the healthier eating establishments may not be open late at night. Basketball players need to be educated on food choices to optimize performance, and expedite recovery, and need to be given guidelines on easy to prepare meals and snacks to increase fuel stores and prevent fatigue. For athletes who desire to gain or lose weight, regular eating episodes are an important component of attaining body composition goals. In addition, athletes often look for the quick fix, gravitating towards the supplements that serve as meal replacements, energy boosters, or anabolics. Athletes need to be aware that none of these products are replacements for the benefits of food, and should be used as an adjunct to eating, not a substitute for meals and snacks.

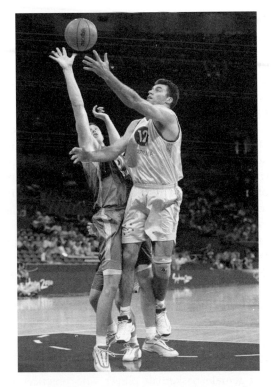

Fig. 3.1 Multiple practice sessions and contests each week require careful planning regarding food intake before, during and after vigorous activity. Photo © Getty Images/Andy Lyons.

Nutrition guidelines

Due to the nature of the game, the primary fuel substrate utilized during play is carbohydrate. In order to have enough energy to play at a high level throughout the entire game, the athlete must be eating enough overall calories, and the majority of those calories should come from carbohydrate-containing foods. Many athletes are unsure as to what constitutes a carbohydrate food, and instead may self-select foods that have a high fat to carbohydrate ratio. The athlete who chooses a doughnut over a bagel is consuming a food item that is 40% carbohydrate, 40% fat, compared to the bagel which is 90% carbohydrate, 2% fat. Carbohydrate is the fuel source used for basketball, so it is in the athlete's best interest to consume pre-exercise foods that can be used more efficiently during physical activity. Nutrition education regarding types of foods, and preferred nutrient sources for exercise and recovery should be a component of training.

The overall type, quantity and timing of nutrients are essential components of sports nutrition for all athletes. Nutritional goals need to be individualized, and the athletes need to be involved in the process. A coach, athletic trainer, team physican, or dietician cannot force the athlete to eat or drink, but can provide suggestions for food and fluid choices, and work with the athlete to implement an eating schedule. The coaching, training and medical staff should regularly reinforce the importance of proper nutrition and hydration, and address these topics with the team. Educational materials should be posted in the locker room, and visual reminders, such as water bottles, and snack items can help to remind athletes that they need to fuel to perform.

Nutritional requirements for basketball players include establishing calories guidelines, macro-, and micronutrient guidelines. The energy expenditure for basketball is 0.586 kJ·kg⁻¹·min⁻¹ of exercise.

Examples

59 kg female basketball player who practices for 120 min:

$59 \times 0.586 = 34.6 \text{ kJ·min}^{-1} \times 120 = 4149 \text{ kJ}$
expended during a 2-h practice

91 kg male basketball player practicing for 120 min:

$91 \times 0.586 = 53.3 \text{ kJ·min}^{-1} \times 120 = 6399 \text{ kJ}$
expended during a 2-h practice

In general, the guidelines for calorie requirements to maintain weight and provide adequate fuel for exercise are:
Males: >209 kJ·kg⁻¹·day⁻¹
Females: 188–209 kJ·kg⁻¹·day⁻¹.
Calorie needs are based upon body weight, and need to be adjusted accordingly, especially for the athlete who desires weight loss or expresses an interest in increasing mass. Smaller, more frequent eating episodes, where the athlete has a chance to fuel throughout the day, instead of eating infrequently, will provide a more constant source of available energy to the body, to enhance performance and expedite recovery. Athletes who eat infrequently often find that they tire more easily during practices and competition.

Basketball players need to establish a routine for meals, and pregame eating. The pre-exercise meal should provide enough fuel to prevent hypoglycemia, and to serve as an additional energy substrate during practices and games. The athlete who comes to practice or games on an empty stomach may not be comfortable eating a large meal before activity, but can learn to add in some foods gradually, and can determine his/her individual tolerance level.

Specific nutrient requirements

Basketball utilizes the three energy systems; ATP, lactic acid, and aerobic. The ATP and lactic acid energy systems allow the athlete to have the quick bursts of power required for fast breaks and jump shots. Slower paced play is fueled by the aerobic energy system. Carbohydrate is the only fuel substrate used for the ATP and lactic acid energy systems, and contributes 50% of the fuel source for the aerobic energy system, the other 50% is derived from fat. Protein contributes minimally as a fuel source during exercise, and should not be the main food source in pre-exercise meals. Emphasis on carbohydrate, as 50% or more of the pre-exercise meal, will optimize performance during activity. The recommendation for the macronutrient composition for a sports diet for basketball is:

Macronutrient	Composition (%)
Carbohydrate	50–60
Protein	15–20
Fat	20–30

Athletes need to be educated about the best food sources within each nutrient category. The carbohydrate foods eaten before exercise may differ from the ones chosen on rest days. Certainly, athletes should be encouraged to include foods that they enjoy, in order to maximize intake and fulfill nutrient needs. Food preferences, intolerances, cultural and religious food influences, the athlete's own beliefs regarding foods eaten before exercise, food availability and accessibility are all important considerations in planning a realistic and feasible sports diet.

Carbohydrate requirements

Much has been written regarding the types of carbohydrate that the athlete should consume. Players should be encouraged to select a variety of carbohydrate-containing foods to minimize taste fatigue and maximize the nutritional quality of the diet. Table 3.1 lists carbohydrate food sources.

Carbohydrate-containing foods should comprise two-thirds of the plate at every meal and snack. Half of the carbohydrate should be a starch-type food (bread, cereal, rice, pasta) and the other half as fruit and/or vegetable. Higher fat carbohydrate food sources such as chips, doughnuts, muffins and fried potatoes are not used as efficiently as a fuel source during exercise, but could be part of the post game food choices.

Some athletes have been told to limit certain types of carbohydrates before exercise due to the belief that sugar-containing foods could lower blood glucose levels before exercise and induce hypoglycemia, and impair performance. Recent studies have shown that unless the athlete suffers from hypoglycemia, the type of carbohydrate consumed before exercise does not negatively impact performance. For the hypoglycemic or diabetic player, individualized meal plans can help to regulate blood glucose during exercise, but carbohydrate foods are still a very important component of the pre-activity meal.

Although fruit and fruit juices are nutritionally dense foods, they may not always be the best pre-exercise choice. Citrus fruits and juices, apple juice, prune juice, and dried fruit may cause gastrointestinal distress if eaten before exercise. Athletes need to experiment to determine a comfort level with fruit and juices. Fiber is very important for normal bowel function, but high fiber food choices, such as legumes, bran, or cabbage family vegetables can cause gastrointestinal stress if eaten before physical activity. Players should be encouraged to include all types of fruits, vegetables, grains and dried beans and peas in their diet, but should be advised to eat the higher fiber foods, or drink fruit juices after exercise instead of prior to physical activity.

Table 3.1 Carbohydrate food sources.

Fruits	Juices	Fruit drinks†	Sports drinks
Carbonated beverages†	Vegetables	Vegetable juices	
Tomato sauces	Potatoes	Legumes	
Bread	Cold cereal	Hot cereal	Pasta
Rice	Millet	Kasha	Buckwheat
Quinoa	Bagels	Muffins*	Crackers*
Chips*	Pretzels	Popcorn*	Cookies*
Cake*	Pie*	Pastries*	Ice cream*
Frozen yogurt	Sorbet	Sherbet	
Fruit ices	Sugar†	Honey†	Syrup†
Molasses†	Candy†*	High carbohydrate sports beverages	
Sports bars	Granola*	Granola bars	Sports gels
Milk*	Yogurt*		

† Higher in simple sugars; * higher in fat content.

Athletes with early morning practices or conditioning sessions often complain of the lack of time for an adequate meal, and an aversion to eating before early morning exercise. After an overnight fast, the body needs fuel to replace liver glycogen stores, and to provide an energy substrate for exercise. Athletes who do not like to eat a full meal in the morning, can still benefit from a small amount of food, in a solid or liquid form. Listed below are some examples:

A banana and a handful of dry cereal

A cereal bar and a container of yoghurt

A bagel with a light spread of peanut butter

A sports gel or small packet of honey and a glass of water

A glass of juice and a sports bar (not a high protein type)

A high carbohydrate sports beverage (Gatorade® energy drink, UltraFuel®)

The recommendations for carbohydrate intake are $7\text{--}10 \text{ g·kg}^{-1} \text{ BW·day}^{-1}$ or approximately $500\text{--}600 \text{ g}$ of carbohydrate per day. The athlete who skips meals, or regularly eats only 1–2 times a day will find it a challenge to fulfill his/her carbohydrate needs. Athletes should be encouraged to consume both solid and liquid sources of carbohydrates. Juices, sports drinks, high carbohydrate sports beverages, and fruit drinks are excellent ways to both take in carbohydrate and hydrate the body.

Protein

Protein-containing foods provide a maximum of 10% of the fuel utilized during exercise. The major role of protein is for muscle growth and repair as well as immune system function. Many basketball players believe that protein should be the major focus of the diet, especially if they are interested in gaining muscle mass. This can lead to an eating plan that is carbohydrate deficient, resulting in impaired performance, delayed recovery, and an inability to synthesize new muscle tissue.

High protein diet plans have become increasingly popular. This is evident not only in meal plans, but in the vast array of high protein, low carbohydrate sports bars, drinks and other food items available in the marketplace. The attraction is a rapid weight

Table 3.2 Protein sources.

Beef	Pork	Veal	Lamb
Chicken	Duck	Turkey	Eggs
Fish	Shellfish	Milk	Cheese
Cottage cheese	Yogurt	Soy foods*	Nuts*
Nut butters*	Seeds*	Legumes*	Grains*
Vegetables*			

* Plant-based protein foods.

loss and appetite suppressing effect. The weight loss is due to water loss, which can impair performance, and the loss of appetite can result in inadequate calorie intake, which can result in earlier fatigue during exercise. The athlete who loses weight, but ends up feeling weak, tired, and unable to compete is a liability to himself/herself, and the team. In addition to dehydration, the excess protein in these diets can lead to calcium and electrolyte loss.

Protein is also an essential component of the diet for the vegetarian player. The athlete who opts to avoid animal-based protein sources needs to be educated about the importance of protein in the diet, and steered towards appropriate sources of plant protein. The only foods that do not supply protein are fruits, beverages (except milk), fats (oils, spreads) and sweets. Animal protein sources such as meat, poultry, fish, eggs and dairy products supply all of the essential amino acids and are labeled as complete proteins. Soy foods are the only plant protein source that provides all of the essential amino acids. Plant-based protein sources such as grains, vegetables, nuts, seeds, and legumes are incomplete protein sources since they do not provide all of the essential amino acids. However, these items are often eaten in combination, e.g., beans and rice, or peanut butter on bread, or with complete proteins, e.g., cereal and milk, so it is possible for vegetarians to fulfill their protein requirements. Table 3.2 lists protein-containing foods.

Protein requirements

Protein requirements are higher for athletes than sedentary individuals, but there is a maximal daily amount of protein that the physically active can effectively utilize.

Adult protein requirements for basketball: 1.7 $g \cdot kg^{-1}$ BW

Adolescent protein requirements for basketball: 2.0 $g \cdot kg^{-1}$ BW

Many athletes assume that the more protein they consume, the more mass they will gain. There is an upper limit with regards to the amount of protein the body can use. The formula is

$$\text{Weight (kg)} \times 2.2 = \text{Maximum number of grams of protein daily}$$

Protein consumed in excess of this amount can result in increased body fat deposition instead of an increase in lean muscle mass.

Fat requirements

Fat intake varies widely in different cultures. Some basketball players routinely eat a low-fat diet consisting of traditional food choices, while others make a conscious effort to restrict fat intake by minimizing the use of added fats, fried foods, and higher fat snack items. Fat is used as a fuel substrate for endurance exercise, and is important for lubrication, thermoregulation and transporting fat soluble vitamins. Some athletes wrongly believe that eating fat-containing foods will lead to excess body fat. If the player eats more calories than his/her body can effectively use, the excess will be stored as body fat whether the food item is derived from protein, carbohydrate, or fat. Fat-containing foods do promote between-meal satiety, which can be advantageous for the athlete who is trying to lose weight. The athlete who restricts fat intake must rely more heavily on carbohydrate stores as the fuel for exercise, which can lead to more rapid muscle and liver glycogen depletion resulting in earlier fatigue and impaired performance.

Fat is a concentrated source of energy, so one does not have to eat a lot to get a significant source of calories. This can be helpful for the athlete who loses weight during the season, but finds it difficult to ingest large quantities of food. Nuts, seeds, or nut butters can provide a good source of fat and protein to add extra calories without having to eat large amounts of food.

Guidelines have been written with regard to the best types of fat to include for health promotion and disease risk reduction. The type of fat is not as important on the playing field, as all fats will be used as a fuel substrate, but it is certainly in the best interest of the athlete to make recommendations as to the healthiest types of fats to include in the daily meal plan. Saturated fats (fat on meats, fattier cuts of meat, skin on poultry, high fat dairy products, coconut, coconut and palm oils, and hydrogenated oils) have been associated with increased cardiovascular disease and cancer risk. Unsaturated fats such as oils, nuts, nut butters, avocado, fatty fish, and flaxseed may have disease-risk reducing potential, and should be the primary fat sources in the diet. Table 3.3 lists sources of fat.

Since fat is a concentrated calorie source, it should be used moderately. Fat-containing foods take longer to digest than either carbohydrate or protein, and a high fat meal before exercise can result in gastrointestinal distress. It is prudent to recommend that athletes minimize the intake of fried foods, or creamy sauces before exercise, and use these foods as part of post exercise refueling.

Since basketball players expend more calories than sedentary individuals, they can afford to eat a diet that provides between 20 and 30% of the total calories as fat. The recommendations for fat intake are 1.0–1.2 $g \cdot kg^{-1}$ $BW \cdot day^{-1}$.

Table 3.3 Fat sources.

Butter*	Cream*	Cream cheese*	Bacon/sausage*
Oil	Olives	Coconut/oil*	Palm kernel oil*
Stick margarine*	Shortening*	Tub margarine	
Creamy salad dressings*	Oil-based salad dressings	Mayonnaise	
Flaxseed	Avocado		

* Sources of saturated fat.

Table 3.4 Hidden fats.

Ice cream	Pastries	Cookies	Chocolate
Sausage	Bacon	Pepperoni	Lunchmeats
Crackers	Chips	Muffins	Biscuits
Cheeses	Milk	Fat on meats	Poultry skin
Fried potatoes	Fried meats	Fried vegetables	

54 kg female would require 54–65 g of fat per day
91 kg male would require 91–110 g of fat per day
A tablespoon of oil provides 14 g of fat
$^1/_2$ cup of nuts provides 38 g of fat
2 tablespoons of salad dressing provides 12 g of fat
2 tablespoons of peanut butter provides 16 g of fat
1 tablespoon of butter has 12 g of fat

In addition, most grains and cereals contain small amounts of fat, as do meats, eggs and dairy products, unless they are fat free. The challenge is that many foods contain hidden fats, which can contribute to the daily overall fat content of the diet. Some of these are listed in Table 3.4.

Vitamin-mineral requirements

Many athletes think that vitamin-mineral supplements will provide energy and can be taken in place of meals. Vitamin-mineral supplements are an addition to, not a replacement for eating. An athlete who eats infrequently and consumes an unbalanced diet but takes supplements will end up with a well-supplemented, subpar diet.

Vitamin-mineral requirements are higher for a basketball player than a sedentary individual, but these additional needs can be met through food. There is no need for athletes to take high potency vitamin-mineral supplements. They are expensive, and still do not provide the active individual with the necessary fuel substrate. Vitamins do assist in the digestion and metabolism of nutrients, but are not a direct source of fuel for the body. Vitamin needs can be met through foods. Table 3.5 lists food sources of vitamins and the DRIs (dietary reference intakes).

If the athlete chooses to take a supplement, the following guidelines can help to direct him or her to an appropriate product:
1 Take a product with 100% of the RDA/DRI.
2 There is no need to buy a costly supplement.
3 Purchase a multivitamin-mineral supplement, instead of individual formulations, unless advised by one's physician.
4 A natural product is not necessarily superior, but may cost more.
5 Supplements should be taken daily, and with meals.

Athletes who regularly consume fortified cereals, sports bars, and protein powders may already be meeting their daily requirements, and would not benefit from a supplement.

Table 3.5 Vitamin sources.

Vitamin	Dietary reference intake (DRI)	Food source
B vitamins		Enriched grains and cereals, whole grain
Thiamin	1.1–1.2 mg	Leafy greens
Riboflavin	1.1–1.3 mg	
Niacin	14–16 mg/day NE	Protein-containing foods
Pyridoxine	1.3 mg·day^{-1}	Whole grains, leafy greens
Folate	400 µg	Enriched grains, leafy greens, lentils
Vitamin B$_{12}$	2.4 µg	Animal foods
Vitamin A	1000 RE/3333 IU	Liver, egg yolk, fortified dairy products
Beta-carotene	5000 IU	Deep orange fruits and vegetables, tomatoes/tomato products, deep green vegetables
Vitamin C	75–90 mg	Citrus fruits/juices, tropical fruits, berries, broccoli, tomato products
Vitamin D	200 IU	Sunshine, egg yolk, fortified dairy products
Vitamin E	15 mg/22.4 IU	Oils, nuts, seeds
Vitamin K	55–80 µg	Deep green leafy vegetables

Table 3.6 Mineral sources.

Mineral	Dietary reference intake (DRI)	Food sources
Calcium	1000 mg	Dairy foods, canned fish w/bones, fortified soy products, fortified juices, dark green leafy vegetables
Phosphorus	700 mg	Dairy foods, canned fish
Magnesium	310–400 mg	Whole grains, nuts, chocolate
Zinc	12–15 mg	Oysters, liver, barley, soy, nuts
Iron	10–15 mg	Red meat, fortified cereals, liver
Manganese	ESADDI: 2–5 mg†	Whole grains, leafy vegetables, nuts, beans, tea
Selenium	55 µg	Fish/shellfish, meat, eggs, fish, nuts
Chromium	ESADDI: 50–200 µg†	Whole grains, organ meats, beer, mushrooms, nuts
Sodium	EMR: 500 mg*	Salt, canned foods, condiments, pickles, sports drinks, snack crackers, chips, pretzels
Potassium	EMR: 2000 mg*	Fruits/juices, vegetables/juices, tomato products, yogurt, milk, nuts, legumes

† Estimated safe and adequate dietary intakes; * estimated minimum requirements.

Minerals

Minerals, especially calcium, magnesium, and phosphorus, are involved in muscle and nervous system function as well as bone health. Minerals are needed in much smaller quantities than vitamins, with the exception of calcium. Care must be taken to ensure that players do not overdo it when it comes to mineral supplementation. With the abundance of supplements available, in addition to fortified foods and beverages, and the belief that more is better, it would be fairly easy for an athlete to exceed his/her daily mineral requirements. Mineral requirements can be met through food sources. For the athlete who does not like or cannot tolerate dairy products, a calcium supplement may be warranted to ensure optimal bone health. Again, a supplement is not a replacement for food, so even if the athlete takes a daily supplement, frequent and balanced meals are a vital part of the athlete's well-being. Mineral requirements can be met through foods. Table 3.6 lists food sources of minerals and the DRIs (dietary reference intakes).

The electrolytes sodium and potassium are important for maintaining optimal hydration status and cardiovascular function, and preventing cramps. Athletes should not overly restrict the use of salt, unless advised by a health care professional. Consuming lightly salted foods or using sodium-containing condiments before a game, as well as making use of sports drinks during exercise can help to prevent sodium loss. Fruits, juices, and sports drinks are excellent sources of potassium, that can be used during and post exercise, as well as the night before games to ensure optimal potassium levels. Some post exercise electrolyte replacement techniques include consuming:
Salted nuts and orange juice
A banana and pretzels
A trail mix of dried fruit, cereal and nuts
Yogurt with cereal added.

Timing eating to exercise

Athletes need to be encouraged to eat prior to play. Basketball requires bursts of activity throughout the duration of the game. The player who is suboptimally nourished will not be able to finish strong. Since practices are frequent and intense, the athlete needs to view fueling as a 7 day a week endeavor. Fueling guidelines are divided into pre-, during, and post exercise recommendations.

Pre-exercise

Studies have shown that athletes who eat a moderately high carbohydrate, low fat, low protein meal

3 h before exercise may notice enhanced performance during exercise. A meal eaten 6 h before exercise will not confer any advantage during play. It is important to remind the athlete that late night eating is not a replacement for the morning meal. After an overnight fast, the body needs to refuel. Many athletes assume that if they eat before they go to bed, the body can use the fuel from late night eating for early morning activity. Athletes need to be encouraged to eat or drink something to provide energy for early morning practices and/or conditioning sessions.

Since the timing of pregame meals varies widely among teams, it may be necessary to encourage athletes to have a snack before games, especially if the pregame meal is more than 3 h before tip-off. The team manager and/or athletic trainer should have some items on hand for hungry players to ensure that athletes are optimally fueled for competition.

Good pregame meals place an emphasis on carbohydrate, with moderate amounts of protein, and a small amount of fat. Examples include:
Pasta with a tomato or broth-based sauce (with very lean ground meat, poultry, or seafood)
A turkey sandwich
Stir fry with chicken, lean meat, or seafood and vegetables over rice
Rice and beans
Chicken, seafood or vegetable curries with rice
Cereal
Waffles, pancakes, French toast
Eggs and bagels with fresh fruit.

If the pregame meal is >3 h before the game, the players should be encouraged to eat a pregame snack about 30–60 min before tip-off. Appropriate snacks include:
Cereal bars
Low fat, low protein sports bars
Fruit (if the player tolerates it)
A high carbohydrate sports beverage
Crackers
Dry cereal
Yogurt
Pretzels.

During exercise

During exercise, the body needs to be fueled to maintain a high level of play. The recommendation for energy intake during exercise is for the athlete to consume 30–60 g of carbohydrate per hour of play. This can be done by recommending any of the following:
Sports drink: 24 ounces per hour
Honey: 2 tablespoons
Sports gel: 1 ounce packet
Sweetened cereal: 1 cup
Gummy type candy/jelly beans: $1/4$ cup
Dried fruit: $1/4$ cup
Cereal bar or granola bar.

Post exercise

The timing and amount of post exercise fuel is critical for optimal and rapid recovery. The window of opportunity for maximal glycogen resynthesis is within 30 min post exercise. The goal is for the athlete to ingest 1–1.5 g of carbohydrate/kg body weight within this time period. Recommending high carbohydrate fluids will not only refuel, but also rehydrate the athlete. Players should be encouraged to bring a snack to practice to consume before they leave the gym or weight room. After games, food and fluid should be available for all players. Appropriate post exercise snacks include:
Lemonade or fruit punch (athletes can bring a powdered drink mix, and just add to water)
Fruit juice
Yogurt
Bagels
Sports bars.

Fluid requirements

One of the biggest challenges for basketball players is maintaining optimal hydration status. Dehydration can significantly affect muscle strength, speed, and stamina, as well as energy levels and concentration. Athletes need to learn to drink on schedule beyond the point of thirst, and to monitor hydration status. Recommendations for achieving optimal hydration status include:
1 Have fluids available and accessible during practice and games.

Table 3.7 Fluid guidelines for basketball.

Time of day	Fluid (amount)
Resting fluid needs	10–12 cups (2.5–3 L)
Pre-exercise (2 h before)	2 cups (0.5 L)
During exercise (every 15 min)	5–10 ounces
Post exercise	53 ounces (1.6 L) of fluid for every kg lost during exercise

2 Encourage use of sports drinks and foods with high liquid content (fruit, popsicles, fruit ices).

3 Schedule drinking breaks, recommending that the player consume 5–10 ounces of fluid every 15–20 min.

4 Have athletes record sweat rates by weighing pre and post exercise to determine the amount of fluid the body loses during exercise. The athlete should aim to replace at least 50% of fluid loss daily.

5 Teach athletes which types of fluids work best:
Decaffeinated beverages
Beverages without guarana, mate, or kola nut
Noncarbonated beverages
Nonalcoholic beverages.

6 Have a water bottle for each player.

7 Have flavored, cool liquids available.

8 Have athletes monitor urine for volume and color.

9 Make drinking a part of the game plan.

Table 3.7 lists specific fluid guidelines for basketball.

The athlete who loses 2 kg during exercise would have to drink 106 ounces of fluid in the hours after exercise to replenish fluid losses.

Since caffeine and alcohol are both diuretics, they will result in fluid loss, and do not effectively hydrate the athlete. Herbal sources of caffeine, such as guarana, mate, and kola nut will have the same effect. Carbonated beverages often give the sensation of fullness before the athlete has satisfied hydration requirements. After a victory, recommend sports drinks, juices and fruit punch first, before the athlete goes out to celebrate. Table 3.8 summarizes the recommendations for fuel and fluid for exercise.

Supplements

Nutritional ergogenic aides or performance enhancing supplements have been used historically in all sports. The business of sports supplements is a multi-million dollar industry worldwide, and athletes are not immune to the sales tactics and marketing ads for products that promise improved fitness, endurance and recovery. For Olympic athletes, there are special concerns about products that may cause the player to fail a drug test. Since there are so many products on the marketplace, issues of supplement safety, purity, legality and effectiveness are of importance to the athlete. Health care professionals and the training and coaching staff need to know what their players are taking and provide appropriate guidelines for product use, as well as the safety implications.

In general, basketball players are most likely to choose from the following types of supplements:

Table 3.8 Timing and amount of fuel for exercise.

Type of athlete	Carbohydrate	Fluid
Player who trains hard daily	7–10 g·kg^{-1} BW	10–12 cups
Player who trains < 1 h daily	5–7 g·kg^{-1} BW	10–12 cups
Time of meal		
Pre-exercise		
1 h before	1 g·kg^{-1} BW	17 ounces (0.5 L)
2 h before	2 g·kg^{-1} BW	2 h before exercise
3 h before	3 g·kg^{-1} BW	
4 h before	4 g·kg^{-1} BW	
During exercise	30–60 g·h^{-1}	5–10 ounces every 15 min
Post exercise	1.0–1.5 g·kg^{-1} BW post exercise and every 2 h post exercise	53 ounces (1.6 L) of fluid for every kg lost within 2 h post exercise

1 Products that increase mass
2 Products that promise weight loss
3 Products that increase energy
4 Products that alleviate pain
5 Products that support a healthy immune system
6 Products that enhance recovery
7 Supplements that improve mental clarity.

Athletes need to be educated on the use of products, so that the end result is performance enhancing, not performance detracting. The training and medical staff should address these issues with the team, and if necessary, on an individual basis with players. The following points are worth reviewing with each player so that supplements can be used responsibly and effectively.

1 The training and medical staff should encourage the athlete to bring in the product(s) that he/she takes, with the label.
2 The athlete needs to know that more is not better.
3 Athletes should avoid mixing or "stacking" products.
4 Athletes should report any unusual side-effects that could be associated with supplement use, and should discontinue using the product(s) immediately.
5 Athletes should look for products that are standardized.
6 Athletes should not exceed the dose on the product.
7 Athletes should not take any supplement if they are on prescription medications without first speaking with their health care professionals.
8 Athletes need to know what products are harmful and banned.

Table 3.9 lists products by claims.

The ergogenic effectiveness of many of the supplements is unknown, and may vary widely among athletes. Supplements are never a substitute for training, diet and hydration, and their use must be carefully monitored, especially in athletes with underlying medical issues and/or those on prescribed medications.

Purity and safety issues need to be addressed with all athletes. Supplement manufacturers are not subject to the same standards as those for prescription medications, so product purity, dosage, and ingredients may not accurately reflect what is in the product. Players need to know that natural and safe are not synonymous terms. Supplements are not just available in a pill, capsule, or extract form, but

Table 3.9 Supplements.

Claims	Product
Anabolic	Creatine
	Protein powders
	Amino acid supplements
	Boron
	Tribulus*
	Androstenedione*/Norandro*
	DHEA*
	GHB/GBL*
	Yohimbe †
	Smilax
	Moomiyo
Weight loss/fat burning	Ephedra*
	HCA*
	Cayenne
	Caffeine*
	Guarana
	Mate
	Kola nut
	White willow bark
Energy boosting	Ginseng
	Ephedra*
Anti-inflammatory	White willow bark
	Boswellia
	Digestive enzymes
	Sam-e
	MSM
	Phosphatidylserine
	Glucosamine
	Chondroitin sulfate
	Turmeric
Immune system	Ginseng
	Astragalus
	Echinacea
Recovery	Glutamine
	Ginseng
Mental clarity	Ginkgo

* Banned substances; † dangerous substances.

are frequently added to beverages, sports bars, and protein powders. Players need to look closely at the labels on these products to determine what they contain. Some products contain supplements that have a laxative or diuretic effect, which can cause dehydration. Others may cause significant gastrointestinal distress, while others can potentiate or decrease the effectiveness of a prescription medication. Guarana, a herbal form of caffeine, can interfere with the absorption of calcium, magnesium and iron supplements.

Table 3.10 Banned nutritional supplements.

Caffeine (urine concentration >12 µg·mL⁻¹)
Ephedrines (urine concentration >10 µg·mL⁻¹)
Pseudoephedrine (urine concentration >25 µg·mL⁻¹)
Nandrolone
19-Norandrostenediol and 19-norandrostenedione
  (>2 ng·mL⁻¹ in males) (>5 ng·mL⁻¹ in females)
Androstenedione and androstenediol
Dehydroepiandrosterone (DHEA)
Growth hormone
Insulin-like growth factor
Insulin (unless athlete is a certified insulin dependent diabetic)
Furosemide*

* Can be present in some herbal products.

Insist that athletes fill out a supplement sheet, which may need to be updated several times throughout the year, and keep this information on file for every player.

Banned substances

In the quest for the "edge", athletes may be tempted to try products that are banned by the International Olympic Committee (IOC). Athletes who take these products and fail a drug test will be banned from competition. Players need to be educated on a regular basis as to what products are banned. This list should be posted in the locker room, the team physician's office, athletic trainer's office, coach's office, and every player should receive a copy as well.

The complete list of prohibited classes of substances and prohibited methods is available on the IOC website. Table 3.10 lists nutritional supplements which are banned.

Weight considerations

Due to the intense physical exertion required for basketball, and the lengthy season, coaches often complain of their players' inability to maintain weight throughout the season. Players may complain of fatigue and staleness due to their inability to eat enough for performance and recovery as the season progresses. The basketball player needs to establish an eating schedule before the season begins, rather than waiting until competition has already begun. The timing of games, and late-night eating can present a challenge for the athlete interested in weight goals. Oftentimes athletes have misconceptions about appropriate weight goals, body composition, and the most effective methods for achieving results. Athletes often want the quick fix, whether they are trying to build muscle, or lose body fat, and need to be encouraged to make changes gradually, in order to be successful.

Weight gain techniques

For the athlete who complains of an inability to gain or maintain weight, frequency of meals should be the primary focus. The player who eats sporadically, with only 1–2 eating episodes per day will not be able to meet normal physiological demands, let alone the increased energy requirements for sport. The answer is not just to have the player increase intake of high fat, high calorie food, but to encourage more frequent eating episodes and creative suggestions for boosting calories without causing the athlete to feel stuffed and uncomfortable. In general, maximal lean muscle weight gain occurs at a rate of about 0.225 kg per week. Athletes need to realize that weight gain does not happen overnight, and does require change in eating habits and food choices in order to achieve one's goals. The weight-gain products that are commercially available are protein powders with some flavoring agents added. Many athletes find them to be quire unpalatable, and they are very costly as well. Recommendations for weight gain include:

1 Try to include three meals per day with snacks in between.

2 Include beverages with calories, instead of just water. Choose more often: milk, juice, sports drinks, fruit drinks, instead of water, plain coffee, tea, or diet beverages.

3 Choose cereals, other grains and breads with a higher calorie content.

4 Use nuts/seeds as a snack, or added to cereal or salads.

5 Aim to increase the portion size of each meal by one-fourth more food.

6 Add a little more fat to food, i.e., oil, spreads, nut butters, salad dressings.

7 Adding extra food needs to be a 7-day a week plan in order to see weight gain.

8 Rely on food, not supplements for weight gain. If a weight gain beverage is desired, encourage the athlete to make his/her own with milk, ice cream, fruit juice and fruit to add some extra calories.

Weight loss strategies

For the athlete who is interested in weight loss, there are several fad diets and gimmicks commercially available, which all promise the easy way to weight loss. Unfortunately, the consumer's definition of the word "diet" implies restrictive eating patterns and food choices, which can have a deleterious effect on performance. An overzealous player, attempting to please the coach by dropping weight quickly may resort to meal skipping, nutrient restriction, excessive exercise, and inadequate fluids. All of these methods will significantly impair the athlete's strength, speed, stamina and cognitive abilities.

Achieving weight-loss goals can be difficult due to the hectic schedule, frequent travel, late-night games, and limited access to healthy, lower calorie meal items.

It is very important to set appropriate weight-loss goals, based upon body composition, not just body weight. Measuring body fat percentage should be the starting point for determining weight goals.

Example

A male basketball player weighs 91 kg and has 21% body fat.
He would like to lower body fat to 15%

91 kg × 0.21 = 19 kg of body fat
91–19 = 72 kg of lean muscle mass

To determine weight goals:

72 kg divided by 0.85 (for desired body fat of 15%)
= 85 kg

This athlete would need to lose 6 kg to achieve a desired body fat of 15%.

Since the body typically loses body fat at a rate of approximately 0.225–0.34 kg·week^{-1}, it would take this athlete about 4 months to lose the extra body fat.

Determining body fat and setting weight goals well in advance of the season can help the athlete to achieve his/her goals before the pressure of competition begins.

It is important for athletes and coaches to realize that there is nothing magical about a body fat percentage, nor is a certain number a guarantee of optimal performance. Oftentimes, the process of weight loss, when done appropriately, is enough to make the athlete feel better about himself/herself, even if the weight recommendation is not achieved. The athlete needs to be encouraged to focus on eating habits, not just food choices. The main reason diets fail is because they advocate drastic changes in food choices, but do not address the underlying eating habits that often contribute to excess weight.

Foods should not be labeled as "good" or "bad". Eating plans that recommend restricting or eliminating entire groups of foods should be discouraged. Players need to realize that there are not magical combinations of foods that produce weight loss. The bottom line is that the athlete needs to consume fewer calories than he/she expends for the body to lose weight.

The use of over-the-counter (OTC) weight-loss products should be strongly discouraged. Some of these products are banned substances, i.e., ephedrines, caffeine (in large doses). Others have a significant laxative or diuretic effect (senna, cascara, hydroxycitric acid) and others are ineffective for weight loss (chitin, quercetin, L-carnitine).

For the player who is interested in losing weight, the process should begin at the end of the season, when the athlete has time to focus on the goals, and make changes to current eating patterns and food choices. Suggestions for weight loss include:

1 Encourage the athlete to eat on a regular schedule. Athletes who skip meals will find that losing weight is much more difficult as they will be more hungry.

2 Recommend that the athlete consume the majority of calories prior to the evening meal.

3 Suggest that the majority of calories come from food, not liquids, as beverages are not as satisfying.

4 Athletes need to be conscious of what they eat, and should make an attempt to eat without the distraction of television, video games or the computer.

5 Recommend that athletes who eat out regularly request normal-sized portions, not super size items. Athletes can also request smaller portions of entrees in restaurants.

6 Players should be aware of what they add to foods. Salad dressings, sauces, gravies and spreads can add a significant number of calories. In restaurants, these items should be served on the side.

7 Players should include foods that promote satiety to help the athlete to feel fuller for longer. Protein-containing foods tend to be more satisfying and should be part of every meal. Including foods that require more chewing, or have a higher liquid content can also help to add a feeling of fullness. These include: fruits, vegetables, salads, whole grains, and soups.

8 Athletes should make gradual changes to eating, cutting back slowly on the amount of food at a meal to prevent feeling overly hungry.

Conclusion

Nutrition recommendations for the basketball player can result in an athlete with more energy, fewer injuries, successful weight management and quicker recovery. Make eating a priority for athletes, with reminders to eat and drink on schedule and to refuel after practices and games. Educate athletes about the appropriate use of supplements, and how to effectively achieve weight goals. The time spent in these endeavors will produce an athlete at the top of his/her game.

Further reading

Antonio, J. & Stout, J.R. (2001) *Sports Supplements*. Philadelphia: Lippincott Williams & Wilkins.

Bernardot, D. (2000) *Nutrition for Serious Athletes*. Champaign, IL: Human Kinetics.

Burke, L. (1995) *The Complete Guide to Food for Sports Performance*, 2nd edn. St Leonards, Australia: Allen & Unwin.

Gatorade Sports Science Institute website: www.gssiweb.com.

Hendler, S.S. & Rorvik, D. (2001) *PDR for Nutritional Supplements*. Montvale: Medical Economics Company.

International Journal of Sport Nutrition and Exercise Metabolism. Champaign, IL: Human Kinetics.

Manore, M. & Thompson, J. (eds) (2000) *Sport Nutrition for Health and Performance*. Champaign, IL: Human Kinetics.

Maughan, R.J. (ed.) (2000) *Nutrition in Sport*. Oxford: Blackwell Science.

PDR for Herbal Medicines, 2nd edn. (2000) Montvale: Medical Economics Company.

Rosenbloom, C. (ed.) (2000) *Sports Nutrition: A Guide for the Professional Working with Active People*, 3rd edn. Chicago: American Dietetic Association.

Williams, M. (1998) *The Ergogenics Edge*. Champaign, IL: Human Kinetics.

Chapter 4
Preventive medicine in basketball

Thomas J. Mackowiak

The sport of basketball is categorized as a contact sport. The *U.S. Trends in Team Sports* (2000) reported that with nearly 40 million active male and female participants yearly, basketball is America's most popular team sport. The prevention of athletic injuries should continue to be a major focus for all health care programs overseeing recreational and athletic competition. Injuries are inevitable in all recreational, practice, and game venues. During the 1990s, a recent trend revealing the increases in the incidence of basketball injuries began to develop. The increasing popularity of the sport of basketball, combined with gradual amplified playing aggressiveness, officials' rule interpretations, coaching styles, and intense style of play, has led to more frequent and severe injuries.

The most common reported injury in basketball is the ankle sprain. This inversion and plantar flexed mechanism is normally caused by a sharp cutting movement, pivoting, or landing on another player's foot or ankle complex. Numerous studies and current research have reported the increased frequency of anterior cruciate ligament (ACL) knee injuries in female basketball players in comparison to male basketball players. Kirkendall *et al.* (2000), Ireland *et al.* (1990), and numerous others have reported that females are two to six times more susceptible than males to sustaining an ACL knee injury in basketball. The reported data shows that the ACL injury normally occurs in noncontact situations. Flanders and Mohandas (1995) reported that basketball players sustain facial injuries at a higher rate than any other reported sport except baseball. They continued to report that 90% of the facial injuries inflicted upon the mouth and teeth regions were by contact with an opponent's head, hands, shoulders, or arms.

Prior, during, and after athletic competition, the sports medicine team works collaboratively to offer immediate triage-type services on the injured athlete. Immediate injury evaluation techniques, initial first aid, therapeutic treatments, follow-up rehabilitation, and functional reconditioning programs are used in conjunction with proper planning strategies to return the athlete back safely and quickly to competition.

Injury reduction and prevention strategies begin with the preparticipation physical examination (PPE). This comprehensive medical health awareness proponent combines the proper medical evaluative procedures and physical fitness profiles. Additionally, sport-specific reconditioning corrective exercises for the hip, knee, and ankle musculoskeletal regions must emphasize a total body rehabilitation approach (Fig. 4.1). The reconditioning programs must pertain to correcting muscular imbalances in the quadriceps/hamstrings muscle groups, especially in female basketball players. Sport-specific plyometric exercises instructing proper landing knee mechanics to decrease the impact of the landing forces, strength training programs, functional multiplane jumping activities, and proprioception balance training are recommended to prevent possible anterior cruciate ligament knee injuries. In athletics, the sports medicine team pursues an aggressive, safe treatment and rehabilitation criteria for the injured athlete in many postinjury situations. Within the

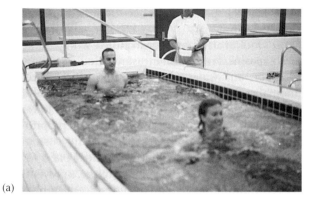

(a)

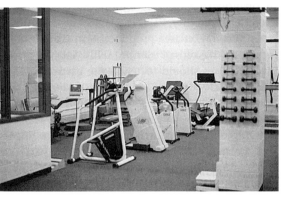

(b)

Fig. 4.1 (a) Swim-ex rehab and cardiovascular conditioning/functional training sessions. (b) General rehabilitation equipment.

past decade, the philosophical acceptance has pursued an aggressive emphasis on preventive maintenance programs.

Why should coaching or medical staff wait for an athlete to become injured or ill, if potential injury circumstances that directly or indirectly predispose the player to injury or illness can be controlled or minimized? The sports medicine team must maintain an awareness and knowledge of the epidemiological injury factors prevalent in the sport of basketball. The implementation of preventive medicine programs is challenging, time-consuming, and individually oriented. Injury prevention strategies impact and involve:

1 regular safety checks of facilities, equipment, and surroundings inside and outside courtside structures;
2 designing protective equipment to prevent injury or re-injury situations;

3 awareness and implementation of universal precautions;
4 designing and implementing year-round conditioning programs to develop and maintain strength, endurance, flexibility, and agility;
5 medical coverage strategies;
6 emergency planning designs;
7 travel factors;
8 seasonal and environmental concerns;
9 daily communication, observation, and awareness of the athlete's physical and mental well-being.

The sport of basketball incorporates anaerobic and aerobic endurance, muscular strength and power, flexibility, speed, balance, muscular endurance, agility, explosiveness, and mental toughness. What type of exercises could be initiated in preventing potential injuries? The current emphasis on strength training and cardiovascular conditioning (aerobic and anaerobic endurance) has improved physical strength and stamina issues throughout the sport. Sport-specific strength training protocols, flexibility exercises, balancing drills, coaching techniques, nutritional programs, structural evaluations, and biomechanical analysis assist as a preventive screening device for future, potential injury patterns.

Basketball injuries can be directly related to a lack of strength in supporting muscle groups. Strength exercises should be directed at muscles supporting the ankle, knee, and lower back regions. Players should be evaluated to identify specific muscular weaknesses or imbalances, which can be corrected through strength training (Stone & Steingard 1993) (Fig. 4.2).

Coaching philosophies, enhanced performance issues, and injury prevention programs have encouraged the athlete to maintain year-round conditioning programs. The implementation of strength and conditioning macro/micro cycle programs are designed to gradually intensify the athlete's performance with the intent of attaining and maintaining a healthy, high level of fitness during the competitive season. Studies have supported the contention that preconditioning reduces the incidence of sports injuries (Stone & Steingard 1993). The preseason, in-season, postseason, and off-season programs all emphasize unique components enabling the basketball player to compete longer, more intensely, with less fatigue, and less susceptibility to injury.

international athletic governing organizations. The local, on-site basketball game officials are responsible for the interpretation and enforcement of the protective equipment criteria rules.

The National Collegiate Athletic Association (NCAA) has specific rules governing special postinjury or protective equipment for men's and women's basketball (NCAA 2000). These rules include:
• Elbow, hand, finger, wrist, or forearm guards, casts or braces made of fiberglass, plaster, metal or any other nonpliable substance shall be prohibited.
• Pliable (flexible or easily bent) material covered on all exterior sides and edges with no less than 0.5 inch thickness of a slow-rebounding foam shall be used to immobilize and/or protect an injury.
• The prohibition of the use of hard-substance material does not apply to the upper arm, shoulder, thigh, or lower leg if the material is padded so as not to create a hazard for other players.
• Equipment that could cut or cause an injury to another player is prohibited, regardless of the hardness of the equipment.
• Equipment that, in the referee's judgement, is dangerous to other players may not be worn.

Unauthorized "equipment" worn for convenience or comfort that could generate injury during basketball activity are rings, earrings, necklaces, and eyeglasses. Basketball players who wear rings during activity can catch them within the basketball net, on the rim, or on an opponent's jersey inflicting serious injury to the digits and surrounding soft tissue area. Necklaces can become entangled in opponent's hands/fingers, clothes or equipment, or cause cervical neck injury. Improper fitting or breakable lenses or rims of eyeglasses can shatter upon contact. These scenarios can create lacerations or severe trauma to the athlete's eye, lid, or facial region. Earrings must be removed or covered prior to competition to prevent serious ear trauma or lacerations to competing players. The sports medicine team should maintain an awareness and knowledge of the athletes with any other body piercings, with specific attention to the face and tongue.

Equipment for basketball

Currently, many basketball players incorporate a variety of preventive and postinjury type equipment during playing sessions. Additional body support protectors include: head bands, finger "buddy" protectors, wrist bands, elbow neoprene sleeves, elbow pads, knee neoprene sleeves, patellar-femoral braces, knee pads, compression shorts, shoulder braces, thigh protectors, goggles, orthotics, mouthpieces, and ankle braces. Basketball shoes offer various styles, support, and designs for the competitive and non-competitive basketball player.

Factors that may influence the selection, purchase and wearing of equipment are safety or protection, social factors, cost, influential peer recommendations, peer attitudes and recent trends, and the perceived influence on performance.

Construction of protective and supportive equipment

The sport of basketball involves a high incidence for collision and impact forces at various speeds. Protective equipment ranges from preventive to postinjury, from prefabricated to unique, individually constructed protective devices. The selection and design of protective equipment is based on the optimal level of impact intensity afforded by the given thickness, density, and temperature of energy-absorbing material (Anderson et al. 2000). Many different materials offer soft or hard-density protection (Fig. 4.5).

Soft or low-density materials, such as neoprene, foam, gauze, cotton, and felt are available in varying thicknesses, densities, cushioning effects, and com-

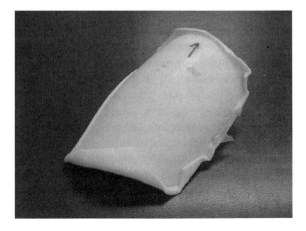

Fig. 4.5 Aquaplast thigh protection.

pressive forces. Firm, nonyielding high-density materials are constructed to absorb more energy during impact. These materials consist of thermoldable plastics and casting materials. Thermoplastics are divided into two categories: plastic and rubber. Specific categories to consider when designing the protection or splint devices are conformity to the body part, stiffness, memory, and durability. Several heat-forming plastic materials are aquaplast, thermoplast, and orthoplast. These materials can be molded and formed into the desired shape for protection. The heat-forming plastics are heated to 140–180°F for 1–2 min, depending on the material. The material is shaped and molded over the body part for 3–4 min before the hardened state of the material returns. A soft, adhesive-type of padding is applied directly to the outside shell of the constructed pad to allow legal clearance and opponent's protection during activity. The protected pad is held in position by tape, moleskin, or an elastic wrap. The pad must be functional and nonrestrictive during activity for the athlete.

Rubber silicone cast protection offers a safe protective, playing alternative compared to fiberglass plaster protection. The rubber splint protection may allow the basketball player to return to competition quickly and safely, compared to other protective alternatives. Medical personnel must evaluate and clear the athlete to safely participate while wearing silicone bracing protection in contact situations. The silicone splint maintains the limb in an immobilized, protected playable state while allowing for proper healing time. RTV-11 material is widely used as the alternative silicone rubber casting protection application. The semirigid rubber silicone support can be molded to protect various body structures including the forearm, wrist, hand, or fingers (Fig. 4.6). Possible injury application uses include forearm fractures, hand fractures, ulnar collateral ligament sprains, scaphoid fractures, or wrist sprains. Medical and playing clearance should be observed, evaluated, and completed by the game officials. National, state or local agencies should be contacted prior to competition to procure clearance for athletic activity.

Protection for facial/nasal/eye injuries

The facial region, especially the nose and eye, are exposed to potential, unprotected contact and

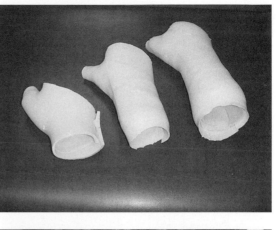

(a)

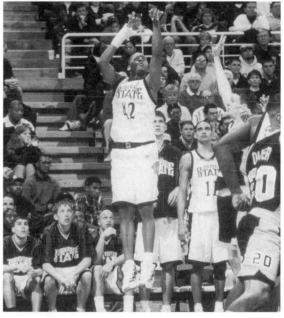

(b)

Fig. 4.6 (a) Silicone wrist/hand splints. (b) Player is completing a jump shot while wearing a right wrist silicone protective splint for a scaphoid fracture on non-shooting hand.

trauma conditions during athletic activity. The game of basketball involves the potential injury trauma situations including facial fractures, facial lacerations, eyelid/eyebrow lacerations, corneal abrasions, blunt trauma injuries, and soft tissue contusions. The recommended eye protection devices are lightweight, polycarbonate eye protector goggles. Only eye protectors that meet the standards established by the American Society for Testing and Materials

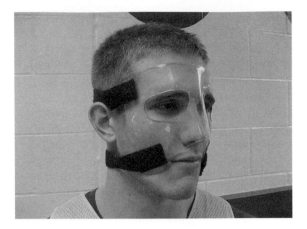

Fig. 4.7 Facial and nasal polycarbonate protection for return to activity.

(ASTM) or parallel the Canadian Standards Association (CSA) standards, offer enough protection for a sport participant (Anderson *et al.* 2000). Zagelbaum *et al.* (1995) recommend protective eye wear in preventing eye injuries following their epidemiological study of eye injuries sustained by professional basketball players in the National Basketball Association (NBA). The study gathered data from February, 1992 until June, 1993 during practices and game competition. Frequent physical contact in professional basketball players leaves them at a great risk for sustaining eye injuries (Zagelbaum *et al.* 1995).

Facial trauma can cause zygomatic, orbital, mandibular, maxillary, and nasal fractures. Acute injuries can also inflict facial/nasal contusions, facial lacerations, lip/mouth lacerations, or tooth luxations or fractures. Physicians will recommend return to competition with facial protection for nasal and facial fractures recommending a polycarbonate facial shield or nasal protector (Fig. 4.7). The nasal protector's failings in the sport of basketball are directed at the athlete's restricted field of vision and the ability to sustain unprotected lateral physical contact to the nose region. The polycarbonate facial shield was devised to eliminate visual field complications, while allowing for full facial protection. The custom fit facial shield is constructed from a plaster mold of the injured athlete's facial structures and fitted according to specified medical recommendations.

Protection for mouth/teeth: mouth guards

The usage of mouth guards in basketball, though strongly recommended by sports medicine teams, has not been accepted as common practice in the sport. There is common agreement among the health care providers of the Michigan Governor's Council on Physical Fitness, Health, and Sports (2000) that the mandatory use of mouth guards by basketball players would markedly reduce the frequency of chipped and fractured teeth, lacerations of the lips and internal structures of the mouth, fractured jaws, and concussions. Despite the overwhelming evidence that basketball players are more likely to sustain facial injuries than athletes in any other sports except baseball (Hewett *et al.* 1996), there is no general mandate to require facial protection as part of the protective equipment for basketball players. Facial injuries in basketball are likely to affect the teeth 90% of the time and nearly 80% are caused by contact with the head, hands, arms, and shoulder of another player. For this reason, medical personnel believe that the frequency and severity of facial injuries in basketball could be drastically reduced by the mandatory use of mouth guards (Flanders & Mohandas 1995). The American Dental Association (ADA) has urged the mandatory use of mouth guards for those engaged in athletic activities that involve body contact and endorse their use in sporting activities where a significant risk of oral injury may occur (NCAA 2000) (Fig. 4.8).

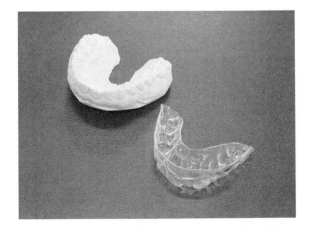

Fig. 4.8 Mouthpiece and plaster mold.

The sports medicine team needs to work closely with the designated team dentist in educating athletes, instituting, and handling of orofacial injuries in the sport of basketball. The action of a mouthpiece is to act as a shock absorber, tooth barrier protector, and a stabilizer for the mandible region. Studies (Flanders & Mohandas 1995) conducted reveal that properly fitted mouthpieces could:

1 reduce potential chipping of tooth enamel surfaces and reduce fractures of teeth, roots, or bones;
2 protect the lip and cheek tissues from being impacted and lacerated against tooth edges;
3 reduce the incidence of a fractured jaw caused by a blow delivered to the chin or head;
4 could reduce the incidence of brain injury (concussion) by possibly absorbing energy from a blow to the chin or head;
5 provide protection to toothless spaces, so support is given to the missing dentition of the athlete (NCAA 2000).

The game of basketball does not make it mandatory for its athletes to wear mouthpieces during competition. However, most dental or associated injuries can be prevented or lessened by the use of the mouthpiece. Two to 16 percent of all injuries involving the mouth result in an avulsed, luxated, or fractured tooth. A significant number of teeth are avulsed each year. Arguments in opposition to the wearing of mouth guards during activity include discomfort to the wearer, restricted breathing opportunities, problems with hygiene, reduced communication among wearers, and the belief of invincibility among athletes. However, many of these concerns have been accepted and overcome by athletes in such sports as football and ice hockey, where the mandated and strongly encouraged use of facial protection has resulted in a simultaneous, drastic reduction in orofacial injuries.

Custom fitted, stock, and mouth formed are three types of mouth guards recognized by the American Dental Association. The stock mouth guard is the least expensive and least satisfactory of the mouth protection equipment. These guards are all one size that do not require individual fitting. The mouth-formed guards are molded to the athlete's bite following a boiling immersion and a brief cooling period in cold water. The athlete molds the mouth guard to the teeth with a gentle biting motion. The custom-fitted mouth guard is recommended for athletes who must communicate clearly during competition and/or those wearing braces or prosthetic teeth. A well fitting mouth guard should be easily inserted, adequately retained, well adapted to oral tissues, and allow for the ease of breathing and speech. The custom-fitted type of intraoral mouth guard is far preferable in basketball players than a stock mouth protector.

The plastic laminate mouth guard material can be fabricated from the athlete's impression through a heating and vacuum type of process. The plastic mouth guard is custom fabricated to the dental arch by heating and vacuum processing. This type of guard allows the athlete to speak, breathe, and drink without difficulty. Retention of the mouth guard in the mouth with activity is good and the guard is comfortable to wear.

The athletic medical staff should work closely with the team physician, team dentist, athletic trainer, and athletes in screening players for potential problems that may require further dental attention. It is recommended to continue educating the players on the benefits and long-term preventive protection of mouth guard usage in the contact sport of basketball.

Protection for the upper extremity

The design of special pads and braces for the upper body needs to offer maximum protection while allowing a functional range of motion of the injured body part. Special pads and braces are created to protect the shoulder region, anterior/posterior chest wall regions, ribs, sternum, breasts, upper arms, elbows, forearms, wrists, hands, and fingers. Pad fabrication can be devised from soft or hard padding, foams, or thermomoldable plastic materials. These materials are suggested for upper body contusions that require firm, yet unyielding protection during competition. Common upper body injuries that require postinjury protection include shoulder separations, shoulder subluxations, chronic dislocations, rib contusions, upper arm contusions, wrist sprains, wrist fractures, thumb sprains, hand fractures or contusions, or finger fractures or sprains. Commercially made braces are available for shoulder injuries, rib injuries, or finger/thumb sprains.

Protection for the lower extremity

Lower body injuries require the use of commercial braces which offer preventive and postinjury protection to the knee, lower leg, ankle, and foot regions. Common injuries sustained to the lower body in basketball include groin/hip/hamstring strains, quadriceps contusions, knee sprains, patellar-femoral dysfunctions, lower leg overuse injuries, stress fractures, ankle sprains, and foot overuse injuries. Hip flexor and adductor groin soft tissue injuries may appear in early season practice sessions until the basketball player adapts to the sharp cutting and sliding movements customary with the sport.

Protection of these injuries range from commercial braces, fabricated pad protection devices, elastic wrap supports, biker shorts, orthotic in-sole devices, and prophylactic taping techniques. A combination of protective devices may be necessary to alleviate general muscle soreness-type injuries.

Knee/patellar-femoral protection

Protection of the knee and patellar region has been classified into three types of braces: prophylactic, functional, and rehabilitative. The preventive or postinjury functional knee braces are commonly used to assist in anterior cruciate ligament (ACL) postsurgical reconstruction, collateral ligament sprains, or rotational-type injuries (Fig. 4.9). The functional brace may affect tibial translation, rotational stresses, and/or flexion/extension limitations for return to sport performance by the athlete. Patellar-femoral braces are recommended to improve patellar tracking, maintain patellar alignment, and decrease forces of infrapatellar or suprapatellar forces. The term commonly referred to as "jumper's knee" or patellar-femoral dysfunction injury, will require the wearing of patellar-femoral braces, infrapatellar straps, neoprene sleeves, or McConnell taping techniques to improve tracking problems. The McConnell taping system encourages the combination of passive taping of the patella in conjunction with neuromuscular control and quadriceps strengthening rehabilitation programs. The McConnell taping will assist in correcting the patellar position and tracking during functional knee movements.

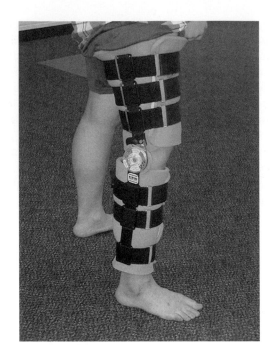

Fig. 4.9 Post injury stabilizing hinged knee brace.

Lower leg/ankle protection

Commercial ankle braces can be used either alone or in combination with ankle taping, to prevent or support an injured ankle joint structure. Recent studies of basketball-related injuries have identified the ankle joint as a gender-specific, rather than sport-specific source of potential injuries in the foot and ankle region. Hosea *et al.* (2000) studied 4940 female and 6840 male interscholastic and intercollegiate basketball players over two seasons and found 25% greater risk of Grade I ankle sprains in females than in males. These findings also indicated that these gender differences were unremarkable in comparison to Grade II and Grade III ankle sprains, ankle fractures, or syndesmotic ankle joint sprains. Because of similarities in schedules, playing surfaces, and reporting of injuries, the authors attributed the differences in ankle sprains to lack of long-term conditioning by female basketball players (Michigan Governor's Council on Physical Fitness, Health and Sports 2000).

Inappropriate footwear magnifies the problem of ankle sprains in basketball (Boitano 1992; Sitler

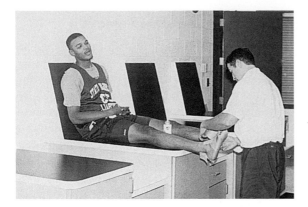

Fig. 4.10 Preventive ankle taping.

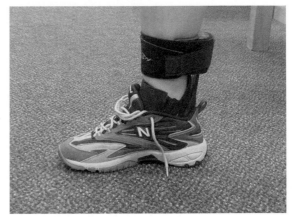

Fig. 4.11 Ankle ligament protector (DonJoy).

et al. 1994). The landing forces from dunking, shooting lay-ins, or rebounding may be five times the athlete's body weight. The shoes worn by many basketball players lack adequate protection to absorb such forces or to restrain the inversion stresses if the landing is on the lateral sides of the feet (Michigan Governor's Council on Physical Fitness, Health and Sports 2000).

Prophylactic taping procedures, wearing three-quarter or high-top basketball shoes, or commercial lace-up ankle stabilizers, strengthening exercises, flexibility, and proprioception drills have been popular in attempting to prevent ankle injuries. Finding a suitable solution to ankle injuries is problematic because the support required to protect the ankle from injury varies with individual and playing conditions (Sitler *et al.* 1994). Numerous studies have revealed that during preventive ankle taping procedures, a maximal loss of support is noted in both inversion and eversion movements following 20 minutes or more of exercise (Fig. 4.10). Numerous studies have been completed in evaluating the efficacy of ankle taping and ankle bracing. The supportive qualities of semirigid and lace-up design braces have been reported as being comparable and superior, respectively, to that of tape (McDermott 1993; Sitler *et al.* 1994) (Fig. 4.11). Ottaviani *et al.* (1995) reported that subjects could generate nearly 30% greater resistance to ankle inversion with a firmly laced three-quarter shoe than with a low-top shoe. Ottaviani *et al.* (1995) found that neither low or three-quarter-top basketball shoes prevented eversion stresses of the ankle at any angle of plantar

flexion. The three-quarter-top shoe significantly increased maximal resistance to inversion stresses at 0, 16, and 32 degrees. The authors concluded that the high-top shoe improved resistance to ankle inversion, especially during the early phases of a potential ankle sprain. Sitler *et al.* (1994) reported that the risk of sustaining an ankle injury was three times greater in a control group than in an experimental group wearing ankle stabilizers when playing in an intramural basketball program at the West Point Military Academy (Michigan Governor's Council on Physical Fitness, Health and Sports 2000). Ricard *et al.* (2000) reported that a reduction in the amount and rate of inversion may allow the body's protective mechanisms time to respond, and depending on the conditions of loading, may reduce the potential for ankle sprains. When the rate of a loading mechanism is slower compared to a faster loading mechanism rate, the body has sufficient time to react and prevent injury. Thus, the preventive conditioning program of peroneal strengthening, balance training, and proprioceptive activities may assist in decreasing possible injury situations (Figs 4.12 & 4.13).

The Michigan Governor's Council on Physical Fitness, Health, and Sports (2000) recommended the following strategies in reducing ankle injuries in basketball players: (1) that new shoes, designed specifically for basketball, provide the lateral support needed to prevent ankle sprains; (2) shoes with high ankle support in combination with taping or

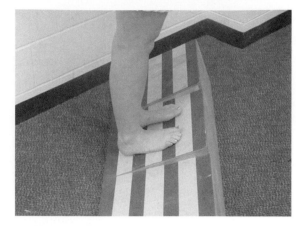

Fig. 4.12 Incline board stretching posterior ankle complex.

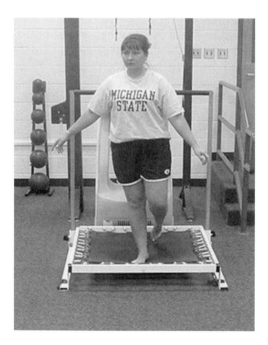

Fig. 4.13 Trampoline and single leg balance training.

orthoses reduce the likelihood of ankle sprains; and (3) semirigid ankle stabilizers are effective in reducing the incidence of ankle injuries when worn in combination with high-top basketball shoes (Sitler *et al.* 1994). They conclude by stating that a majority of the studies confirm that devices or shoes that prevent inversion of the plantar-flexed ankle are useful in preventing ankle sprains.

Foot protection/shoe selection

Specific foot conditions prevalent in basketball are medial, longitudinal, and metatarsal arch injuries, medial tibial stress syndrome stresses, posterior/anterior tibial tendonitis, lower leg stress fractures, acute foot and stress-related fractures, fifth metatarsal or "Jone's fractures", plantar fasciitis, Achilles tendonitis/bursitis, and turf-toe injuries. Every basketball player has a unique history of past medical injury, unique biomechanical demands, motion control and stability needs, shock absorption qualities, and personal preferences to be considerd when being fitted for basketball shoes. Shoe selection should focus on personal playing style, foot biomechanics, and preventive injury pattern needs, rather than style, media recommendations, or promotional influences. The basketball player must maintain the awareness that the selection and wearing of basketball shoes will affect more than foot and ankle stability. The player must acknowledge that biomechanical controls on the foot will gradually influence the forces and potential injuries at the lower leg, knee, hip, and low back regions.

The proper fitting shoe type may reduce the incidence of overuse injuries by controlling faulty foot mechanics. A pes cavus foot more typically may lead to potential problems, as well as the pes planus-type foot. Other mechanical weaknesses that may predispose the basketball player to ankle sprains is a weakness in the peroneal longus, excessive tibial varum, internal tibial torsion, and plantar-flexed first ray. An observation of an athlete walking and jogging will reveal possible hyper-pronation or under-pronation gait restrictions. An athlete who hyper-pronates may exhibit callus build-up under the first, second, or third toes with low arch patterns. The under-pronator will exhibit tendencies of a high, rigid arch with tight lower leg musculature and callus build-up on the lateral structures of the foot. The muscles that work on the strengthening control of the subtalar joint are the tibialis posterior, flexor digitorum longus, flexor hallucis longus, gastrocnemius, soleus, tibialis anterior, extensor digitorum longus, and the peroneus brevis. The tibialis posterior eccentrically functions to decelerate pronation of the ankle joint during the contact phase of the player's running gait. The gastrocnemius muscle group will provide supination of the subtalar

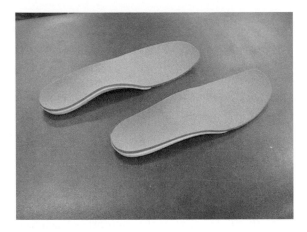

Fig. 4.14 Off shelf insoles.

joint during the push-off phase. An adequate amount of plantarflexion must be maintained to allow the first metatarsal head and medial cuneiform (first ray) to maintain ground contact as the foot moves into an inversion position. The position of the first ray is necessary for proper forefoot movements and control. A proper biomechanical evaluation and a supervised rehabilitation program will assist in correcting many of these mechanical foot deficiencies.

Shoe selection should be based on motion control, stability factors, and arch support and cushioning construction. The central focus should be a review of the midsole and heel counter control factors necessary for individual athletes. The motion control shoe will assist with hyper-pronation problems. This shoe will assist with a solid, stable heel counter to prevent the rearfoot from excessive pronation movements. A medial posting may be added to control for further pronation control problems. A shoe that offers a firm midsole will offer shock absorption qualities that combine to offer foot/ankle control and cushioning characteristics (Fig. 4.14).

Shoe construction combined with ankle/foot control knowledge, will prevent future over-use stresses to the lower leg and foot regions. Due to the constant, repetitive actions of jumping and bounding, the number of floor contacts and foot touches, and the accumulated stresses to the lower body, overuse injuries are prevalent in the competitive and recreational basketball player. A continued communication and awareness of lower body biomechanics,

the proper fitting motion control shoe, the possible implementation of orthotic control, and lower leg flexibility, strength, and neuro-control exercises, may prevent the basketball player from incurring an overuse, stress-type injury.

Universal precautions

Universal precautions are defined as a group of safety and hygienic guidelines used in the handling of potentially infectious bodily fluids in order to prevent or minimize transmission of pathogens. Athletes participating in organized sports are subject to procedures and policies relating to transmission of blood-borne pathogens. The National Athletic Trainers' Association (NATA), U.S. Olympic Committee (USOC), National Collegiate Athletic Association (NCAA), National Federation of State High School Athletic Associations (NFSHSAA), National Basketball Association (NBA), National Hockey League (NHL), National Football League (NFL), and Major League Baseball (MLB) all have established policies to help prevent transmission of blood-borne pathogens (Arnheim & Prentice 2000). The awareness and knowledge of these diseases have increased nationally for all health care providers throughout the past decade. Prevention strategies are recommended for all medical personnel, health care givers, athletes, coaches, and game officials.

Blood-borne pathogens are disease-causing microorganisms that may be present in human blood and may be transmitted through exposure to blood. The two blood-borne pathogens of significance include hepatitis B virus (HBV) and human immunodeficiency virus (HIV). Other blood-borne diseases include hepatitis C, hepatitis D, and syphilis. The particular blood-borne pathogen HIV is transmitted through sexual contact (heterosexual and homosexual), direct contact with infected blood or blood components, intravenous drug use with contaminated needles, and perinatally from mother to baby. In addition, behaviors such as body piercing and tattoos may place the student-athlete at some risk of contracting HBV, HIV, or hepatitis C. The emphasis for the student-athlete and the athletic health care team should be placed on education and concern about these traditional routes of transmission from behaviors off the athletic field. Experts have concurred that the risk of transmission on the athletic fields is minimal (NCAA 2000).

Neither the NCAA or the Centers of Disease Control and Prevention recommends that institutions conduct mandatory testing of student-athletes for either HBV or HIV for participation purposes (NCAA 2000). Mandatory testing for HIV may not be allowed because of legal reasons related to the American with Disabilities Act (Arnheim & Prentice 2000). Athletes who engage in high-risk activities should be encouraged to seek voluntary anonymous testing for HIV. All individuals who desire voluntary testing for personal reasons should be assisted in obtaining the necessary services from local public health care officials. State laws have been instituted to protect the confidentiality and anonymity of the HIV-infected individual. The International Olympic Committee (IOC) categorizes the sport of basketball as a moderate risk transmission sport similar to field hockey, hockey, soccer, team handball, and judo. Boxing, wrestling, and taekwondo pose the greatest risk according to the IOC.

The Occupational Safety and Health Administration (OSHA) is a consumer rights organization established to assist healthcare workers and protect them from occupational hazards. OSHA has recommended several prevention workplace standard strategies for minimizing exposure to blood-borne pathogens in the workplace. The blood-borne pathogen precautions emphasized in basketball practice and game situations should include:

1 A written detailed description of tasks and procedures, for occupations such as physicians, athletic trainers, physical therapists, equipment managers, athletes, and ballboys/ballgirls.

2 The placement of sharps containers, hand washing facilities, eye stations, and biohazards bags and labels within the team locker room and bench locations. Hand washing following blood contact or exposure should be conducted immediately or as soon as possible after removal of gloves. Contaminated needles should not be bent or recapped after procedures. Shearing or breaking of needles is prohibited. Sharp containers should be properly discarded.

3 All medical staff and/or coaching personnel should be supplied with personal protective equipment which includes latex gloves, masks, gowns, aprons, goggles, and/or face shields used to protect from contamination of skin, mucous membranes, or puncture wounds.

4 The basketball locker room, court, or athletic training room should focus on a concept of universal precautions in treating all blood and certain bodily fluids as if they were contaminated with HIV, HBV, or other possible blood-borne pathogens. All soiled towels and linen should be bagged and washed separately in hot water and chlorine bleach. All gauze pads and soiled medical items must be placed into a marked biohazard container. The sharps container of disposable needles, scalpels, etc. must be disposed of instituting the appropriate hazardous waste company procedures. An appropriate germicide cleanser should be available courtside for potential blood spills and clean-up.

5 An educational training program should be offered for all basketball staff, medical personnel, and equipment managers regarding potential blood-borne contact and a review of the exposure plans.

6 All medical personnel, equipment managers, and basketball staff are strongly recommended to receive a hepatitis B vaccination.

The various body fluids listed below contain very high to high risk of HIV transmission. Universal precautions apply to the potential transmission and exposure of these materials:

• Blood
• Semen
• Vaginal secretions
• Cerebrospinal fluid
• Synovial fluid
• Pleural fluid
• Any body fluid with visible blood
• Any unidentifiable body fluid
• Saliva from dental procedures.

Universal precautions do not apply to the following body fluids unless they contain visible blood. These various body fluids are considered to be very low to no risk. Health-care officials recommend continued precautions incorporating glove usage, hand cleansing, and site clean-up procedures after exposure to the any of the following materials:

• Feces
• Nasal secretions
• Sputum

- Sweat
- Tears
- Urine
- Vomitus.

Health care awareness and universal precaution responsibilities are recommended by the NCAA *Sports Medicine Handbook* (2000). Specific recommendations for the sport of basketball include:

1 Pre-event preparation and appropriate coverage of wounds, abrasions, cuts, and weeping wounds that may serve as a source of bleeding or as a port of entry for blood-borne pathogens.

2 The necessary equipment/supplies should be available for caregivers. These supplies include appropriate gloves, disinfectant bleach, antiseptics, designated receptacles for soiled equipment/uniforms, bandages or dressings, and a sharps container for the appropriate disposal of needles, syringes, or scalpels.

3 When an athlete is bleeding, the bleeding must be stopped and the open wound is covered and protected to withstand the demands of the participation. Current NCAA policy mandates the immediate, aggressive treatment of open wounds deemed potential risks of transmission of the disease. Participants with active bleeding should be removed from the event as soon as is practical. Return to play is determined by the appropriate medical staff personnel. Any participant whose uniform is *saturated* with blood, regardless, must have that uniform evaluated by appropriate medical personnel for potential infectivity and changed if necessary before return to participation.

4 During an event, recognition of uncontrolled bleeding is the responsibility of officials, athletes, coaches, and medical personnel.

5 Personnel must follow the universal precaution guidelines. Latex gloves should be worn for direct contact with blood or bodily fluids with blood. Gloves should be changed after treating each individual participant and hands should be washed following the glove removal.

6 Any surface contaminated with spilled blood should be cleaned with the following procedure: with gloves on, the spill should be contained in as small an area as possible. After the blood is removed, the surface area of concern should be cleaned with an appropriate decontaminate.

7 Proper disposal procedures should be practiced.

8 After the contest, all equipment or uniforms soiled with blood should be handled and laundered with hygienic methods normally used for treatment of soiled clothing.

9 All personnel involved with sports should be trained in basic first aid and infection control, including the preventive measures discussed.

The following items are required and recommended for all potential blood-borne pathogen exposure situations and to be on-site for all practices and competitions. The items are latex gloves, biohazard bags, sterile gauze pads, 10% bleach solution or suitable germicide spray, disposable towels, coban/medi-rip, or similar products for securing the wound. An effective exposure plan should be communicated and implemented for all life threatening or blood-borne pathogen exposures. An effective plan involves placing the necessary blood-borne supplies at an available, close location near the basketball court and in the athletic training room for quick and prompt access. All bleeding should be stopped prior to allowing the athlete to return to activity. Direct pressure and/or further medical steps (sutures, steri-strips, butterfly's) must be completed prior to returning to participation. The wound area must be completely covered. The wound region must be secured and continue to allow the athlete to be functional for the game of basketball.

Special attention must be given to allow full, normal range of motion for those wounds located on the hinge-type joints, such as elbow, knee, wrist, or fingers. Be prepared for wounds located on the face and head to bleed profusely. Appropriate care and time must be taken to allow adequate bleeding control of the wound. An awareness of the proper body location and the potential for perspiration, affecting the materials chosen to cover and secure the wound, need to taken into consideration before the athlete returns to play. A tape adherent spray should be applied directly and/or locally around the wound (avoid the wound and eyes) to secure the bandage prior to the return to competition. The medical personnel should be prepared and equipped for this situation at all times during practice and games, since time of return for the athlete is crucial. Medical personnel should carry gloves, gauze, various band-aids, betadine swabs, and coban type material to quickly secure the dressing. All contaminated materials should be discarded into a biohazard bag, sealed, and disposed of properly. The medical personnel must properly cleanse hands after exposure. Any remaining blood on the uniform must be disinfected with 10% bleach solution or medically approved germicide before returning to competition. If the uniform is deemed saturated with blood by the team physician or medical personnel, the athlete must return to play with a fresh, clean jersey or shorts.

Facility concerns

The awareness of the basketball facilities, court, and surrounding playing area is essential in the continued pursuit of preventive medical measures. A visual inspection of the surrounding facilities should be completed before all basketball practices and games by the assigned medical personnel or coaching staff.

Observation of the playing floor can be conducted by walking on the surface and looking for cracked, soft, or slick playing surfaces. The playing surface should be dust mopped and properly cleansed prior to any type of shooting and cutting activities. Personnel should be assigned to mop or wipe up wetness or perspiration from the playing surfaces immediately during the game or practice competition. The hardness of the floor can increase the landing impact forces and affect lower body stresses. Injury statistical documentation can assist in determining if the playing surface may be detrimental to specific injury patterns. Outdoor courts should be swept and cleaned of all sand, rocks, and debris prior to activity. Outside surfaces should be noted for cracks, holes, or damaged pavement. Slick surfaces caused by rain or environmental causes should be inspected for potential injury-causing situations.

Checking for adequate padding on the backboard and the base of basket should be completed before all practices and competitions. Inspection of the backboards, baskets, and rims should ensure compliance with existing codes and standards. The basketball rim should be constructed with a break-a-way hinge support system and show no visible signs of sharp metal edges. The basket and backboard system should be properly stable and secured with the backboard exhibiting shatterproof capabilities. Adequate, approved, and proper padding should be added to walls/poles that are located too close to the baselines underneath the basket region. This padding should be examined and changed when deemed necessary. The scorer's table and bench area should be adequately padded and positioned a safe distance from the playing surface.

Safety within and around the court of participation is often neglected due to time, ignorance, awareness, and practicality. Possible concerns include inadequate space related to the court's sideline and baseline areas. The placement of spectators, cheerleaders, ballboys/ballgirls, and media along the baselines add to the safety concerns for the players. Proper enforcement of allowing adequate landing and running space for the basketball players is crucial in preventing upper or lower body injuries caused by slippage and/or contact with these individuals during competition. Proper ventilation and temperature controls will assist in the prevention of heat and hydration issues on inside courts for basketball. Each basketball facility should attempt to plan for proper awareness, observation, and supervision of the playing court and surrounding equipment. Many potential injury problems can be noted, addressed, and simply rectified prior to a possible injury scenario. These preventive injury situations must be identified, addressed, and enforced daily in both the practice and game situations. Proper maintenance and awareness of the playing facilities and equipment should be implemented for the improved effectiveness of preventing injuries in the game of basketball.

Medical coverage of basketball competition

Sports medicine involves an interdisciplinary approach encompassing many specialty fields in medicine and health care. The team physicians and certified athletic trainers are immediately responsible for prevention, recognition, management, rehabilitation, and education of athletic injuries. The team physician and certified athletic trainer are an integral part of the sports medicine team in the

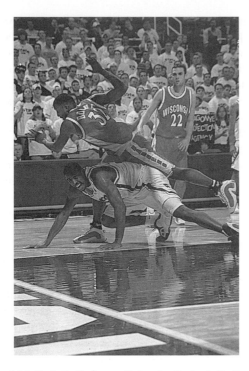

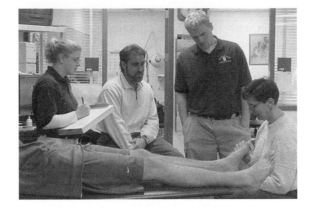

Fig. 4.16 Sports medicine team approach is encouraged in evaluating and collaborating on a lower extremity injury and future consultation.

Fig. 4.15 Basketball players diving for the basketball and contact injury mechanism possibilities.

not necessarily on-site but readily accessible to the primary sports medicine team, also contribute their specialized knowledge and expertise. These may include the orthopedic surgeons, physical therapists, emergency medical technicians (EMT), podiatrists, exercise physiologists, nutritionists, sports psychologists, biomechanists, dentists, ophthalmologists, and various medical specialists (Fig. 4.16).

Medical coverage and responsibilities prior to competition

Members of the sports medicine team work together in researching, organizing, planning, and implementing daily practice and game competition medical coverage. Athletic injuries occur in all sports during both practice and game situations. Medical coverage should be prepared for any type of life threatening and nonlife-threatening injury/illness situations during basketball practices or competitions. Early recognition, proper decision-making skills, appropriate treatment plans, and knowledgeable rehabilitation strategies are all keys for providing quality medical care. The sports medicine team's comprehensive medical care continues to include the preparticipation physical examination, on-site coordination of practice/game medical coverage, implementation of emergency planning strategies, proper determination of the athlete's readiness to return to play, appropriate follow-up injury evaluation and daily treatment plans, overseeing proper

overall physical and mental well-being of the competitive or recreational athlete. In the absence of the team physician or certified athletic trainer, the coach or designated supervisor of the sport-related activity must assume the role of the immediate health care provider (Anderson *et al*. 2000) (Fig. 4.15).

The team approach towards preventing, recognizing, assessing, managing, and rehabilitating injuries or illnesses related to sport, exercise, or recreational activity is an enormous responsibility. The team approach has proven to be the most successful method of addressing health care for sports participants (Anderson *et al*. 2000). The primary members of the sports medicine team provide the immediate daily health care and decision-making skills for proper and safe health care. These members include the primary care physician or designated team physician, certified athletic trainer, coach or sports supervisor in the absence of the physician and athletic trainer, and the athlete. The certified athletic trainer is the primary individual responsible for daily on-site health care. Other professionals, and safe rehabilitation programs, and daily communication with the athletes, coaches, administrators, and sports medicine staff members. The primary concern supporting all these decisions is the proper and ethical safety considerations for the athlete.

Planning, preparation, and organization for all levels of athletic participation need to be reviewed and implemented prior to the season by the sports medicine staff. Planning must simulate all possible injury scenarios and locations. The planning must incorporate the team physician, certified athletic trainer, coach, manager, administrators, and student assistants in communicating roles and expectations of the emergency scene.

The planning environment must take into account the availability or nonavailability of the planning team's members at the time of an injury situation. Since the majority of injuries occur in practice venues and the team physician may not be present, the certified athletic trainer is responsible for the planning, identification, and appropriate decision making as the first responder in assessing the acute injury situation. Many times, however, the coach may be the first and only responder to these situations. This means that the first task of the team physician and sports medicine staff is to upgrade the coach's ability to handle injuries, especially those that are potentially catastrophic. Currently, many institutions and organizations are implementing a yearly mandatory provision that all coaches become educated and certified in first aid and cardiopulmonary resuscitation (CPR), life threatening emergency skills, and are instructed on the proper methods for handling emergency situations with written and documented planning directives.

Proper organization and planning should be completed for all life threatening and nonlife-threatening injury situations. Life threatening emergency situations (see Emergency plans, p. 60) should be discussed prior to the start of the basketball season. The discussions should involve all appropriate medical personnel regarding the immediate care, appropriate equipment, and proper transportation of the injured athlete. The roles are defined and delegated to all emergency medical handlers involved in the care of the injured athlete beforehand. These roles are specific and practiced throughout the season to ensure the appropriate health-care and proper emergency transportation, if the life threatening situation arises. It is imperative that all members of the sports medicine team understand their role during this emergency situation and have a clear understanding of responsibilities. The initial preseason role involves contacting the local emergency medical services for event day coverage and determining the level of care provided by the service. This visitation with the EMS system should discuss the following: (i) introductions and strategy with the on-site medical personnel present if a life threatening injury develops; (ii) the emergency equipment available on-site; (iii) if they will not be on-site, the response time to the competition site; (iv) transportation to local hospital and if they are equipped for emergency or catastrophic situations; (v) the most accessible location of entrance/exit from the facility; and (vi) possible planning of workshops or seminars to review management and protocol of handling life threatening injuries.

Specific sports medicine team members or assistant roles may include: (i) acting as the on-site individual supervisor completing the initial assessment; (ii) assigning the delegated leader of the triage team (physician, certified athletic trainer, coach, or delegated medical personnel); (iii) person instructed to initiate telephone contact appropriate for emergency medical services; (iv) person who gathers appropriate emergency equipment; (v) person who meets the emergency medical service team and directs them to the injury location; (vi) person delegated for record keeping; (vii) the individuals responsible for crowd control and containment; and (viii) appropriate public relations and communication responses to the proper administrator or media member delegated for the role. Confidentiality and discrete responses are necessary items for this role. The emergency equipment should be checked, updated and current, and in proper working order. All instructions and telephone numbers should be posted in several easily identifiable locations in and around the athletic training room, locker room, and gymnasium facilities.

The medical coverage and emergency planning situations need to be well defined, organized, structured, and communicated to offer quick and proper responses for all levels of athletic injuries. An organized, well-communicated emergency plan is critical. The plan needs proper implementation strategies for both home and away competition sites. Standard available emergency equipment should include a spine board, stretcher, sandbags and/or towels, cervical immobilizer, splinting materials, crutches, slings, ice, compression dressings and elastic wraps, cardiopulmonary resuscitation (CPR) equipment, and if possible, an automated external defibrillator (AED). The team physician should have a trauma kit and medical emergency equipment prepared with emergency medications and intravenous fluids. The certified athletic trainer should maintain a sports medicine bag of necessary first aid and injury management supplies (see pp. 58–59).

Advanced communication should be completed prior to any away or international competitions. This advanced communication stresses knowledge of the local resources including ambulance coverage, EMS resources, on-site emergency equipment of away team and ambulance crew, response times, accessible telephones, hospital locations, and local physician coverage. Will the local ambulance or EMS team be on-site or on-call? Is the local hospital or medical facility equipped to handle a catastrophic injury? If international competition, the team physician will be required to become acquainted with the local medical facilities, emergency medical transportation availability, and the local hospital emergency resources on-site.

Medical coverage and responsibilities during competition

Perhaps no role is more important than that provided by the team physician when he or she assumes the care of athletes during athletic competition. Although the incidence of catastrophic injury in basketball is minimal, the potential for serious injury always exists. Therefore, it is essential that appropriate planning, communication, and implementation policies be undertaken to guarantee an effective and efficient response to any emergency situation. The sports medicine team works together in overseeing and preparing for game day competition medical coverage. All planning strategies involving the emergency injury system should be reviewed prior to and on game day activities. All medical equipment, splints, and supplies are checked and placed in an accessible location for quick access to the basketball court. All members should know the location and the proper use of the medical equipment and supplies. The emergency medical services transportation personnel should be visited upon their arrival or contacted, if off-site. An introduction from the team physician and/or certified athletic trainer to the emergency medical team should include personal introductions, a review of the equipment available, a re-introduction of the chain of command policies involving the team physician and certified athletic trainer, the communication system used to summons the EMS services, and review of entrance/exit off the basketball court (Fig. 4.17).

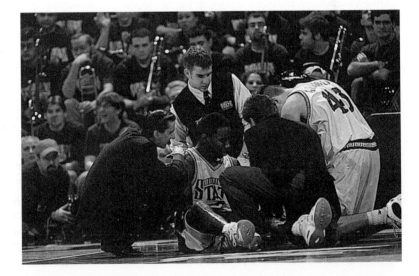

Fig. 4.17 Medical injury evaluation post collision during game.

A review of the OSHA rules regarding open wounds and blood-borne pathogens concerning an athlete, the uniform, towels, or the basketball court is discussed. The certified athletic trainer or assigned health care personnel checks on the necessary equipment and cleansing items needed for a blood spill. Ballboys and ballgirls are informed about the usage of gloves when wiping up the floor for perspiration, water, or blood. Recommendations include the usage of mops wrapped in washable towels to wipe up water or perspiration on a basketball court. Disposable paper towels or wipes should be used to remove blood from the court area. The proper biohazard materials for cleansing and discarding should be located at an appropriate location on each team's designated bench. Water, cups, and ice are placed on the bench for each team to use for proper hydration and injury management situations. For all home competitions, general introductions including a review of emergency injury policies, equipment, facilities, and location of nearest medical facilities should be completed with the basketball game officials, visiting team certified athletic trainer, team physician, or designated medical personnel. If the visiting team has not traveled with appropriate medical personnel, the visiting coach should be informed of the appropriate medical services offered and made available by the home team, if an injury arises.

A review of roles and delegated tasks are completed with the appropriate sports medicine team members prior to the game's competition. Communication is critical and a review of the emergency plan is essential in a life threatening injury situation. A checklist is used to chart and review the planning strategies for game day medical coverage (Fig. 4.18).

The team physician and certified athletic trainer should have close and rapid access to the playing court. The sports medicine team must maintain constant observation and attentiveness for potential injury situations. The primary responsibility of the team physician and/or certified athletic trainer is to determine the extent of any injury or illness occurring during a game and to determine the player's specific medical needs. A decision is made to decide if the athlete can return to play. If the athlete cannot return immediately, a decision must be

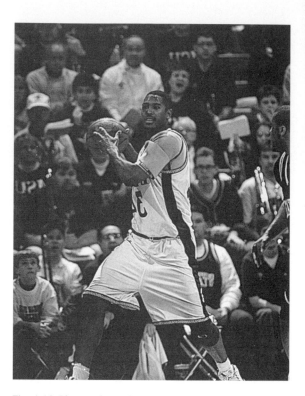

Fig. 4.18 Player rebounding wearing Sully shoulder brace.

made about how the athlete should be transported from the sideline or to the locker room and what initial treatment should be implemented.

Once an acute injury is sustained, immediate assessment is necessary to evaluate the significance of the injury and observe for signs of catastrophic injury. Signs of emergency trauma injury include, but are not limited to: loss or inability to breathe, respiratory failure, severe shock, loss of consciousness, suspected head/neck trauma or spinal cord injury, severe pain, neurological complaints, or deficits, significant bleeding, obvious open wounds and/or fractures, or significant loss of joint/muscle function. The protocols to determine whether an on-the-field assessment of injury is of moderate or serious potential, are presented below (Anderson *et al.* 2000). The on-the-field evaluation should address the following emergency injury prioritized issues:
• Life threatening trauma to the head
• Spinal cord injury with abnormal or absent neurologic signs
• Massive hemorrhage

- Fractures with gross deformity
- Joint dislocations
- Other soft tissue injuries.

The initial evaluation involves observing the position of the player while noticing for consciousness, body and chest movements, breathing, or obvious deformity. The primary survey is conducted to assess and evaluate the athlete's level of responsiveness, airway, breathing, and circulation (ABC). The physician or athletic trainer must initiate or execute the emergency planning procedures if a life threatening injury or another medical emergency is determined. The emergency plan is activated if the signs or symptoms of a life threatening injury or inappropriate vital signs exist. The proper emergency medical services (EMS) system should be contacted for transportation to the nearest medical facility. If the player is conscious, begin asking the player general history questions while continuing a primary survey of the scene. Continue to calm and reassure the athlete, observe for abnormalities, and assess for the severity of the injury. The history questions should involve how it happened, where the pain is located, sounds heard or felt, past history, and the type of pain felt. A specific clinical evaluation is conducted focusing on observation, palpation, joint stress integrity testing, muscular testing, neurological findings, vascular conditions, and functional testing of the athlete. Immediate care of this situation may involve the stabilization and immobilization of the injured musculoskeletal or joint region and application of the appropriate first aid dependent upon the clinical assessment findings. Next, the appropriate transportation procedures for the injured player are assessed and implemented using an ambulance and EMT response team, stretcher, spine board, ambulatory assistance walking, manual conveyance, or walking safely under their own control.

The athlete may be transported to the athletic training room, locker room, or medical facilities for a more thorough and confidential evaluation, or return to the team bench for further observation. If the athlete remains on the bench area, frequent clinical evaluations and observations will be completed. The athlete may return to participation following a qualified medical assessment by the sports medicine team. The sports medicine team will make the final decision on the athlete's full return to play. Specific return to participation criteria must be achieved and the team physician must conclude that the athlete will not sustain further harm or injury upon return to play.

Medical coverage and responsibilities after competition

The team physician and medical personnel complete any general follow-up evaluations and communications with the injured player after the competition is completed. The assigned medical personnel confer with the visiting team on any immediate or pertinent issues prior to their departure.

All injuries sustained by the home team must be re-evaluated prior to the next day. This evaluation period will allow the sports medicine team the opportunity to plan accordingly on the urgency and proper handling of all acute injury situations. Any necessary referrals to specialists or other sports medicine team members, diagnostic recommendations, or therapeutic treatment/rehabilitation plans will be developed and implemented. A proper treatment plan will include record keeping with short-term and long-term goal development, for the quick and safe return of the athlete to competition. Communication must be completed to include the coach, athlete, parents/guardians, media, and sports medicine team members regarding the acute injury situation.

Supplies necessary for coverage

Medical supplies necessary for athletic coverage may vary depending on the level of participation, team, sport, physician, and certified athletic trainer. The athletic medicine team must be prepared for all injury situations that will affect the player while competing on the basketball floor. Acute injuries received on the court, chronic performance restricting injuries, illnesses, travel conditions, and international travel situations all require various supplies and medications. The athletic medicine team must communicate to ensure that appropriate equipment and medical supplies are available for both home and away events.

Emergency medical supplies necessary for the coverage of basketball competition include:

- Spine board/cervical collars
- Stretcher/chair
- Oxygen
- Vacuum immobilizer splints/air splints
- Blood pressure cuff
- Stethoscope
- Crutches
- CPR barrier pocket mask
- Biohazard equipment including latex gloves, sterile gauze, waste disposal containers, sharps containers, spill kits, face shields
- Penlight
- Towels
- Splint bag with assorted splints, pads, elastic wraps, and slings
- Automated external defibrillator (AED).

Athletic training medical supplies (Anderson *et al.* 2000, Arnheim & Prentice 2000) recommended for the coverage of basketball competition include:
- Acetaminophen tablets
- Adhesive tape:
    $^1/_2$ inch, 1 inch, $1^1/_2$ inch, 2 inch
    1 inch elastic, 2 inch elastic, 3 inch elastic
    2 inch stretch tape, 3 inch stretch
    Dermicel, Dermiclear
    McConnell Patellar Femoral Tape, Hypafix
- Aqua-plast, orthoplast
- Alcohol pads
- Adaptic dressings
- Epinephrine chloride solution (epinephrine nasal topical solution)
- Afrin nasal spray
- Ankle braces (tie-up/air-casts)
- Antacid (liquid and tablets)
- Antifungal (powder and spray)
- Antibiotic (topical ointment)
- Antiseptic hand cleanser
- Bacitracin/Neosporin
- Betadine (topical swabs, surgical scrub solutions)
- Biohazard materials (waste containers, spill control kits, protective equipment)
- Blood pressure cuff
- Casting materials
- Cervical collars (small, medium, large)
- Contact lens (cleanser, solution, wetting solution, lens case, mirror)
- Cotton tipped applicators
- CPR pocket masks

- Crutches
- Elastic wraps (2′, 3′, 4′, 6′, 4′ double, 6′ double)
- Electrolyte drink
- Emergency packet: emergency telephone numbers, medical center/hospital numbers, athlete's health history and information, injury reports, athlete's insurance information
- Epsom salts
- Eyepatches (sterile)
- Eyewash and eye cup
- Felt/foam (adhesive and nonadhesive) ($^1/_4$ inch, $^1/_2$ inch, 1 inch) (firm, soft) (memory foam)
- Finger splints (aluminum/stack)
- Fingernail/toenail clippers
- Fingernail drill
- Fluorescein sterile ophthalmic strips/cobalt blue light
- Forceps (tweezers)
- Gauze pads (sterile/nonsterile) (3×3, 4×4)
- Heel and lace pads
- Heel cups
- Hydrogen peroxide
- Ibuprofen tablets
- Ice bags
- Immobilizer splints (knee, ankle, wrist, hand, thumb)
- Insoles
- Kleenex
- Knee pads/elbow pads
- Latex gloves (sterile/nonsterile)
- Massage lotion
- Mastisol liquid adhesive
- Mirror
- Moleskin
- Mouthpiece material
- Nasal plugs
- Nasal protector
- Neoprene sleeves (thigh, knee, elbow, low back)
- Oral thermometer
- Otoscope/ophthalmoscope
- Paper, pen, pencil
- Patellar-femoral braces
- Penlight
- Petroleum jelly
- Ring cutter
- RTV-11 silicone rubber material
- Save-a-tooth kit
- Scalpel blades (disposable)

- Scissors ($5^1/2$ inch, 7 inch)
- Second Skin
- Silver nitrate applicators
- Skin lubricant
- Slings (sling/sling and swathe)
- Steri-strips ($^1/8$ inch, $^1/4$ inch, $^1/2$ inch)
- Stelie saline
- Stethoscope
- Suture kits
- Tape adherent
- Tape cutter
- Tape remover
- Telfa pads (nonstick guaze)
- Tweezers
- Underwrap
- Vacuum splints
- Water and cups/bottles/coolers
- Zinc oxide
- Zorbicide germicide spray

Emergency plans

Injuries occurring in basketball practices, competitive games, pick-up games, and playground activities are inevitable. Due to the increasing nature of physical contact, quickness, strength, jumping ability, intensity, and athletic ability in the sport of basketball, the incidence of injury has also increased. Fortunately, emergency life threatening situations are rather rare. With the increasing number of participants in sport, however, emergency injury situations and related physical problems may gradually increase. In the United States, basketball-related injuries causing death are extremely rare. In the United States from 1984 to 1998 within the 0–19 years age group, the Consumer Products Safety Commission (1999) reported 69 deaths in baseball, 63 in football, 26 in horseback sports, and 25 in soccer. The CPSC reported 26 basketball-related deaths with 24 of the basketball-related deaths involving males. Nine of these deaths were attributed to cardiac arrest. Of the 24 reported related deaths, 10 involved blunt trauma to the head, either from goals falling on players or impact with walls, floors, or other players (Consumer Products Safety Commission 1999). Therefore due to the possible uncertainty of athletic-

related injuries, an expedient response plan must be implemented if life threatening injuries or emergency trauma in the recreational or competitive player develop.

The planning, development, and implementation of an emergency plan should be created to assist with the emergence of an emergency and/or life threatening situation.

> Athletic organizations have a duty to develop an emergency plan that may be implemented immediately when necessary and to provide appropriate standards of health care to all sport participants. The sports medicine team must be prepared. Preparation involves formulation of an emergency plan, proper coverage of events, maintenance of appropriate emergency equipment and supplies, utilization of appropriate emergency medical personnel, and continuing education in the area of emergency medicine (R. Courson).

Preventive medicine focuses on careful and competent screening of potential life threatening conditions noted in the preparticipation histories and physical examinations, adequate practice and competition medical coverage, proper coaching techniques, proper and adequate conditioning programs, consistent and proper officiating enforcement, and continual planning and preparation for emergency situations. A thorough and well-organized emergency plan consists of defined roles and responsibilities for all appropriate personnel, accessibility to a telephone for emergency medical contacts, properly trained and supervised emergency medical personnel, appropriate emergency equipment, and reliable and appropriate medical transportation.

The team physician may not be present at many practices or noncompetitive situations. A member of the sports medicine team, the certified athletic trainer, or a coach, most typically may be your first responder to an emergency and/or life threatening situation. A coach should be encouraged to be educated and certified in cardiopulmonary resuscitation (CPR) techniques, first aid, disease prevention (universal precautions), and emergency planning implementation strategies.

An emergency plan must be formulated prior to the season to include team physicians, emergency medical personnel, certified athletic trainers, coaches, managers, administrators, and students. Each member of the response team has specific delegated responsibilities associated with the emergency medical care offered. Prior to the season, practice, and home/away competition, all members of the emergency planning team should review emergency procedures, signals, equipment, and supplies. This plan must be communicated and shared with all possible medical assistors. Due to the variance in athletic venues, facilities, equipment, and personnel, planning must be reviewed and practiced often before each practice and competitive situation. Time, organization, and communication are crucial elements during this emergency period.

The first and foremost concern during any emergency and/or life threatening situation is the immediate safety and care for the athlete. The team physician or qualified medical coordinator, if present, should provide the immediate direction, decision making, triage, and leadership skills appropriate for the injury scenario as the group leader. If a team physician or qualified medical coordinator is not present, the most qualified and experienced personnel on-site should direct and coordinate the emergency situation. The group leader should immediately activate the emergency medical system (911) or contact the appropriate local police or fire department. The individual sent to activate the emergency system should be reliable, calm, and articulate in communicating. If the emergency transportation and personnel are not available at the scene of the injury, the individual contacting the medical personnel must state the following on the telephone: (a) name, address, and telephone number of the location of the injury; (b) the possible injury/condition of the athlete and type of emergency situation; (c) the immediate first aid initiated by the first responder and who is present at the scene; (d) specific directions to the location and entrance to enter the scene; and (e) they must remain on the telephone to answer any remaining questions regarding the situation. If the emergency transportation is located on site, a prior designated location, signal, and access to the site should be preplanned to allow an expedient entrance and exit from the location. Access to a telephone should be confirmed prior to any activity. Any cellular telephone, public telephone, or press row, locker room or training room telephone should be located and have prearranged usage prior to the competition or practice.

The next appropriate role is to gather and retrieve any necessary emergency equipment. The emergency equipment should be located in an easily accessible location close to the proximity of the competition. All equipment should be checked regularly and be in proper working order. Emergency equipment may include stretchers, backboards, splints, oxygen, cervical collars/sandbags, and the possible availability of automated external defibrillators (AED).

After the emergency medical system is activated, another individual is sent immediately to meet and direct the activated medical personnel to the proper entrance of the facility. The proper emergency entrance should provide a quick, efficient, and safe access into the facility. This access entrance should be discussed and coordinated during the preseason planning period.

Communication and planning are the most important elements in delivering safe and organized care in the emergency and/or life threatening situations. Proper development, planning, organization, preparation, and implementation of an emergency plan are necessary for the life threatening situations. Communication must be planned and discussed prior to the beginning of each season, practice, or competition. Open dialogue and communication must be continuously maintained with physicians, certified athletic trainers, physiotherapists, emergency medical personnel, coaches, managers, and students.

Travel considerations

Physical and mental fatigue factors may be present in athletes following exposure to significant travel distances or frequencies. Jet lag, loss of sleep, fatigue, headaches, and decreased performance factors are all potential results of the demands of frequent intense competition and increased travel opportunities.

Time differences

The challenging travel schedule for the sport of

basketball forces many athletes to exhibit flexible and adaptable personal habits. The travel schedule of a basketball player will challenge time zones, rest patterns, sleep habits, and general body fatigue. The basketball player's travel demands will result in a disruption of normal sleep patterns, dietary factors, hydration maintenance, and body rhythms. Changes in body rhythms may result in digestive and gastrointestinal problems, headaches, changes in endocrine secretions and hormone release, blood pressure, heart rate, breathing patterns, bowel habits, and general physiological and mental fatigue symptoms. Significant athletic performance factors affected by travel are reaction times, immune systems, fatigue, energy levels, coordination, anxiety, and motivational factors.

Circadian rhythm refers to one's internal clock controlling various physiological functions. A disruption in an athlete's circadian rhythm will impair exercise performance, sleep patterns, and lifestyle adjustment periods. Symptoms of jet lag may include a reduction of appetite, sleep loss, general fatigue, or a reduction in psychomotor movements. An individual adapts more easily to a westward travel flight due to an endogenous clock of 25 h in our body's systems and the longer time of day encountered. Circadian rhythms normally require one day per time zone traveled to return, adapt, and synchronize the body's regulatory system to normal functional response levels. An individual's internal or biological clock will generate different rhythms with greater difficulty. The research on melatonin as an alternative for treating or preventing jet lag or fatigue is presently being researched. Studies have indicated that melatonin can play a role in the treatment of sleep disorder symptoms or jet lag. However, the exact dosage and individual recommendations are variable and subject to medical interpretation and dispensation.

Athletic medical staff, athletes, and coaches should remain aware of the physical and mental stresses, muscular and psychological fatigue factors, and adequate recovery time needed for a consistent athletic basketball performance. The preventive planning strategies should consider a commonsense and practical approach to travel situations. Athletes need to maintain good hydration principles, consistent and balanced dietary habits, consistent sleep habits, and allow adequate physical and mental recovery time throughout the long, arduous season. Steingard (1993) and Starkey (2000) recommended these practical considerations for the NBA teams:

1 realistic travel schedules and comfortable flight seating;
2 realistic practice schedules recognizing time changes and allowing for fatigue;
3 abstaining from alcohol immediately before and during these flights;
4 comfortable and quiet sleeping accommodations once the players have arrived at their destination.

Seasonal concerns

The sport of basketball has become a year-round activity. The competitive season may encompass the fall, winter, spring, or summer seasons. All levels of basketball competition encourage basketball playing year round to remain competitive. Off-season activities encourage cardiovascular, strength training, flexibility, and basketball drill programs to improve on weaknesses. As the athlete competes year round, various seasonal concerns may develop.

Seasonal affective disorder

As athletic competition intensifies and the demand for enhanced performance increases, athletes must master not only the mechanical aspects of their sport, but also the psychological variables that affect their performance and susceptibility to injury. The prevalence of seasonal affective disorder (SAD) in the United States varies from 1.4% in southern latitudes, to 9.7% in the north-eastern states (Rosen *et al.* 1996). The current review of the literature reveals minimal information regarding SAD in competitive athletics.

The key to diagnosing and distinguishing SAD from other forms of depressive behavior is the pattern, an occurrence, disappearance, and re-occurrence, year after year of similar symptoms of lack of energy, hopelessness, and unexplained sadness. Research on seasonal affective disorder syndrome (SADS) does not reveal the existence of a genetic link; however, most sufferers of SADS tend to show strong family histories of seasonal problems, or other potential mood disorders. Rosen and co-workers discussed the disturbing fact of mood disorders having a significant effect on athletic performance and the potential for injury. Rosen *et al.* (1996) noted the unrecognized factors, such as anxiousness, fearfulness, or depression that can play a destructive role in the athlete's personal and professional life. Their studies on SAD examined patterns of decreased energy, fatigue, decreased physical capacity, affected sleep and mood patterns, increased appetite (particularly carbohydrates), decreased libido, and hypersomnia. These significant mood disorders can affect the seasonal fall and winter basketball player's physical performance displayed on the court. Rosen *et al.* (1996) reported a prevalence rate of subsyndromal SAD as 25% in the athletic population for hockey. Rosen *et al.* (1996) concluded by stating:

> an athlete who competes in a sport in which winning and losing can be measured in milliseconds, and who must be able to maintain intensity, speed, and strength throughout a contest can ill afford to concede even a mild decrement in function, let alone a major impairment in the parameters affected by a seasonal mood disorder.

Following review of a screening device questionnaire, personal history, sport activity physical and psychological concerns, and medical evaluation, specific recommendations for a diagnosis and treatment plan are developed. The recommended treatment for SADS is phototherapy. The researchers at the National Institute of Mental Health in Bethesda, Maryland first administered bright white light therapy in 1980 to offset the lost daylight effects on the body. Formal studies report success rates of 75% to 90%. This 30–45 minute phototherapy session (the higher intensity, the shorter the session) restores normal mental and physical functioning in most individuals. The basic light box is usually portable, weighing 10–20 pounds, a few inches deep, and from 1–2 feet high to 2–3 feet wide.

Rosen's study emphasizes the need for the athletic medical staff to maintain a preventive awareness and critical observation of their athletes. By observing daily for the athlete's changes of energy levels, mood variances, appetite patterns, sleep disturb-

ances, and social interactions, the athletic medical staff may prevent further physical or psychological disturbances. The medical staff's opportunity for an early identification and treatment of a physically and psychologically struggling athlete is crucial. The medical specialist needs to address both the physical and psychological factors when evaluating an athlete for decreased performance patterns and mood changes.

Influenza

Influenza is an acute seasonal systemic respiratory illness caused by influenza viruses A and B transmitted by coughing or sneezing. General influenza symptoms include headache, fever, runny nose, muscle aches, sore throat, dry cough, and fatigue or lack of energy. Basketball athletes are highly susceptible to influenza due to their winter sports seasons, close physical contact, shared water bottles, and possible body fatigue. The recommended treatment of influenza is prevention. The influenza vaccine issued in October through November each fall season, provides adequate protection from the identical strains each winter season. Use of the oral antiviral agents help shorten the duration of the illness and are most effective when prescribed within 24–48 h of the onset of symptoms. Other preventive measures include frequent hand washing, avoiding frequent hand shaking, individual water bottles, increased fluids, and improved resting habits.

Upper respiratory infections (URI) and the common cold are two of the most prevalent seasonal illnesses sustained by basketball players during the fall and winter months. Symptoms of the common cold may include body aches, mild sore throat, nasal stuffiness, nonproductive cough, and possibly a low-grade temperature. Further medical diagnostic tests should be pursued following physical concerns of lingering fever, productive cough, tender palpable sinuses, consistent nasal irritation or drainage, ear soreness, or positive sounds on lung auscultation. Diagnostics may include laboratory blood work, nasal swabs, allergy testing, chest X-rays, nutritional consultation, stress related awareness, and possible review of playing and conditioning training habits or overtraining syndrome identification.

Vitamin C and zinc gluconate are two current vitamins recommended for the treatment of the common cold. The benefits of vitamin C remain controversial, while zinc gluconate lozenges have been proved somewhat effective in reducing cold symptoms if initiated early within the illness. The benefits of vitamin C and zinc lozenges, increased and improved rest, with an increase of clear fluids including water, clear juices and caffeine free teas, have proven to reduce the duration of symptoms.

Heat illness

Hot and humid environmental conditions pose potential problems for basketball players. Heat-related injuries are a concern and susceptibility increases for athletes who report a past history of heat illness, show an excessive amount of body fat, minimal levels of acclimatization, decreased aerobic capacity, inadequate re-hydration, a febrile athlete, and those who regularly push themselves to maximum levels of exercise. A continued awareness of prescription and over-the-counter medications, such as antihistamines and pseudoephedrine, may increase the risk of heat illness (NCAA 2001).

The game of basketball, though considered an indoor sport, needs to be aware of climatic environmental and adequate hydration conditions. The inside/outside environment of basketball practices/games must plan for comfortable, cool playing conditions. Proper education on acclimatization protocols and increased fluid intake before, during, and after activity are critical factors in preventing heat illness conditions.

Acclimatization through moderate gradual adaptation to heat and conditioning exposures in hot temperatures, are probably the most effective methods of avoiding heat injuries. Major acclimatization to the new environmental conditions occurs during the first 7 to 10 days of heat exposures. Gradual progressive increases in duration and intensity after 10 days will allow for a decreased heart rate and body temperature, thus producing an increase in the sweating mechanism and decreased blood flow to the skin regions. The increased perspiration rate over a longer period of time decreases the skin temperature and allows for less vasodilation in the skin and improved cooling of blood throughout the skin tissue.

Fluid replacement is essential to maintain adequate levels of plasma volume, stroke volume, optimum sweating mechanism levels, maintained cardiac function, normal kidney functions, peripheral blood flow, and proper circulatory levels. Low levels of dehydration (e.g., less than two percent loss of body weight) impair cardiovascular and thermoregulatory response and reduce the capacity for exercise (Murray 1996). Fluids must be ingested and absorbed by the body to replace substantial losses of fluid by the body and to prevent dehydration. Cold liquids tend to empty significantly faster from the stomach and small intestines than warmer drinks. The observance of a light to clear colored urine of above normal volume is a good indicator of substantial fluid hydration. One of the primary reasons for fatigue in basketball players is dehydration. Research has reported that benefits of activity are assisted by the consumption of properly formulated carbohydrate–electrolyte beverages before, during, and after activity. Electrolyte drinks will assist with delaying the deterioration of sport-specific motor skills and psychological concentration skills during activity. Research has revealed that a high-concentrated carbohydrate–electrolyte drink will assist and speed up the replacement of the muscle glycogen, thus improving the players' long-term performance factors.

In order of severity, heat syncope, heat cramps, heat exhaustion, and heat stroke, are typical heat illnesses individuals can exhibit. Early signs of fatigue, dizziness, thirst, fainting, and nausea may develop. Heat cramps are painful, involuntary muscle spasms often occurring in the calf, abdomen, or large muscle groups. The cramping is caused excessive electrolyte and water loss during intense activity. The athlete who is in fairly good condition and acclimatized and who overexerts in activity may be more susceptible to this condition. Clinical signs of heat exhaustion include headache, dizziness, fatigue, profuse sweating, rapid and weak pulse, cool and clammy skin, low blood pressure, and hyperventilation. The athlete may appear pale and ashen during intense bouts of early season activities. The athlete needs to be removed from the heated environment and rapidly cooled with cool water. A major ingestion and increase of fluids is necessary with possible intravenous replacement of fluids. Heat stroke is a serious life threatening condition. Clinical signs include disorientation, unsteady gait, initial stages of profuse sweating leading to cessation of the sweating mechanism, hot, dry, and red skin, rapid and strong pulse, and a significant increased core body temperature. The emergency medical system should be activated. An effective cooling method of ice water immersion in conjunction with cool wet towel applications to the neck, axilla, and groin regions will need to be implemented as soon as possible. The longer the body temperature is elevated to 106°F or higher, the greater the potential chance for death.

In conclusion, heat illnesses are preventable, controllable situations. Education, awareness, and strong management skills are essential in adequate fluid and electrolyte hydration principles, acclimatization and conditioning protocols, and proper nutritional and clothing issues. Potential informational and educational sessions include:

1 Assigning each player with a personal water bottle for all activities. The bottle will decrease the possibility of spreading infections, emphasize the importance of hydration, and allow the medical staff the opportunity to monitor the player for proper fluid hydration.

2 Continue to educate the players on the importance of monitoring the color of their urine. Clear, odorless urine is a good indicator of good hydration during activity and dark urine suggests possible dehydration signs.

3 Continue to promote hydration and force the fluids by training the athletes to drink.

This educational message of continuous hydration and electrolyte drinking must be enforced on a consistent basis by all members of the coaching, medical, and strength and conditioning staffs (Burns *et al.* 1999). Through awareness and understanding of potential environmental conditions, the medical personnel can be influential in acknowledging a life threatening situation. The sports medicine team must continue to be aware of the following factors which may also be affected by environmental heat related conditions in the athlete: current illnesses, obesity, hydration levels, acclimatization, training and conditioning levels, age and gender issues, and the duration and intensity of exercise.

Conclusion

All health care personnel must continue to focus on the athlete as a "whole" individual. Prevention of injuries/illnesses should not focus solely on musculoskeletal systems. A continued open line of communication between the health care staff and the athlete may allow for an early intervention program that may decrease the risk factors influencing the rate of injury. Hidden psychological crisis may cause increased stress, fatigue, and depressive factors. An athlete's decreased immune system opens the body to an increased risk of disease due to a lack of infection-fighting defenses which can be exacerbated by too much exercise, over-training signs and symptoms, lack of rest and inconsistent sleep habits, and improper nutritional habits.

References

Anderson, M., Hall, S. & Martin, M. (2000) *Sports Injury Management*. Philadelphia: Lippincott, Williams & Wilkins.

Arendt, E. (1996) Common musculoskeletal injuries in women. *Phys Sportsmed* **24**, 39–48.

Arnheim, D. & Prentice, W. (2000) *Principles of Athletic Training*. McGraw-Hill Higher Education.

Boitano, M.A. (1992) Subtalar dislocations in basketball players: Possible contributing factors. *Phys Sportsmed* **20**, 59–67.

Burns, J., Davis, J.M., Craig, D.H. & Satterwhite, Y. (1999) Conditioning and nutritional tips for basketball. *Sports Sci Exchange Roundtable* **10** (4), 1–4.

Consumer Products Safety Commission Data (1999) http://www.info.cpse.gov, February.

Courson, R. Example template: sports medicine emergency plan, http://www.ncaa.org/sports_sciences/emergency_plan.html.

Crosby, L. (1989) Subtalar dislocation in a basketball player. *Phys Sportsmed* **17**, 145–148.

Flanders, R.Z. & Mohandas, A. (1995) The incidence of oral facial injuries in sport: a pilot study in Illinois. *J Am Dental Assoc* **126**, 491–496.

Hewett, T., Stroupe, A., Nance, T. & Noyes, F. (1996) Plyometric training in female athletes. *Am J Sports Med* **24**, 765–773.

Hosea, T., Carey, C. & Harrer, M. (2000) The gender issue. Epidemiology of ankle injuries in athletes who participate in basketball. *Clin Orthopedics Related Res* **372**, 45–49.

Ireland, M.L. & Wall, C. (1990) Epidemioogy and comparison of knee injuries in elite male and female United States basketball athletes. *Med Sci Sports Exerc* **22**, S82.

Kirkendall, D. & Garrett, W. (2000) The anterior cruciate ligament enigma. *Clin Orthopedics Related Res* **372**, 64–68.

McDermott, E.P. (1993) Basketball injuries of the foot and ankle. *Clin Sports Med* **12**, 373–393.

Michigan Governor's Council on Physical Fitness, Health, and Sports (2000) *Position Statement: The Prevention of Injuries in Basketball.*

Murray, R. (1996) Dehydration, hyperthermia, and athletes: science and practice. *J Athletic Training* **31** (3), 248.

National Collegiate Athletic Association (NCAA) (2001) *Sports Medicine Handbook, 2000–2001.*

Ottavieni, R.A., Ashton-Miller, J.A., Kothari, S.U. & Wojtys, E.M. (1995) Basketball shoe height and the maximal muscular resistance to applied ankle inversion and eversion moments. *Am J Sports Med* **23**, 418–423.

Ricard, M.D., Schulties, S.S. & Saret, J.J. (2000) Effects of high-top and low-top shoes on ankle inversion. *J Athletic Training* **35**, 38–43.

Rosen, L.W., Smokler, C., Carrier, D., Shafer, C.L. & McKeag, D. (1996) Seasonal mood disturbances in collegiate hockey players. *J Athletic Training* **31**, 225–228.

Sitler, M., Ryan, J., Wheeler, B., McBride, J., Arciero, R., Anderson, J. & Horodyski, M. (1994) The efficacy of a semirigid ankle stabilizer to reduce ankle injuries in basketball. *Am J Sports Med* **22**, 454–461.

Starkey, C. (2000) Injuries and illnesses in the National Basketball Association: a 10-year perspective. *J Athletic Training* **35**, 161–167.

Steingard, P.M. (1993) *Clinics in Sports Medicine: Basketball Injuries*, Vol. 12, Number 2. Philadelphia: W.B. Saunders.

Stone, W.J. & Steingard, P.M. (1993) Year-round conditioning for basketball. *Clin Sports Med* **12**, 173–191.

U.S. Trends in Team Sports (2000) Sporting Goods Manufacturer Association, North Palm Beach, FL.

Zagelbaum, B.M., Starkey, C., Hersh, P.S., Donnenfeld, E.D., Perry, H.D. & Jeffers, J.B. (1995) The National Basketball Association eye injury study. *Am J Sports Med* **113**, 749–752.

Chapter 5
Preparticipation screening and the basketball player

Andrew L. Pipe

Introduction

The medical examination of athletes before they become involved in training or competition is a fundamental responsibility of the sport medicine practitioner. The approach to be taken in ensuring that athletes are healthy enough to participate in competitive basketball (and in particular have no evidence of significant cardiovascular or other conditions that might be life threatening), and free of pre-existing injury or illness will vary tremendously between communities and sport settings. The "preparticipation examinations" mandated in many settings (e.g., some European countries and American schools and colleges) may be appropriate in those situations—but time, facilities, and resources will differ markedly throughout the basketball world. Sport authorities and medical officers will be most familiar with their own unique situations, and best placed to develop preparticipation and other screening strategies appropriate to their community's needs. Some have suggested that the utility of such examinations in identifying problems of clinical significance is questionable and not supported by evidence in the medical literature. This perspective presupposes, however, that the purpose of such examinations is solely to discover previously unknown pathology. In truth the preparticipation evaluation, particularly in a sport like basketball, allows the physician to develop an array of information about an athlete's health status, discuss a broad array of other relevant health and behavioral issues, and in

the most fundamental way begin the development of an ongoing relationship with an athlete.

The elements of the preparticipation examination

Irrespective of the level of competition or the sophistication of a basketball programme's medical services, the aims of initial screening strategies are identical. It is hoped that by learning of the personal and family medical history of an athlete, performing a medical examination and conducting an appropriately focused interview that a specific understanding of the athlete's medical needs or problems will permit timely and appropriate medical intervention. Such interventions, it has already been noted, may permit the identification of dangerous or disqualifying medical conditions; allow the treatment or rehabilitation of existing illness or injury; and facilitate the development of a personal and professional relationship between athlete and sport medicine practitioner. Many physicians may have little experience with athletes or other vigorously active, seemingly healthy young people and the need for medical scrutiny of such a population may not be obvious. Nevertheless, it is the case that athletes may have had minimal previous contact with a medical system, unrecognized or unmet medical needs (e.g., basic immunizations and tetanus prophylaxis), personal or family medical histories of relevance to their participation in sport, and a need to discuss health or other issues of particular personal significance unrelated to sport participation.

The history

"Listen to your patient", advised Sir William Osler "he is giving you the diagnosis". His dictum is especially relevant in assessing the health status of athletes inasmuch as more is likely to be gleaned from a carefully taken, appropriately focused history than from any other element of the preparticipation evaluation. The majority of musculoskeletal and medical conditions in athletes are detected on the basis of history taking rather than in the course of a physical examination. Pressures of time and numbers usually dictate that obtaining a history is best accomplished with the use of a carefully constructed questionnaire followed by a brief interview to clarify or amplify issues identified in its completion. In some settings, the questionnaire can be completed in advance using Internet technology, which also affords the opportunity to develop an initial electronic record. Sport medicine practitioners worldwide may wish to visit the Stanford University Department of Sportsmedicine website (www.stanford.edu/dept/sportsmed) to view the questionnaire developed for that institution—it can easily be adapted to any setting and provides an ideal outline for a screening history. Alternately readers may prefer to apply the template devised by a taskforce of the American Academy of Family Physicians on the Preparticipation Physical Examination (PPE) (Fig. 5.1). Irrespective of the sophistication of the approach it is of fundamental importance that the questionnaire identify (a) any familial illnesses, tendencies or traits; (b) any history of sudden or premature deaths; (c) any pre-existing medical conditions; (d) all previous injuries, hospitalizations and surgical procedures; and (e) all medication use.

Physicians caring for female athletes must be particularly sensitive to their unique health needs and problems. Such sensitivity must be reflected in questionnaires, interviews, and physical examinations. The alterations of menstrual function, disorders of eating, and changes in bone density now identified as the "female athlete triad" warrant particular care and thoughtful management. The

Table 5.1 Cardiovascular considerations: critical questions in the preparticipation evaluation. Adapted from American Heart Association (1996) Cardiovascular preparticipation screening of competitive athletes. *JAMA* 94, 850–856.

---

1 Is there a history of chest pain or shortness of breath?
2 Is there a history of syncope or unexpected fatigue while, or shortly after exercising?
3 Has anyone ever detected a heart murmur or evidence of high blood pressure?
4 Is there any family history of heart abnormalities?
5 Has anyone in your close family (including aunts or uncles) died suddenly at a young age?
6 Has anyone in your close family (including aunts or uncles) had serious heart disease at a young age?

---

preparticipation evaluation provides an ideal opportunity for careful attention to menstrual and dietary history, and a sensitive exploration of training practices and weight-control strategies that are of profound significance to the health of any female athlete.

The identification of that very, very small number of athletes who may be at risk of exercise-associated sudden cardiac death (calculated to range from one in 150 000 to one in several million) is best accomplished by identifying all who have a family history of sudden or premature death, a personal history of exercise-associated syncope, or the constellation of physical features that are suggestive of Marfan syndrome (Table 5.1). It cannot be emphasized too often that physicians caring for athletes in a sport which preferentially attracts tall athletes *must* be constantly aware of the potential likelihood of encountering individuals with this syndrome, or incompletely expressed variants. The presence of any of these findings must lead to closer scrutiny, careful physical examination, and appropriate investigations (see Chapter 11).

The significance of so-called minor head injuries is now appreciated by sport medicine physicians; the importance of documenting previous head trauma, loss of consciousness and concussion is self-evident. Many teams and physicians now include simple neuro-psychological testing of their athletes; the results of such testing can serve as a benchmark in case of subsequent head injury, providing objective indication of subtle changes in function that might

Preparticipation Physical Evaluation

HISTORY

Date of examination _____

Name _____ Sex _____ Age _____ Date of birth _____

Grade _____ School _____ Sport(s) _____

Address _____ Phone _____

Personal physician _____

In case of emergency, contact

Name _____ Relationship _____ Phone (H) _____ (W) _____

Circle questions you don't know the answers to. Explain "Yes" answers below.

	Yes	No
1. Have you had a medical illness or injury since your last checkup or sports physical?	☐	☐
2. Have you ever been hospitalized overnight?	☐	☐
Have you ever had surgery?	☐	☐
3. Are you currently taking any prescription or nonprescription (over-the-counter) medications or pills or using an inhaler?	☐	☐
Have you ever taken any supplements or vitamins to help you gain or lose weight or improve your performance?	☐	☐
4. Do you have any allergies (for example, to pollen, medicine, food or stinging insects)?	☐	☐
Have you ever had a rash or hives develop during or after exercise?	☐	☐
5. Have you ever passed out during or after exercise?	☐	☐
Have you ever been dizzy during or after exercise?	☐	☐
Have you ever had chest pain during or after exercise?	☐	☐
Do you get tired more quickly than your friends do during exercise?	☐	☐
Have you ever had racing of your heart or skipped heartbeats?	☐	☐
Have you had high blood pressure or high cholesterol?	☐	☐
Have you ever been told you have a heart murmur?	☐	☐
Has any family member or relative died of heart problems or of sudden death before age 50?	☐	☐
Have you had a severe viral infection (for example, myocarditis or mononucleosis) within the past month?	☐	☐
Has a physician ever denied or restricted your participation in sports for any heart problems?	☐	☐
6. Do you have any current skin problems (for example, itching, rashes, acne, warts, fungus or blisters)?	☐	☐
7. Have you ever had a head injury or concussion?	☐	☐
Have you ever been knocked out, become unconscious or lost your memory?	☐	☐
Have you ever had a seizure?	☐	☐
Do you have frequent or severe headaches?	☐	☐
Have you ever had numbness or tingling in your arms, hands, legs or feet?	☐	☐
Have you ever had a stinger, burner or pinched nerve?	☐	☐
8. Have you ever become ill from exercising in the heat?	☐	☐
9. Do you cough, wheeze or have trouble breathing during or after activity?	☐	☐
Do you have asthma?	☐	☐
Do you have seasonal allergies that require medical treatment?	☐	☐

	Yes	No
10. Do you use any special protective or corrective equipment or devices that aren't usually used for your sport or position (for example, knee brace, special neck roll, foot orthotics, retainer on your teeth or hearing aid)?	☐	☐
11. Have you had any problems with your eyes or vision?	☐	☐
12. Have you ever had a sprain, strain or swelling after injury?	☐	☐
Have you broken or fractured any bones or dislocated any joints?	☐	☐
Have you had any other problems with pain or swelling in muscles, tendons, bones or joints?	☐	☐

☐ Head	☐ Elbow	☐ Thigh
☐ Neck	☐ Forearm	☐ Knee
☐ Back	☐ Wrist	☐ Shin/calf
☐ Chest	☐ Hand	☐ Ankle
☐ Shoulder	☐ Finger	☐ Foot
☐ Upper arm	☐ Hip	

If yes, check appropriate box and explain below.

	Yes	No
13. Do you want to weigh more or less than you do now?	☐	☐
Do you lose weight regularly to meet weight requirements for your sport?	☐	☐
14. Do you feel stressed out?	☐	☐

15. Record the dates of your most recent immunizations (shots) for:

Tetanus _____ Measles _____

Hepatitis B _____ Chickenpox _____

Females Only

16. When was your first menstrual period? _____

When was your most recent menstrual period? _____

How much time do you usually have from the start of one period to the start of another? _____

How many periods have you had in the past year? _____

What was the longest time between periods in the past year? _____

Explain "Yes" answers here: _____

_____

_____

_____

_____

I hereby state that, to the best of my knowledge, my answers to the above questions are complete and correct. Furthermore, I consent to the performance of a sports physical exam, and I hereby authorize the athletic director, school nurse, or their designated agents to access and utilize my complete preparticipation physical evaluation.

Signature of athlete _____ Signature of parent/guardian _____ Date _____

Fig. 5.1 The preparticipation physical evaluation (PPE) form can be copied and used for each examination of student athletes. Using this form can help ensure that examining physicians consider the components of the cardiac evaluation recommended by the PPE Task Force. (Adapted with permission from Smith, D.M. (1997) *Preparticipation Physical Evaluation*, 2nd edn. American Academy of Family Physicians, Physician Sportsmedicine, Minneapolis.)

NATIONAL MEN'S BASKETBALL TEAM
DECLARATION REGARDING DRUG USE AND SPORT
-Athlete-

I acknowledge that I, _____ have today discussed the issue of Drug Use in Sport with the team physician of the Canadian National Men's Basketball Team. I am aware of my obligations as an athlete and a member of the Canadian National Men's Basketball Team to abide by the rules and regulations regarding drug use in sport as they have been developed and are applied by the International Olympic committee, World Anti-doping Agency, FIBA, Canada Basketball, Sport Canada and the Canadian Centre for Ethics in Sport. I am aware that I am subject to year-round drug testing including short-notice drug testing. I am committed to the pursuit of excellence using fair and ethical approaches to sport.

In Particular, I am aware of the necessity to verify the acceptability, insofar as the rules and regulations concerning drug use in sport are concerned, of any medication, nutritional supplement, vitamin preparation or any related product, preparation or compound which I am using or contemplating using with the team physician or a member of the team medical staff. I understand that the team physician will document all such enquiries and the specific advice provided in each instance.

I am further aware that the use of nutritional supplements may pose significant risk for athletes because such products may contain banned or harmful substances.

_____
Athlete

_____
Witness & Team Physician

_____
Location and Date

Fig. 5.2 An agreement regarding drug and supplement use signed by members of an elite basketball team at the time of their preparticipation evaluation.

otherwise go unnoticed and permitting withdrawal and return-to-play decisions to be made with more confidence.

It is of particular importance to identify all dietary supplements, "ergogenic" aids, homeopathic preparations, vitamins or other products that an athlete might be consuming. Many commonly available supplements may contain compounds whose use is hazardous and/or banned according to the antidoping rules of sport, e.g., ephedra. A cautionary note for team physicians and other medical officials: it is important to document the declarations of athletes in this regard. It has been my practice for several years to have players sign a document noting their responsibility to be aware of: (i) the hazards of supplement use in sport; and (ii) their obligation to review the use of such products with team officials.

Such an approach serves to impress upon both athletes and medical officials the need for extreme care in the use of these problematic compounds (Fig. 5.2).

While there is an obvious interest in detecting the presence of conditions that might limit participation or serve as prelude to injury, it is important to recognize that among teenagers and young adults (the age groups most commonly represented in sport), a variety of hazardous behaviors may be commonly expressed. There is some evidence that male athletes in team sports may have a higher incidence of hazardous behaviors than their nonathletic counterparts. Noting the use of alcohol and "social" drugs, a history of unprotected sexual activity, and episodes of irresponsible driving or other risk-taking behaviors may be more relevant to the health of the athlete than eliciting a history of nonspecific, activity-related knee pain. It is often the case that the most significant revelations that occur in the process of obtaining and refining a medical history in an athletic population are those pertaining to psychiatric, social, or behavioral issues. The athlete with undiagnosed depression or other psychiatric disorder, the teenager from an abusing household, the point-guard with a history of binge drinking, and the anorexic and bulimic young woman are all examples of problems of profound personal significance that can come to light in the context of a properly, and sensitively taken history.

Additional concerns

While musculoskeletal findings are the most common reasons for restriction from sport activities, it is important to identify other common conditions whose management is of significance in any sport setting. The presence of anemia in athletes from countries where malaria is endemic, or the identification of the sickle cell trait in black competitors may be overlooked, or revealed only at the time of a preparticipation medical examination. Athletes with the sickle cell trait require instruction in the need to maintain hydration and counseling regarding the problems that may occur at altitude.

Those with a history of convulsive disorder must be identified and their management and well-being assured. Asthma and exercise induced bronchospasm (EIB) are increasingly common in many communities and it is important that athletes with these conditions are appropriately diagnosed and managed with inhaled corticosteroids and beta-agonists. Diabetic athletes have particular and obvious needs, not the least of which are an ability of all involved in the care of the athlete to recognize and respond to hypoglycemic states. A history of heat-related illness will stimulate medical officials to be both vigilant in permitting participation in competition and training only at appropriate temperatures. Athletes with single organs must be advised of the particular risks of competition—basketball is contraindicated for the individual with one kidney if that kidney is polycystic or abnormally located; protective eyewear is mandatory for basketballers

Table 5.2 Conditions in which sport participation is contraindicated. Adapted from Smith, D. (1997) *Preparticipation Physical Evaluation* (2nd edn). Minneapolis: Physician and Sportsmedicine.

Acute myocarditis or pericarditis
Hypertrophic cardiomyopathy
Severe hypertension
Suspected coronary artery disease until appropriately evaluated
Long QT syndrome
History of recent concussion
Poorly controlled convulsive disorder
Instability of cervical spine
Sickle cell disease
Eating disorder where athlete is not compliant with therapy or
    follow-up
Hepatomegaly
Splenomegaly

with monocular vision. The sport physician should be aware of those conditions that are grounds for disqualification from sport (Table 5.2).

A thoughtfully constructed, carefully reviewed questionnaire supplemented with focused questioning of an athlete will permit all of these important issues to be identified efficiently. A careful review and sensitive interview will facilitate an appropriate physical examination.

The physical examination

Much has been written about the physical examination of athletes. The limitations of such examinations have been noted by many authors; a consensus remains, however, that the examination may permit the identification of abnormalities or problems that will be of assistance to the athlete in competing optimally and comfortably. Some of these problems may seem trivial (I'm always surprised to see florid tinea pedis in many elite level basketballers—its treatment is generally straightforward and highly appreciated—and yet it is seldom brought to my attention spontaneously!), others can have life-long significance (I frequently identify essential hypertension in young, black athletes). The application of a stethoscope to a chest and other manifestations of the examination process provide a tangible, and important, expression of care to the athlete!

Sport physicians will have developed their own routines and approaches to the examination of the athletes under their care. Screening examinations are sometimes performed using the services of a number of physicians or other health professionals —an approach which is both efficient and effective. It is important for the basketball team physician to assume ultimate responsibility for the review of all positive findings to ensure that they are properly addressed with further examinations, referrals, and special investigations when such are indicated.

In some settings (e.g., professional or elite basketball) it may be possible to involve specialist assistance in the performance of part of the examination. Dentists and ophthalmologists or optometrists may be present, podiatrists and orthotists involved, and sport psychologists available or an integral part of the review process. This is, however, highly atypical and for the overwhelming majority of players in organized basketball not a reality. The challenge for the sport medicine professional is to conduct a systematic examination with particular emphasis on systems: (a) identified in the course of the history taking; and/or (b) of critical importance to the health of the athlete.

The physical examination must include measurement of the pulse and blood pressure and an assessment of visual acuity. A careful, systematic examination of the cardiovascular system is mandatory in all basketball players. Clear guidelines for the conduct of cardiovascular screening of competitive athletes have been prepared by the American Heart Association and include: (1) auscultation of the heart in both standing and supine positions; (2) palpation of both femoral pulses; (3) a search for the findings of Marfan syndrome; and (4) measurement of the blood pressure in the supine position. Note that the routine use of electrocardiograms is not recommended.

Most physicians are familiar with an approach to the examination of the musculoskeletal system and have undoubtedly developed their own routine; in the setting of preparticipation examinations the use of a systematic screening approach may be very helpful in ensuring the best use of time and facilities. The preparticipation examination routine published by the American Academy of Family Physicians may be particularly helpful and permit the development of a systematic approach to the musculoskeletal examination of athletes (Fig. 5.3).

Basketball players commonly experience injuries of the lower limbs (particularly the ankle) and fingers. Documentation of the range of movement and any deformities of the fingers is important. Female basketballers experience injuries of the anterior cruciate ligaments more frequently than do males. Particular attention should be paid to the lower limbs with an emphasis on careful examination of the mass and strength of the quadriceps and the stability of the knee. Palpation of the lower pole of the patella, the proximal patellar tendon and the anterior tibial apophysis will often reveal the typical tenderness of patellar tendinopathy or "jumper's knee" (almost universal in elite players with little opportunity for appropriate rest and recovery and often responsive to a prolonged and tenacious program of eccentric quadriceps training.) An assessment of the ankle ligaments is important and will typically reveal laxity of an anterior talo fibular (ATF) ligament as a result of previous ankle sprains. The presence of a "drawer sign" in the ankle is indicative of a complete rupture of the ATF ligament. (An appropriate point to discuss the utility of ankle braces in the prevention of further ankle injuries!) Many basketball players have high, cavus feet—frequently accompanied by deformities of the toes—with understandable implications for the proper fitting of footwear and the use of orthotics. Stress fractures of the tarsal and metatarsal bones are common basketball injuries and the identification of suggestive symptoms especially in association with dynamic loading of the foot may indicate the need for further investigations. Predictably, many basketballers experience episodic low back pain and an examination of the lumbo-sacral spine provides an excellent opportunity for a discussion about the importance of core strength and other important approaches to the prevention of back discomfort. The elbow is a common site—and source—of injury. Basketballers frequently experience facial lacerations, nasal fractures, and dental injuries because of a collision with an opponent's elbow. The use of mouth guards should be encouraged and there is no better

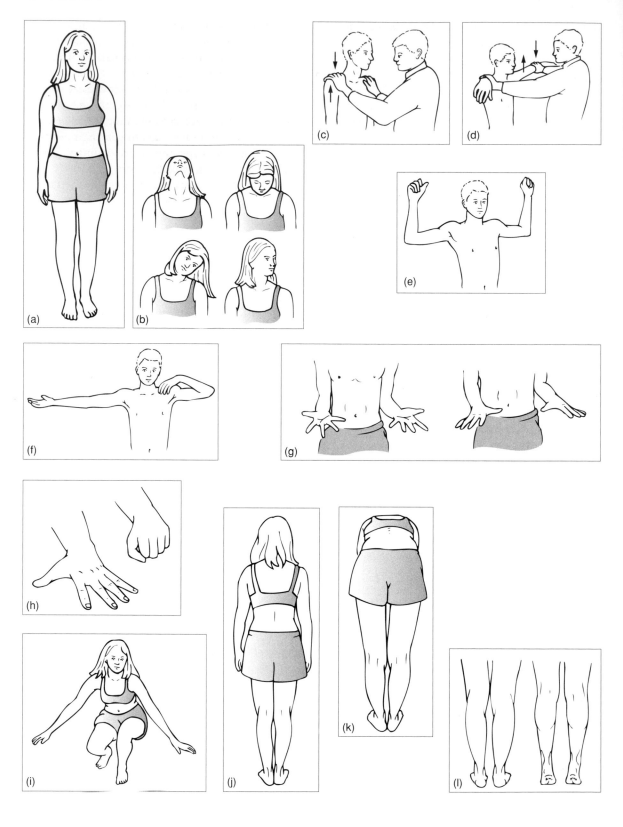

time to address this issue than when examining the head, neck and oropharynx!

Laboratory and other investigations

There is little evidence to support the use of a battery of hematological or biochemical investigations in evaluating the health of athletes. Laboratory evidence is most useful when there is a clear clinical reason for requesting it! It has been my practice in almost a quarter of a century of caring for the Canadian men's national basketball team to measure electrolytes, blood urea nitrogen and creatinine, and perform a complete blood count at the time of a preparticipation examination. It would make sense in caring for female athletes to measure serum feritin as a measure of iron storage status when specific concerns are present. Except for research purposes we have not, in the absence of any clinical indications, performed routine electrocardiograms. It is to be anticipated that athletes presenting for preparticipation examinations in other settings may

Fig. 5.3 (*opposite*) The preparticipation examination routine.
(a) Patient stands straight with arms at sides, facing examiner. Normal findings: symmetry of upper and lower extremities and trunk. Common abnormalities include enlarged acromioclavicular joint, enlarged sternoclavicular joint, asymmetric waist (leg-length difference or scoliosis), swollen knee and swollen ankle.
(b) Patient looks at the ceiling, looks at the floor, touches right (and left) ear to shoulder and looks over right (and left) shoulder. Normal findings: patients should be able to touch chin to chest, ears to shoulders and look equally over the shoulders. Common abnormalities, which include loss of flexion, loss of lateral bending and loss of rotation, may indicate previous neck injury.
(c) Patient stands in front of examiner with arms at side. Examiner tries to hold shoulder down while patient tries to shrug. Common abnormalities include atrophy or weakness of muscles indicating shoulder, neck or trapezius nerve abnormalities.
(d) Patient holds arms out from sides horizontally and tries to lift them (while examiner holds arms down). Normal findings: strength should be equal in both arms, and deltoid muscles should be equal in size. Common abnormalities include loss of strength and wasting of the deltoid muscle.
(e) Patient holds arms out from sides with elbows bent at 90 degrees; patient raises hands vertically as far as they will go. Normal findings: hands go back equally and at least to upright vertical position. Common abnormalities: loss of external rotation, which may indicate shoulder problem or old dislocation.
(f) Patient holds arms out from sides, palms up, and completely straightens and bends elbows. Normal findings: motion should be equal on left and right sides. Common abnormalities, which include loss of extension and loss of flexion, may indicate old elbow injury, dislocation, fractures, etc.
(g) Patient holds arms down at sides with elbows bent at 90 degrees, then twists palms up and down. Normal findings: palms should go from facing the ceiling to facing the floor. Common abnormalities, which include lack of full supination and full pronation, may indicate an old injury of the forearm, wrist or elbow.
(h) Patient makes a fist, opens the hand and spreads the fingers. Normal findings: fist should be tight and fingers straight when spread. Common abnormalities, which include a knuckle protruding from the fist and a swollen or crooked finger, may indicate old finger fractures or sprains.
(i) Patient squats on heels, duckwalks four steps and stands up. Normal findings: maneuver is painless, heel-to-buttock distance is equal on left and right sides and knee flexion is equal during the walk. Common abnormalities include inability to fully flex one knee and inability to stand up without twisting or bending to one side.
(j) Patient stands up straight with arms at sides (with back to the examiner). Normal findings: symmetry of shoulders, waist, thighs and calves. Common abnormalities include high shoulder (scoliosis) or low shoulder (muscle loss), prominent rib cage (scoliosis), high hip or asymmetric waist (leg-length difference or scoliosis), and small calf or thigh (weakness from an old injury).
(k) Patient bends forward slowly with knees straight and touches the toes. Normal findings: patient bends forward straightly and smoothly. Common abnormalities include patient twisting to one side (low back pain) and asymmetric back (scoliosis).
(l) Patient stands on the heels and then rises up on the toes. Normal findings: equal elevation on right and left sides, symmetry of calf muscles. Common abnormalities include wasting of calf muscles (Achilles injury or old ankle injury).
Published by the American Academy of Family Physicians.

present with a much wider range of health issues than those whose career has taken them to elite levels of sport. The need for laboratory investigations will still be minimal.

Conclusion

The performance of a preparticipation evaluation of basketballers will not ordinarily result in the detection of significant pathology. It will permit the identification of a range of broad health and behavioral issues and permit the sport physician to develop a professional relationship with the athlete. Sport medicine practitioners must appreciate both the limitations of, and the opportunities presented by the process. The basketball physician must appreciate that individuals with Marfan syndrome may be drawn to this sport and retain a high index of suspicion as they mange the health needs of their tall athletes.

Further reading

Abdulla, A. & Abdulla, F. (2002) The preparticipation evaluation of athletes. *Patient Care Canada* **13**, 85–93.

American Academy of Pediatrics (2000) Assessing health in young female athletes. *Women's Health in Primary Care*, 876–878.

American Heart Association (1996) Cardiovascular preparticipation screening of competitive athletes. *JAMA* **94**, 850–856.

Kurowski, K. & Chandran, S. (2000) The preparticipation athletic evaluation. *Am Fam Physician* **61**, 2683–2690, 2696–2698.

Matheson, G. (1998) Preparticipation screening of athletes. *JAMA* **279**, 1829–1830.

McKeag, D. & Sallis, R. (2000) Factors at play in the athletic preparticipation examination. *Am Fam Physician* **61**, 2617–2618.

Pelz, J., Haskell, W. & Matheson, G. (1999) A comprehensive and cost-effective preparticipation exam implemented on the World Wide Web. *Med Sci Sports Exerc* **31**, 1727–1740.

Smith, D. (1997) *Preparticipation Physical Evaluation*, 2nd edn. Physician and Sportsmedicine, Minneapolis.

Chapter 6
The young basketball player

Kevin B. Gebke and Douglas B. McKeag

Millions of young people around the world are introduced to basketball at an early age. Children initially spend time learning fundamentals and then participate in a variety of activities (Figs 6.1 & 6.2). As young athletes train with increased intensity, there is a concomitant increase in strain on their developing bodies. Injuries are common in young basketball players. This chapter strives to address issues *most pertinent* to young basketball players and includes a discussion of epiphyseal injuries and apophysitis, fluid imbalance and heat-related illness, back problems, and genitourinary and abdominal injuries. Other important issues in the young basketball player include chronic medical conditions such as asthma and diabetes. These issues are addressed in Chapter 8. Also, congenital heart problems must be considered when caring for young athletes and are discussed in Chapter 11.

Epiphyseal injuries and apophysitis

Young athletes' developing bodies place them at risk for a variety of unique injuries. A good example is the "greenstick" forearm fracture suffered by children when falling onto an outstretched hand. An axial load in combination with a torsional load can cause tensile failure of the bony shaft on one side (volar vs. dorsal) and compression failure on the other. Perfect reduction of these injuries is not necessarily required. Children have the ability to remodel forearm fracture deformities and respond well to forearm reduction that would not be considered satisfactory in adults. Other unique bone and cartilage problems in children include epiphyseal injuries and apophysitis. These disorders are seen in the regions of growth.

Growth cartilage is present in the epiphyseal plate (growth plate) and at the apophysis (insertion site of major tendons). In skeletally immature athletes, this region of growing bone represents an area of relative weakness and is more likely to be injured

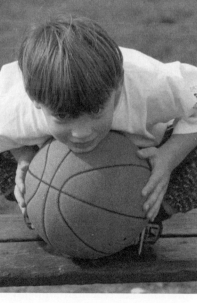

Fig. 6.1 Basketball—the perfect sport . . . for young athletes?

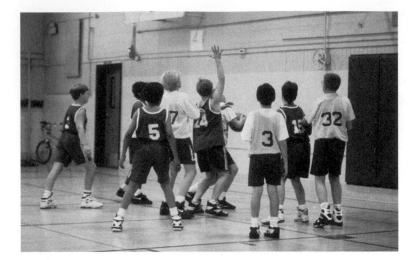

Fig. 6.2 Unique injuries may await young basketball players.

with episodes of repetitive stress or trauma to the musculoskeletal system. A variety of acute and chronic injuries can occur in the epiphyseal plate and at the apophysis.

The epiphyseal plate is predisposed to injury because it is the weak link in the kinetic chain. Growth cartilage is weaker than the supporting ligamentous structures, thus the growth area will fail earlier than the supporting structures when stressed. Consider the case of a young basketball player who suffers an inversion stress to the ankle which subsequently injures the growth plate of the distal fibula while the anterior talofibular, calcaneofibular, and posterior talofibular ligaments remain intact. When direct trauma or secondary mechanical forces are transmitted across the growing cartilage, there is a risk of injury. The following classification system for epiphyseal injuries uses an anatomic description of the fracture to categorize the lesion and determine treatment:

I   Through epiphyseal plate
II Extension into epiphysis
III Extension into the metaphysis
IV Extension into the epiphysis and metaphysis
V   Impaction of the epiphyseal plate.

Complications of epiphyseal injury include a risk for permanent damage to the growth plate that can lead to growth disturbance or arrest. Although any epiphyseal injury can cause growth disturbance, the highest degree of risk is associated with type V injuries. Impaction of the epiphyseal plate can result

in limb-length discrepancy or angular deformity. Distal femur and distal tibial fractures require close follow-up to identify any early disruption of normal growth.

Strength training programs are increasingly prominent in basketball programs. There is a theoretical concern that injury to the growth plate may occur. Studies have demonstrated that prepubescent athletes are *not* at risk for injury from strength training. Strength gains in this population are achieved primarily by neurogenic adaptation (increased recruitment and decreased inhibition). Significant increases in contractile proteins and overall muscle bulk are not seen due to absence of pubertal hormonal changes. An appropriate program should include:

1 Experienced supervisors
2 Warm-up and cool-down periods
3 Proper technique
4 One set of high repetition (15) with low weight
5 Machines sized to young athletes.

Weight training with maximal loads is not recommended and may risk injury in the young basketball player.

Minimizing untoward effects of epiphyseal injury requires proper early diagnosis and the key to diagnosis is maintaining a high level of suspicion. Diagnosis then determines treatment. Standard radiographs may not reveal a minimally displaced or nondisplaced fracture (Salter type I). In this instance, a presumptive diagnosis of epiphyseal plate

Table 6.1 General treatment recommendation for Salter injuries.

Salter I and II	Closed reduction and immobilization
Salter III	Restore normal anatomic configuration (closed vs. open) and immobilize
Salter IV	Restore normal anatomic configuration (closed vs. open) and immobilize
Salter V	Restore normal anatomic configuration (closed vs. open) and immobilize

injury can be made, and the athlete may be treated conservatively with closed reduction and immobilization (Table 6.1). The vast majority of athletes recover fully and experience no long-term problems after Salter injuries.

Young basketball players will commonly develop pain in the knee, hip, or heel. History and physical exam findings may localize symptoms to the tibial tubercle (Osgood–Schlatter syndrome), calcaneus (Sever's disease), inferior pole of the patella (Sinding–Larson–Johansson syndrome), or iliac crest (iliac apophysitis). This represents inflammation of the growth cartilage where the tendon inserts into the bony structures, also known as the traction apophysis. Repetitive stress at the traction apophysis produces microfractures of the tendon insertion and resultant inflammation. Risk factors for these problems include overuse, lack of flexibility, and biomechanical abnormalities. During rapid growth, bones commonly grow at a faster pace than musculotendinous structures. This leads to loss of flexibility and increased tension on the apophysis.

Osgood–Schlatter syndrome is the most frequently occurring apophysitis. Prevalence is higher in males than females (3 : 2). Bilateral symptoms are seen in about one fourth of cases. Usual presentation is a gradual onset of pain and swelling at the tibial tubercle exacerbated by jumping, running, squatting, kneeling, and direct impact. Physical exam findings include tenderness to palpation of the tibial tubercle and often associated tubercle enlargement. Radiographic findings range from normal to dramatic fragmentation of the tuberosity. Avulsion of the apophysis is a possibility, but, if avulsed, is usually nondisplaced. Treatment includes protection with padding, relative rest, ice, and nonsteroidal, nonaspirin anti-inflammatory medications

as needed. Surgical intervention is rarely necessary unless a displaced avulsion is present. Stretching and strengthening programs and therapeutic modalities are frequently employed with symptomatic improvement. The most important aspect of Osgood–Schlatter syndrome management is an understanding that the course is self-limited. Symptoms typically resolve with a period of rest, and reassurance is important for parents and athletes. Unnecessary restriction from participation is a common management pitfall.

Sinding–Larson–Johansson syndrome manifests with tenderness at the inferior pole of the patella. This is the second, albeit less common, apophysitis affecting the patellofemoral extensor mechanism. Repetitive jumping and forceful knee extension movements have been implicated as causal factors. A continuum between this syndrome and patellar tendinitis has been proposed. The prevalence is higher in males, but occurrence is at a younger age in girls (age 10–13 as opposed to 11–14 in boys). Tenderness to palpation and even bony prominence at the inferior pole of the patella are the standard physical exam findings. Radiographic findings range from normal to a calcified mass separated from the patella. Treatment must focus on the same principles used in Osgood–Schlatter syndrome, which includes protection, rest, ice, and nonaspirin anti-inflammatory medications as needed. Participation in basketball should be titrated according to symptoms. Surgery is rarely necessary, but in recalcitrant cases, tendon debridement and bony loose body removal may be required.

Sever's disease is apophysitis of the Achilles tendon calcaneal insertion. Again, it is considered an overuse injury predisposed by lack of flexibility, varus angulation of the forefoot, valgus angulation of the rearfoot, or pronounced femoral internal rotation. The athlete will typically complain of posterior heel pain with or without the presence of a lump. Physical exam findings may include localized tenderness, palpable fullness over the Achilles insertion site, and poor gastrocnemius–soleus flexibility. Radiographic evaluation is insensitive, but may reveal sclerosis or bony fragmentation. Treatment involves adjustment of the training schedule and addressing any biomechanical predisposing factors. These interventions include correction of foot angulation with shoe orthotics, heel lifts to decrease stress on the Achilles complex, aggressive Achilles stretching in conjunction with strengthening of the foot dorsiflexors, icing, heel lifts, and non-aspirin anti-inflammatory medications. Symptoms are self-limited and usually resolve with conservative therapy.

Apophysitis can also occur at the iliac or ischial apophyses, but less commonly than the aforementioned disorders. The sartorius muscle is a secondary hip flexor and attaches at the anterior superior iliac spine (ASIS); the rectus femoris functions as both a secondary hip flexor and knee extensor and attaches to the anterior inferior iliac spine. These muscles have been implicated in iliac apophysitis. Ischial apophysitis occurs at the ischial tuberosity at the attachment of the hamstring musculature. Young basketball players who present with pain in these locations can be suffering from traction apophysitis. Radiographic findings can demonstrate avulsion, but usually will only confirm that the growth plates remain open. Activity adjustment, relative rest, icing, anti-inflammatory medications, and stretching remain the standard of therapy. Surgical evaluation may be necessary to avoid future disability if a significant avulsion (1–2 cm) is present.

Fluid balance and heat injuries

Oral hydration is a preventive habit that should be taught to all young developing athletes. Simply replacing fluids as dictated by thirst is inadequate and can result in deleterious dehydration that impairs athletic performance. Approximately 75% of the energy expended by the human musculoskeletal system is lost in the form of heat. This heat must then be eliminated from the body to maintain a homeothermic milieu and avoid injury. These principles become even more essential when the sport involved requires constant, high-intensity exertion as is seen in basketball.

Heat is dissipated from the body by a variety of mechanisms including evaporation of sweat, radiation from the skin to the surrounding environment, convection from airflow across the body, and conduction. Evaporation is the most efficient mechanism and can account for over 80% of heat

transference. If these mechanisms are compromised, however, body temperature can mount precipitously. The most important factor involved is hydration status because adequate intravascular volume helps maintain cardiac output and delivery of blood flow to the skin. With dehydration, vascular dilation at the level of the skin and sweating are reduced in an attempt to maintain cardiac output. This, in turn, allows for less dissipation of heat and perpetuation of the cycle.

Recognition of the early signs and symptoms of dehydration are of utmost importance. Multiple game tournaments or contests played outdoors can predispose players to fluid imbalance. Early sequelae include increased thirst, generalized malaise, and a variety of subjective complaints. Failure to act on the initial signs and symptoms can allow for potentiation of fluid depletion and the more severe problems of heat illness.

Differences exist between young athletes and adults that may affect the efficiency of thermoregulation and maintenance of adequate hydration. It has been proposed that children and adolescents are at increased risk for heat illness due to a number of factors. These include increased heat production per mass unit during exercise, lower sweating capacity (fewer sweat glands) leading to decreased evaporation, smaller relative circulatory systems with decreased cardiac output capacity, slowed acclimatization compared to adults, and a faster rate of core body temperature rise during exercise if dehydration is present. It has also been observed that children do not readily drink fluids while exercising. They will only seek fluids when they experience thirst. This practice can predispose to rapid depletion of fluid stores. Fortunately, heat exhaustion is seen infrequently in children and heat stroke is very rare in young people.

The spectrum of fluid imbalance associated with physical exertion is classified according to severity. This ranges from muscle cramping to heat stroke. Initially, athletes will present with painful muscle cramps as hypovolemia begins to manifest. As fluid loss continues, symptoms such as fatigue, dizziness, and even syncope can occur. If these symptoms are ignored and the athlete continues to participate, heat exhaustion may be experienced. It presents with weakness, myalgia, headache, hyperventilation,

Table 6.2 Treatment recommendations for varying degrees of heat illness.

Condition	Body temperature	Signs and symptoms	Physiologic findings	Treatment
Early (2%) dehydration	Normal	Asymptomatic, thirst	Impaired thermoregulation	Oral hydration
Heat cramps (dehydration >2%)	Up to 39.5°C	Muscle cramping	Early relative hyponatremia and hypovolemia	Oral hydration
Heat exhaustion	Up to 40.5°C	Headache, weakness, hyperventilation, anorexia, myalgia	Worsening hyponatremia, and hypovolemia cessation of sweating	Oral hydration, external cooling, removal from competition
Heat stroke	Above 40.5°C	Mental status changes and lack of sweating in addition to heat exhaustion findings	Intravascular depletion, hypotension, potential for protein denaturing at temperatures above 42°C	Intravenous hydration, internal and external cooling, evaluate electrolyte status

anorexia, and persistent muscle cramps. If participation continues, an athlete will lose the ability to sweat secondary to severe intravascular volume depletion. A continuum exists between all of these conditions. When severe dehydration sets in, the athlete is at risk for heat stroke. Heat stroke is an emergency with possible catastrophic outcome. Patients suffer from mental status changes, severe hyperthermia (>40.5°C), and signs of profound dehydration. There is a risk for cardiovascular collapse, disseminated intravascular coagulation (DIC), renal failure, rhabdomyolysis, lactic acidosis, liver damage, and seizures. Treatment is based on fluid replacement in all forms of heat illness (Table 6.2).

Oral hydration with external cooling measures is usually effective in heat cramps and heat exhaustion. In the rare case of heat stroke, more drastic measures are required. These include intravenous hydration, internal and external cooling mechanisms, and evaluation of electrolyte status. Evaluation and observation in a medical facility is necessary for all athletes with heat stroke and those with heat exhaustion who fail to respond to oral hydration and external cooling.

The American College of Sports Medicine (ACSM) and the National Athletic Trainers Association (NATA) have compiled recommendations for fluid replacement that can be applied to any age group (Fig. 6.3). These include the incorporation of a hydration protocol for athletes that addresses sweat rate using pre- and postexercise weight as well as urine

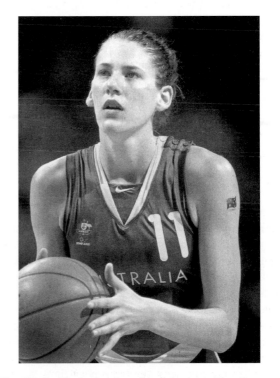

Fig. 6.3 Oral hydration is an important consideration to counter sweat loss for players of all age groups. Photo © Getty Images/Jed Jacobsohn.

dilution. An appropriate fluid replacement program replaces the sweat and urine losses incurred during the activity. This can be roughly estimated by replacing 16 ounces of fluid for every pound of dry weight lost during exercise. Each individual involved in a basketball-training program can be easily assessed before, during, and after activity to determine whether adequate hydration is being maintained. An emphasis should be placed on easy accessibility of fluids during practice and competition. If possible, individual fluid containers with incremental markings should be provided so the athletes can monitor their individual intake and be taught how much should be consumed to maintain appropriate hydration to maximize performance. The importance of pre-exercise hydration should be stressed. Athletes should be encouraged to drink fluids at every opportunity during activity. Thirst should not be used as a guide to hydration because thirst is typically delayed until the athlete has reached a level of fluid depletion sufficient to impair thermoregulatory function (approximately 2% dehydration). For activities lasting longer than 60 minutes, a carbohydrate-containing drink (8% or less) is beneficial to replace glucose stores and preserve liver glycogen. Sodium chloride-containing beverages can help offset sodium losses when activity lasts longer than 4 hours or if the temperature is significantly warmer than the athletes are adapted to. A sodium concentration of 50 mg is ideal, but taste dictates that the majority of sports drinks contain between 10 and 25 mg of sodium (Gatorade® = 20 mg). Post-exercise hydration should correct any fluid loss experienced and ideally should be completed within 2 hours. In addition to water, carbohydrates and electrolytes play an important role in the post-exercise period to assure effective rehydration and return of physiologic function. The biggest obstacle to postexercise fluid replacement is inadequate thirst drive.

A key component in preventing dehydration and heat injury is an effective education program. This includes involvement of athletes and parents, coaches, trainers, and the team physicians. Assessment of hydration status can be taught simply by making the athlete aware of the symptoms suggestive of early dehydration and how to address the problem (see Table 6.2). A basic understanding of the physiologic changes associated with dehydration and the effect on performance can impress upon the athlete and coach the necessity of adherence to a hydration program.

The specific recommendations of the ACSM are summarized below:
1 Well-balanced diet including adequate fluid intake, especially in the period preceding exercise with pregame meal.
2 Fluid intake of 250–500 mL approximately 2 h prior to activity.
3 During exercise, fluid should be consumed at a rate sufficient to replace losses or at the maximal rate tolerable by the athlete.
4 Cool, flavored fluids should be available in containers that allow adequate volumes to be ingested with ease.
5 Addition of carbohydrates and electrolytes for games or practices of 1 h duration or longer.
6 For activities longer than 1 h, 30–60 g of carbohydrate should be ingested per hour to maintain oxidation of carbohydrates and delay fatigue.
7 Inclusion of sodium in rehydration solution for activities of longer than 1 h to enhance palatability, promote fluid retention, and prevent hyponatremia in susceptible individuals.

Back problems

Back pain is not uncommon in young basketball players. Injury is usually secondary to trauma or overuse. Certain sports-related activities predispose athletes to low back injury. Predisposing factors in basketball include repetitive spinal flexion, extension, twisting, and loading. Poor development of abdominal musculature in conjunction with strong paraspinal muscles can allow for added stress on the lumbar spine in hyperextension. Also, athletes with hyperlordosis are at an increased risk for back injury at a young age.

As the intensity and frequency of youth participation increases, so does the incidence of injuries. Children and adolescents suffer from different causes of low back pain than adults, and require a careful evaluation to rule out a significant pathologic source. The following causes of adolescent low back pain were cited by Micheli *et al.* (1995) in a retrospective comparison study with adults: spondylolysis/spondylolisthesis (47%), hyperlordotic mechanical back strain (26%), discogenic (11%), scoliosis (8%), lumbosacral strain (6%), hamstring strain (1%), and trochanteric bursitis (1%). Low back pain in adults is frequently from a discogenic source, which includes lumbar disc herniation and degeneration. Conversely, discogenic back pain is an uncommon etiology of low back pain in young athletes; injuries to the posterior elements of the spine account for a large percentage of injuries in this age group. Spondylolysis and spondylolisthesis should be suspected in any athlete with back pain especially if symptoms have persisted for longer than 2 weeks. A delay in accurate diagnosis can lead to persistent symptoms and exacerbation of the underlying pathology.

Spondylolysis is a loss of continuity of the pars interarticularis (isthmus) of the vertebrae. Stress fracture formation in this region occurs due to repetitive microtrauma. Controversy exists over whether these pars defects are also seen as a congenital malformation. If untreated, this lesion can progress to a complete fracture of the pars with slip of the involved vertebrae (spondylolisthesis). The defect is usually unilateral. The most commonly affected region is L5–S1. Incidence of spondylolysis in the general population is approximately 6%, but studies have shown a much higher incidence in young athletes. Males are more commonly afflicted, but progression of the disease seems to occur more frequently in females. A genetic predisposition has been postulated, and many athletes with spondylolysis are found to have a comorbid spina bifida occulta (not of clinical significance).

Many people with spondylolysis remain asymptomatic. Those who become symptomatic will typically present during the preadolescent rapid growth phase with pain that improves with rest. History will usually reveal exacerbation of pain with certain activities, especially back extension or twisting. High impact trauma is usually not described, but onset of symptoms may coincide with relatively minor trauma. Physical examination may demonstrate spasm of lumbar paraspinal musculature, localized tenderness, increased thoracic kyphosis, lumbar scoliosis, hamstring tightness, or reproduction of symptoms with back hyperextension. Symptoms may also be provoked by having the athlete stand on one leg on the affected side while extending the back. The neurologic examination is usually unremarkable.

Radiographic evaluation of the lumbosacral spine is essential. Plain radiographs should be obtained first including weight-bearing AP, lateral, bilateral oblique, and possibly spot views at the involved level. Advanced spondylolytic lesions can be identified with plain films. The characteristic "Scotty dog collar" may be identified on oblique views. If the defects are bilateral, the lateral view should demonstrate the lesion. Acute pars fractures and stress fractures may not be seen on plain radiographs. Bone scan can be utilized to identify a suspected acute defect if plain films are negative. SPECT (single-photon emission computed tomography) scan can localize an acute lesion if necessary. Finally, computed tomography (CT) can play a role in differentiating a pars defect from other potential causes of a positive bone scan.

Spondylolisthesis occurs when both pars are disrupted at a specific level. This allows for forward displacement of a vertebral body on the body below. Meyerding developed a classification system for spondylolisthesis based on the degree of forward slip. The measurement is obtained by assessing the percentage of displacement of the involved vertebrae on the inferior vertebrae as visualized on the upright lateral radiograph. Grading of spondylolisthesis is as follows:

Grade 0: No slippage
Grade I: Up to 25% slip
Grade II: Up to 50% slip
Grade III: Up to 75% slip
Grade IV: Up to 100% slippage
Grade V: Greater than 100% (spondyloptosis).
Displacement of greater than 50% is considered a high-grade slip.

Athletes with spondylolisthesis may be asymptomatic or have the symptoms described above associated with spondylolysis. In addition, symptoms suggestive of lumbar radiculopathy may be described, especially in the L5 nerve root distribution. Additional physical examination findings in an athlete with spondylolisthesis may include hamstring tightness (majority of subjects), a hip-flexed, knee-flexed gait (Phalen–Dickson sign), step-off deformity of the lumbar spinous processes, or neurologic dysfunction in the L5 nerve root distribution.

Assessment of displacement is identified via standard radiographs. Magnetic resonance imaging is used to evaluate for nerve root compression in athletes with symptoms or physical examination findings suggesting involvement.

Conservative management is appropriate for young basketball players with spondylolysis and low-grade spondylolisthesis. This involves restriction of activities that produce a stress on the lumbar spine typically from hyperextension. Young athletes are at increased risk for progression of slippage during the rapid growth phase of puberty and require more diligent follow-up and restriction. Nonaspirin anti-inflammatory medications can be used to control symptoms early on. If symptoms persist despite removal of stress on the lumbosacral spine, the athlete can be fitted with an antilordotic thoracolumbosacral orthotic. Unfortunately, orthotic devices have proven relatively ineffective. Physical therapy is aimed at strengthening the abdominal musculature and improving flexibility in the paraspinal and hamstring muscles. Return-to-sport is acceptable when symptoms have resolved in cases of grade 0 and I spondylolisthesis. Athletes with grade II and higher lesions should continue to avoid hyperextension stress. Follow-up is recommended at 3-month intervals in skeletally immature athletes of Tanner stages II–IV. Tanner stage V adolescents can be evaluated at 6-month intervals until growth stops, then on an annual basis.

Surgical repair of the pars defect in spondylolysis is an option. This allows for healing of the involved segment. Outcomes are optimal for cases of pars defects without slippage in segments L1–L4. Results are less successful at L5 and repair is rarely performed at this level.

Spinal fusion procedures are indicated if conservative therapy fails to improve symptoms or prevent progression of slip. Spinal fusion is a drastic measure and should be considered a last resort, especially in cases of spondylolysis without slip. Discontinuation of athletic activities should long precede any consideration of surgical fixation. Athletes with high-grade spondylolisthesis should be evaluated for early surgical intervention. Nerve root decompression may be necessary prior to fusion if impingement symptoms are present.

Genitourinary and abdominal injuries

Sports that include some degree of contact carry an inherent risk for injury from blunt trauma. This trauma is usually secondary to collision with another athlete or from a fall. Genitourinary injuries are infrequently seen in basketball players, but must be readily recognized. Other intra-abdominal organs are also at risk. Injuries range from minor contusions to surgical emergencies. A discussion of renal, bladder, scrotal liver, and spleen injuries will be included.

Athletes with documented solitary kidney or single testicle should be identified at the time of the preparticipation physical exam. Exclusion is not the rule and each individual athlete and family should be educated on the risks involved with participation in basketball. Protective devices are available and should be offered to athletes who choose to play. Another dilemma facing those screening athletes is how to approach the urine dip demonstrating microscopic hematuria. It is recommended that any athlete with significant hematuria (2+) should be held from activities for 48 h and rechecked. If the urine dip is normal, clearance should be granted. If hematuria persists, a further work-up is warranted.

The kidney is the most commonly affected organ in genitourinary injuries. In general, renal injuries occur in approximately 5 to 10% of children with blunt trauma. Typically, the blunt trauma involved in basketball is not high impact and the injury rate can be expected to be lower. The kidneys are normally located in a retroperitoneal position bilaterally with protection provided by the lower ribs. A direct blow to the athlete in the region overlying the kidney carries the potential for injury. Ectopic location of the kidneys and congenital renal anomalies may be predisposing factors.

In most cases, the athlete will suffer a renal contusion and may not even report the symptoms. On occasion, the injury is more severe. Possibilities include small parenchymal hematomas, renal parenchymal laceration that may extend into the collecting system, and injury to the vascular pedicle (Fig. 6.4). Hematuria (gross or microscopic) is often present but is not a reliable indicator of the extent

Right kidney (cross-section)

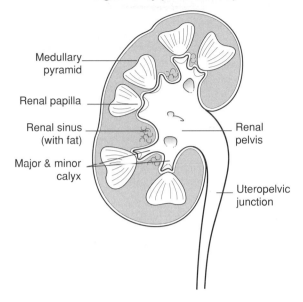

Medullary pyramid

Renal papilla

Renal sinus (with fat)

Major & minor calyx

Renal pelvis

Uteropelvic junction

Fig. 6.4 Kidney schematic.

of injury. The athlete may complain of flank pain and tenderness, display ecchymosis in the costovertebral anyle region, or show signs of shock if vascular injury has occurred and bleeding is present. Immediate evaluation is required. In addition to history and physical exam, CT with contrast is useful in evaluation of the extent of damage to the kidney. Perirenal hematoma or urinoma may be identified if vascular or collecting system injuries have occurred. Immediate surgical intervention is required for athletes displaying signs of hemodynamic instability or with a confirmed pedicle avulsion. Other injuries will typically be observed early in the course of therapy, but may require surgical intervention at a later time.

Bladder injury is significantly less common. Again, most injuries will be mild and are unlikely to be reported. Bladder rupture is possible with high impact blunt abdominal trauma. Approximately 90% of bladder ruptures are associated with pelvic fractures and unrelated to sporting activities. Athletes will present with varying degrees of lower abdominal pain depending on the coexisting injuries. Hematuria or blood at the urethral meatus can be seen. Urethral injury must be ruled out if blood is evident at the meatus. Retrograde cystography, CT, or both can confirm diagnosis of bladder rupture. Depending on the location of the rupture (intraperitoneal vs. extraperitoneal), treatment will vary.

Testicular injuries in young basketball players are most frequently the result of a direct blow to the scrotum causing compression of the testicle against the pubic bones. Scrotal trauma can lead to a number of different injuries including traumatic epididymitis, intratesticular hematoma, laceration of the tunica albuginea, hematocele formation, and testicular torsion.

Traumatic epididymitis can occur after a scrotal trauma. Immediately following the inciting event, the athlete will experience pain that resolves after a short period of time. This is usually followed by a symptom-free interval of a few days. Scrotal pain and tenderness will then recur gradually. Physical exam findings may include an edematous and erythematous scrotum with a tender, indurated epididymis. Urinalysis is typically negative. If available, color Doppler ultrasonography can be employed to rule out a more significant testicular pathology. Hyperemia of the epididymis can also be demonstrated by a Doppler ultrasound study. Treatment is the same as nontraumatic epididymitis and antibiotic coverage is appropriate.

The scrotum is lined by a visceral layer of tunica vaginalis that encapsulates the scrotal contents (Fig. 6.5). Deep to the tunica vaginalis is the tunica albuginea, which is the outer layer of the testes. Trauma to the scrotum can result in intratesticular hematoma formation or laceration of the tunica albuginea. Physical exam will reveal scrotal swelling and tenderness. Testicular transillumination should be employed to screen for possible pathology (bleeding or mass). These injuries can be identified using ultrasonography. If the tunica vaginalis is lacerated, surgical drainage of the hematoma and repair of the laceration is standard therapy. In the absence of a laceration, surgical intervention is unnecessary.

Traumatic scrotal injuries can result in scrotal fullness. Further evaluation is warranted. Blood can be seen on ultrasound as a collection within the tunica vaginalis. Again, the scrotum cannot be transilluminated in the presence of bleeding. This is known as a hematocele. Hematocele formation

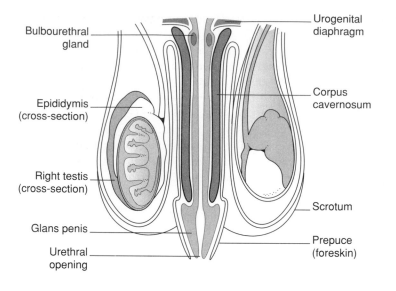

Fig. 6.5 Scrotal content schematic.

should raise concern about severe testicular injury. If a coexisting testicular injury has been ruled out, surgical intervention is not required. Some advocate surgical debridement and drainage of a large hematocele to expedite healing.

Young males are predisposed to testicular torsion if they lack normal testicular attachments to the tunica vaginalis. This anatomic variant allows the testicle to hang freely within the tunica vaginalis and possibly torse. Testicular torsion is an emergent condition that occurs when the spermatic cord twists within the tunica vaginalis and compromises blood flow to the testis. Torsion can occur at rest, during activity, or associated with trauma. An athlete will present with a history of acute-onset testicular pain and tenderness. Often the symptoms have been present for more than an hour by the time medical attention is sought. Physical exam findings include scrotal edema and erythema, a high riding testicle in a transverse position on the affected side, testicular tenderness, absent cremasteric reflex on the affected side, and possibly a palpable fullness in the spermatic cord representing the torsion. Inflammation and edema worsen with time.

Testicular torsion can be confirmed by color Doppler imaging with pulsed Doppler or by nuclear scanning with a sensitivity of 95%. Color Doppler has the advantage of being noninvasive. If testicular blood flow can be confirmed, surgery is not required.

Surgical treatment of testicular torsion includes detorsing the affected testicle if salvage is possible. Intervention within 12 h produces optimal outcomes. After 12 h, salvage rates decline and removal is more likely. Orchiopexy (fixation of the contralateral testicle) is also performed to prevent future torsion of the uninvolved testis.

Inguinal hernias are seen in young people with a persistent processus vaginalis. Intra-abdominal contents can protrude through the internal inguinal ring and into the processus vaginalis (indirect inguinal hernia). Further extension can cause swelling in the groin or scrotum. Athletes or parents may describe intermittent scrotal fullness during the preparticipation evaluation that may not be readily apparent on exam. Doppler ultrasonography can confirm the presence of a hernia by visualization of bowel within the scrotum. Other herniations of the intra-abdominal contents can be seen. These include femoral hernia, ventral hernia, and "sports hernia". Femoral hernias are seen as a fullness of the proximal medial thigh. Ventral hernias are usually through a persistent umbilical defect, but can occur in regions of previous surgery. "Sports hernia" refers to a condition in which an athlete develops chronic groin pain in the absence of a discernible bulge. It is thought to be secondary to weakness of the posterior wall and can progress to a fully developed inguinal hernia (direct hernia).

Young basketball players with hernias are at risk for incarceration. This describes a hernia that is not reducible into the abdominal cavity that may become strangulated. Strangulation is the compromise of blood flow leading to ischemia and necrosis of the trapped loop of bowel. A strangulated hernia requires emergent surgical intervention to free the trapped bowel and prevent necrosis.

The spleen is the most commonly injured solid abdominal organ. Injury is typically secondary to left upper quadrant trauma and is frequently seen in conjunction with rib fracture. Infectious mononucleosis is a risk factor for both spontaneous and traumatic splenic laceration and rupture, especially in the first 21 days of illness. Athletes will present with complaints of left upper quadrant pain or diffuse abdominal pain depending on the degree of injury. Serial abdominal exams may demonstrate increasing intensity of pain or signs of peritoneal irritation. If significant bleeding is present, signs of shock may be apparent. Diagnosis can be confirmed with computed tomography. Conservative management is recommended in an attempt to avoid splenectomy if possible. With severe injuries, emergent splenectomy may be required. Return-to-play is based on normalization of the spleen on physical exam for mild injuries, and CT evidence of splenic injury resolution in more severe injuries. Athletes with documented mononucleosis should refrain from sports for at least 3 weeks to minimize risk of splenic rupture.

The liver is the second most commonly injured solid abdominal organ. Injury is usually secondary to trauma to the right upper quadrant, back, side, or right lower ribs. Athletes will present with generalized abdominal pain, right upper quadrant pain, or shoulder pain. Physical exam findings typically include right upper quadrant tenderness or signs of peritoneal irritation. CT scanning of the abdomen can identify liver injury and any associated injury. Conservative therapy is appropriate in the hemodynamically stable patient. Return-to-play is based on resolution of the hepatic injury as evidenced by imaging studies.

Further reading

Casa, D. *et al.* (2000) National Athletic Trainers' Association Position Statement: fluid replacement for athletes. *Journal of Athletic Training* **35**, 212–219.

Congeni, J., McCulloch, J. & Swanson, K. (1997) Lumbar spondylolysis: a study of natural progression in athletes. *American Journal of Sports Medicine* **25**, 248–253.

Convertino, V.A. *et al.* (1996) *Exercise and Fluid Replacement.* American College of Sports Medicine: Position Stand **28**, 1–11.

Emery, H. (1996) Musculoskeletal medicine: considerations in child and adolescent athletes. *Rheumatic Diseases Clinics of North America* **22**, 499–513.

Greenspan, A. (1996) *Orthopedic Radiology*, 2nd edn. Lippincott-Raven, Philadelphia.

Harries, M. *et al.* (eds) (1998) *Oxford Textbook of Sports Medicine,* 2nd edn. Oxford University Press, New York, p. 957.

Johnson, R. (ed.) (2000) *Sports Medicine in Primary Care.* W.B. Saunders, Philadelphia, p. 363.

Kass, E. & Lundak, B. (1997) Pediatric urology: the acute scrotum. *Pediatric Clinics of North America* **44**, 1251–1266.

Luke, A. & Micheli, L. (1999) Pediatrics in review: emergency assessment and field-side care. *Pediatrics in Review* **20**, 291–302.

Mellman, M. & Podesta, L. (1997) Primary care of the injured athlete, Pt II: common medical problems in sports. *Clinics in Sports Medicine* **16**, 635–663.

Micheli, L.J. & Wood, R. (1995) Back pain in young athletes. *Archives of Pediatrics and Adolescent Medicine* **149**, 15–18.

Myers, A. & Sickles, T. (1998) Adolescent medicine: preparticipation sports examination. *Primary Care: Clinics in Office Practice* **25**, 225–236.

Patel, D. & Nelson, T. (2000) Adolescent medicine: sports injuries in adolescents. *Medical Clinics of North America* **84**, 983–1007.

Rana, E. *et al.* (1997) Pediatric urology: imaging in pediatric urology. *Pediatric Clinics of North America* **44**, 1065–1089.

Smith, J.A. & Hu, S. (1999) Disorders of the pediatric and adolescent spine: management of spondylolysis and spondylolisthesis in the pediatric and adolescent population. *Orthopedic Clinics of North America* **30**, 487–499.

William, E., Garrett, J., Speer, K.P. & Kirkendall, D.T. (eds) (2000) *Principles and Practice of Orthopaedic Sports Medicine.* Lippincott, Williams and Wilkins, Philadelphia, p. 1062.

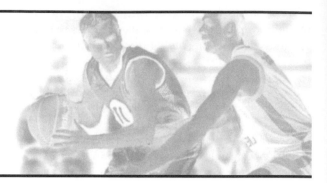

Chapter 7
The female athlete

Margot Putukian

Introduction

Basketball is a sport that has been enjoyed by girls and women for a long time. More recently, however, the opportunities for girls and women to participate have increased significantly (Fig. 7.1). There are a multitude of local programs, high school and college teams from which to choose, and the number of college scholarships are rising giving young women opportunities to participate at a very competitive level. Over a 15-year period ending in 1998, the National Collegiate Athletic Association (NCAA) has demonstrated that the participation rate for women compared to men has increased by 69% vs. 13%, respectively (NCAA 1983–1998). The success of the United States women's national team in international competition and the Olympics, has brought more attention to the athletic prowess of our female players. With the recent formation in the United States of the Women's National Basketball Association (WNBA), women can participate at the professional level. Now, young girls who used to dream about being the next Michael Jordan, can more realistically dream about being the next Cheryl Swoopes, Dawn Staley, or Lisa Leslie.

The positive effects of exercise and sport for girls and women are numerous and far reaching. Involvement in sport promotes healthy lifestyle behaviors that last a lifetime, including a decreased risk for the development of diabetes, hypertension, and obesity (Leon *et al.* 1987; Harris *et al.* 1989). For young girls involved in sports, lower rates of teenage pregnancy, substance use and depression

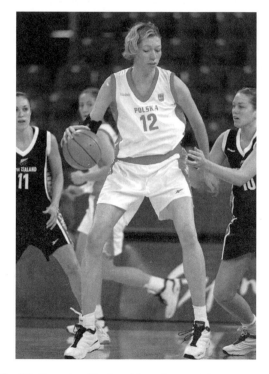

Fig. 7.1 Opportunities for girls and women have markedly increased during recent years in a wide variety of sports. Photo © Getty Images/Jed Jacobsohn.

have been reported (Chalip *et al.* 1980; Colten & Gore 1991). In a study of high school adolescents in western New York, participation in sports for girls was directly associated with reduced frequency of sexual behavior and indirectly to pregnancy risk (Sabo *et al.* 1999). This is in contrast with the male athletes, where the frequency of sexual behavior and involvement in pregnancy was no different than in their nonathlete counterparts. Involvement in sport and exercise also promotes the healthy development of self-esteem and increased self worth for young girls that transcends into adulthood.

Many of the injuries and sport-specific conditioning issues are the same for both male and female players. There are medical issues in the female athlete that are unique: pregnancy, and the female athlete triad (menstrual function, eating disorders and their link to osteoporosis). In addition, there are certain physiologic and nutritional issues that are different in the female athlete compared to their male counterparts. Basketball is a sport that requires cardiovascular training, strength, balance, and sport-specific skills. The sport itself is very similar for both male and female athletes, and the injury profile is similar, though the incidence of certain injuries is higher in women than men. Examples include anterior cruciate ligament (ACL) sprains in the knee, patellofemoral pain, trochanteric bursitis, and stress fractures. ACL injuries are the most severe injury that occurs in basketball, and these are more common in female players. The emphasis of this chapter is to discuss some of the issues in basketball that are specific to the female player.

The female athlete triad

In recent years, there has been concern regarding the incidence of eating disorders and menstrual dysfunction that occurs in the athletic female. These entities have both been associated with premature bone loss and osteoporosis and together have become known as the "female athlete triad". The elements of the triad occur more commonly in athletes than their nonathletic counterparts, and although they are more common in sports that select for leanness or where appearance is important, they occur across all sports. When an athlete is identified as having one component of the triad, it is essential that the other components are assessed for and addressed. The consequences of the triad are significant, they worsen with time, and may be irreversible, underscoring the need for early detection, treatment and, most importantly, prevention.

It is difficult to discern the exact incidence of the female athlete triad. Screening tools for eating disorders are often inadequate, and recognition of menstrual dysfunction is often delayed. As part of a preparticipation exam of 450 Division I college athletes (freshman, transfers, seniors) 60% reported irregular periods, and 30% reported complete cessation for 3 months or more at some point in time (Evans et al. 2000). Of these athletes, 3.4% reported being diagnosed as having an eating disorder (ED), 45.5% were unhappy with their present weight, and 13.4% reported feeling out of control with eating patterns. Methods of weight control behavior included dieting or fasting (16.8%), excessive exercise (12.6%), diet pills (4.1%), vomiting (3.6%), laxatives (2.9%) and diuretics (0.3%). Stress fractures, diagnosed by bone scan or radiographs, were reported in 16% of the athletes screened. These numbers, although not compared with a nonathlete group, demonstrate that the elements of the triad occur at significant rates among collegiate female athletes.

Disordered eating behaviors occur on a spectrum which at their mildest may represent caloric restriction or dietary modifications. Purposeful avoidance of fat ("fat-phobic") is a common example of nutritional modifications that an athlete may experiment with in order to decrease their body weight. Other methods of weight control behavior that an athlete may experiment with include use of diuretics, diet pills, laxatives, self-induced vomiting, and/or excessive exercise. At the other end of the spectrum are the classic eating disorders: anorexia nervosa (AN), bulimia nervosa (BN), and eating disorders not otherwise specified (EDNOS). Definitions for the ED are given in Tables 7.1–7.3.

Table 7.1 Diagnostic criteria for anorexia nervosa.

A. Refusal to maintain body weight at or above 85% of normal weight for age and height
B. Intense fear of gaining weight or becoming fat, although underweight
C. Disturbance in the way in which one's body weight or shape is experienced, undue influence of body weight or shape on self-evaluation, or denial of the seriousness of the current low body weight
D. In postmenarchal females, amenorrhea

Table 7.2 Diagnostic criteria for bulimia nervosa.

A. Recurrent episodes of binge eating. An episode of binge eating is characterized by the following:
    1. Eating, in a discrete period (e.g., within any 2-hour period), an amount of food that is definitely larger than most people would eat during a similar period of time under similar circumstances
    2. A sense of lack of control over eating during the episode (e.g., a feeling that one cannot stop eating or control what or how much one is eating)
B. Recurrent inappropriate compensatory behavior to prevent weight gain, such as self-induced vomiting; misuse of laxatives, diuretics, enemas, or other medications; fasting; or excessive exercise
C. The binge eating and inappropriate compensatory behaviors occur, on average, at least twice a week for 3 months
D. Self-evaluation is unduly influenced by body shape and weight
E. The disturbance does not occur exclusively during episodes of anorexia nervosa

Table 7.3 Criteria for eating disorders not otherwise specified. From American Psychiatric Association (1994) *Diagnostic Criteria from DSM IV*. Washington, DC: American Psychiatric Association, pp. 544–545.

A. For females, all of the criteria for anorexia nervosa are met except that the individual has regular menses
B. All the criteria for anorexia nervosa are met except that, despite significant weight loss, the person's current weight is in the normal range
C. All the criteria for bulimia nervosa are met except that the binge eating and inappropriate compensatory mechanisms occur at a frequency of less than twice a week for a duration of less than 3 months
D. The regular use of inappropriate compensatory behavior by an individual of normal body weight after eating small amounts of food (e.g., self-induced vomiting after the consumption of two cookies)
E. Repeatedly chewing and spitting out, but not swallowing, large amounts of food
F. Binge-eating disorder: recurrent episodes of binge eating in the absence of the regular use of inappropriate compensatory behaviors characteristic of bulimia nervosa

Initially, an athlete may try to control their weight in order to improve their appearance or performance by experimenting in pathogenic weight control behaviors. Many resort to pathogenic weight control behaviors to reach their goals quicker or because they minimize or do not appreciate the negative health effects of these behaviors. Unfortunately, the weight or body composition goals that coaches and athletes have are often unrealistic. The pressure from coaches, parents, teammates and others often results in an athlete who is desperate to lose weight yet who does not have the correct information on how to accomplish these goals in a safe manner. As these behaviors continue, and given the right psychological profile, an ED may develop that progresses and can lead to serious consequences.

In the general population, the incidence of AN and BN have been reported as 0.5–1.0% and 2–5%, respectively (Loucks 1985). In athletes, the numbers have ranged from 15% to 62%, depending on the study (Yates *et al.* 1994). In a study of elite Norwegian athletes, the incidence of AN, BN and subclinical ED was 1.3%, 8.2% and 8.0%, respectively. When compared to nonathletes, the incidence of AN was not different in the athletes, though for BN and subclinical ED, the incidence was higher in athletes than nonathletes. Those participating in aesthetic sports and weight dependent sports were at particularly high risk, a finding that has been demonstrated in several other studies (Rosen *et al.* 1986; Dummer *et al.* 1987; Rosen & Hough 1988; Wilmore 1991; Brownell & Steen 1992; Sundgot-Borgen & Larsen 1993; Sundgot-Borgen 1994; O'Connor *et al.* 1995; Sundgot-Borgen 2000) (Fig. 7.2).

In a study of college female athletes, 32% practiced some form of pathogenic weight control behavior (binging, self-induced vomiting, diuretics, diet pills, laxatives), and an alarming 70% thought these behaviors had no ill-effect (Rosen *et al.* 1986). In a study of college gymnasts, 62% used pathogenic behaviors, and in this study 75% reported that they had been told by their coach to lose weight (Rosen & Hough 1988). In a study of swimmers aged 9–18, 15.4% engaged in pathogenic eating behavior (Dummer *et al.* 1987). These studies demonstrate that the use of pathogenic weight control behaviors is significant, that athletes do not see these behaviors as unhealthy, and that the age at which experimentation starts is quite young.

Athletes are at a greater risk for developing disordered eating than nonathletes, and although no sport is immune, certain sports are associated with an even higher risk. Why athletes are at greater risk is likely multifactorial. Some of the characteristics that describe our best athletes are also characteristics that put athletes at risk for developing eating disorders. Athletes are often goal oriented,

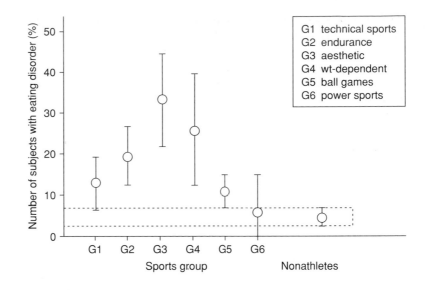

Fig. 7.2 Percentage of athletes with eating disorders.

perfectionists, compulsive, determined, and willing to do "whatever it takes" to reach weight goals that may not be healthy or realistic. They may feel that a certain weight or body composition will give them a competitive edge or improve performance. Unfortunately, they have often gotten this information from those without proper knowledge or experience with athletes.

The other factors that contribute to the risk of developing disordered eating include societal influences, how society treats young girls and women and prizes thinness; and family issues, how girls and women are treated in their family. There is also a biologic response to dieting which can make it more difficult for someone to control their weight because their body has become accustomed to a lower intake of calories. It has been reported that those with disordered eating report a higher incidence of both sexual and physical abuse. One of the most powerful factors that can put someone at risk for disordered eating is self-esteem and control. Often these athletes will feel as though they have no control over their situation. They do not feel good about themselves, and do not feel that they have any control over their situation. They may not be able to control whether they start, what their coaches, teammates or parents think of them, but they *can* control what they eat and what their body looks like. The factors that are felt to lead to ED are given in Table 7.4.

Table 7.4 Origin of eating disorders: where do they come from?

Social climate
Behaviors that contribute to the development of eating disorders have been normalized in western society
Disordered eating perpetuated by our sociocultural norms that prize thinness

Family
Persons with eating disorders often come from families that do not provide them with good coping skills to deal with stressors
Often, women in these families derive self-worth in reflection of others' responses to them, particularly appearance

Biologic
Severe dieting can result in loss of psychological and physiological cues for satiety
Starvation may result in abnormal function of hypothalamic axis
Imbalances in serotonin and endorphin activity? Modulate expression of anorexia nervosa

Response to victimization
20 to 35% of persons with eating disorders report sexual abuse
67% of bulimics report sexual and/or physical abuse

Lack of sense of identity
Externalizing, rather than internalizing, one's identity (self worth based on accomplishments and appearance)
Eating disorder gives athlete sense of identity; something controlled from within

Low self-esteem
Often exacerbated by a stressor: suggestion from coach, an injury, a break-up with boyfriend
Athlete may cope by trying to lose weight: "If only I were thinner . . ."

Role conflict
Child vs. parent (parenting one's parents)
Strong athlete vs. feminine woman

Sundgot-Borgen (1994) addressed risk factors and triggers for ED in elite athletes in Norway. She identified the following as risk factors: prolonged dieting (37%), a new coach (30%), an injury or illness (23%), a casual comment (19%), leaving home or failure at school or work (10%), family problems (7%), family illness or injury (7%), the death of a significant other (4%), and sexual abuse by the coach (4%).

Once an eating disorder starts, much of the concern is due to the medical risks that are associated with it. Nutritional deficiencies are by far the rule, with iron deficiency, and deficiencies in the fat soluble vitamins (A, D, E and K) common. The ability to fight infections and heal wounds is impaired, and these athletes often have nagging injuries or are constantly getting illnesses. If pathogenic weight control behaviors such as vomiting, laxatives or diuretics are used, then electrolyte disturbances are possible with resultant arrhythmias a life-threatening concern. Gastrointestinal problems are also common consequences of ED. Most disturbing are some of the long-term consequences of ED: decreased bone mineral density (BMD), infertility, and psychiatric problems. Depression is a common comorbidity. Eating disorders have been associated with a 6–18% mortality rate, with cardiac disease, starvation, and overwhelming infection all as causes. Sadly, the majority of deaths in ED are due to suicide.

Detection of eating disorders in athletes

The longer an ED has been present, the harder it is to effectively treat the individual suffering from it. Given this, and the consequences of eating disorders, early detection becomes more important. Eating disorders are often difficult to detect because some eating and exercise behaviors have been normalized in competitive athletes. Initially, an athlete's performance may improve as their weight decreases. However, as these athletes become more unhealthy, their performance eventually suffers. Athletes may present with overuse injuries or stress fractures, or may constantly require attention because of illnesses or other medical problems.

Depending on the type of ED that is present, athletes may be easier or harder to detect. The athlete

Table 7.5 Symptoms and signs of disordered eating.

Repeatedly expressed concerns about being fat, even when weight is average or below average
Refusal to maintain a minimal normal weight consistent with the athlete's age, height, body build, and sport
Preoccupation with food, calories, and weight
Increasing criticism of one's body
Consumption of huge amounts of food not consistent with the athlete's weight
Secretly eating or stealing food
Eating large meals, then disappearing/making trips to the bathroom
Bloodshot eyes, especially after trips to the bathroom, swollen parotid glands at jaw angle, giving chipmunk-like appearance
Vomitus, or odor of vomitus in toilet, sink, shower, etc.
Foul breath, poor dental hygiene, frequent sore throats
Wide fluctuations of weight over short time spans
Excess laxative use, use of diet pills
Periods of severe calorie restriction or repeated fasting
Relentless, excessive physical activity that is not part of training regimen
Depressed mood and self-deprecating thoughts after eating
Avoiding situations in which the athlete may be observed while eating (e.g. refusing to eat with teammates on trips)
Appearing preoccupied with the eating behavior of other people such as friends, relatives, and teammates
Mood swings, irritability, poor concentration, fatigue
Wearing baggy or layered clothing
Complaints of bloating or lightheadedness that cannot be attributed to other medical causes

with AN often appears extremely underweight, and thus they are often recognized earlier though they will also have a high level of denial that a problem exists. On the other hand, although individuals with BN may be harder to detect because they are often normal or slightly overweight, they are also more likely to come forward on their own because of their extreme sense of "lack of control" over their behaviors. Having a heightened awareness of the prevalence of this problem in the female athlete is important in detecting these athletes early. Table 7.5 lists some signs and symptoms of ED.

Once an athlete is identified as having an ED, it is important to treat them with an individualized, multidisplinary approach. Psychologic counseling is the cornerstone of treatment and should be the first intervention. Depending on the extent of the ED, additional laboratory testing is often indicated including electrolytes, blood count, a chemistry panel, and an electrocardiogram. If an athlete has concomitant menstrual dysfunction, a work-up is indicated which often includes additional laboratory testing and pelvic examination. Assessing for all elements of the female athlete triad and initiating treatment when indicated is important.

It is important to secure confidentiality, and allow the athlete to continue participation unless performance puts the athlete at risk. This often entails an assessment of the athlete's weight and body composition, determining the extent of their pathogenic weight control behaviors, and determining their overall energy balance and caloric intake. A nutritionist comfortable with working with athletes is often very helpful in making these decisions along with the medical staff. The psychologist, physician, and nutritionist form the basic treatment team, though numerous other specialists may also be helpful.

The athlete should be given the opportunity to make decisions regarding confidentiality and who is made aware of their issues. Depending on the support system available to the athlete, it may be useful to discuss treatment issues with family members, coaching staff or athletic training staff. If an athlete is over the age of 18, however, these issues must be discussed first with the athlete. However, if the athlete cannot participate, or there are significant mental health issues, others may need to be made aware of the situation (e.g. coach, athletic trainer), and these situations can be sensitive and difficult to handle. It is important that the athlete understands these issues as they relate to overall student athlete safety and health.

In some situations, the use of a contract with the athlete can be useful. This allows the athlete to agree to certain terms in order for their continued participation. An example would be that an athlete would agree to attend weekly psychologic counseling, monitoring by the physician, and meeting with the nutritionist. It might also include parameters for participation. A contract can be useful in demonstrating to the athlete the importance of their problem, and the expectations for treatment.

Menstrual function and dysfunction

Normal menstrual cycle function depends on an intact hypothalamic–pituitary–ovarian axis in the setting of normal pelvic organ function. The hormonal signals that regulate normal function are complex and dysfunction at any level can lead to abnormalities in menstrual function. Several changes in menstrual function can occur as a result of training including alterations in the levels of ovarian hormones, testosterone, prolactin, β-endorphin, β-lipoporotein and the catecholamines.

Menstrual dysfunction can be characterized as normal (9–12 cycles per year, eumenorrheic), absent for greater than 3 months or less than 3–6 cycles per year (amenorrheic) or inbetween (6–9 cycles per year or oligomenorrheic). Menstrual dysfunction has also been characterized by whether or not ovulation occurs. Training can lead to alterations in lutel phase length, anovulation, or amenorrhea. Individuals with anovulation may still have menstrual bleeding, and thus these individuals may be difficult to detect. The other abnormalities usually are associated with a disturbance in cycle length such that they are more apparent.

The etiology of menstrual dysfunction is multifactorial, and includes body weight, body composition, nutritional intake (both quality and quantity), training factors, as well as previous menstrual function. Although body weight and composition was initially felt to be the most important and limiting factor, this has subsequently been shown to be less important. Athletes with amenorrhea have higher resting levels of cortisol, and a blunted cortisol response to exercise. Abnormalities in the amplitude and pulsatility of the release of luteinizing hormone (LH) and follicular stimulating hormone (FSH) have been demonstrated in athletes with exercise-associated amenorrhea. These signal hormones released by the hypothalamic–pituitary axis are important in maintaining normal function.

The most convincing theory currently is the energy drain hypothesis, where an athlete expends more energy than they consume; resulting in a negative energy balance. This negative energy balance ultimately leads to a disruption in the LH pulsatility. Several studies have demonstrated the low caloric intake of athletes with menstrual dysfunction. Other research by Dueck (Dueck *et al.* 1996) supports the energy drain hypothesis by demonstrating that when caloric intake is increased, menstrual function returns to normal.

Recently, low estrogen and leptin levels have been measured in athletes with amenorrhea. This was felt to potentially explain why menstrual dysfunction occurred. However, leptin levels have also been shown to be lower in athletes with normal menstrual function compared to nonathletes. In athletes with amenorrhea, however, there is complete suppression of the diurnal release of leptin. In adolescents, hypoleptinemia has been demonstrated in prepubertal gymnasts. However, these athletes were also energy deficient, and were not compared with energy replete athletes. These findings suggest that there may be a threshold of energy availability required to maintain normal menstrual function. More research is needed to elucidate the role of leptin, as well as other hormonal changes in the development of menstrual dysfunction.

Consequences of menstrual dysfunction: the link to bone health

Prior to the early 1980s, there was little concern when an athlete developed menstrual dysfunction. It was often felt to be a natural consequence of training, one that had little long-term sequelae. Athletes generally did not mind losing the monthly discomfort and inconvenience of their menses, and for many it was a sign that they were training adequately.

In 1984, researchers demonstrated that low estrogen levels were seen in runners with amenorrhea (Cann *et al.* 1984; Drinkwater *et al.* 1984). These low estrogen levels were also associated with low bone mineral density (BMD) levels in the vertebral spine. Over the ensuing years, tremendous research has further demonstrated the link between menstrual dysfunction and low BMD, with an increased risk for the development of stress fractures and premature osteoporosis. Drinkwater *et al.* (1990) demonstrated that BMD correlated to menstrual history in a linear manner. Athletes with normal function presently and a history of normal function had the highest BMD, and those with abnormal function, and a history of abnormal function, had the lowest BMD (Fig. 7.3).

Past menstrual history has been shown to be the best predictor of BMD in several studies. Although the initial research assessed the lumbar spine, an area of metabolically active trabecular bone, more

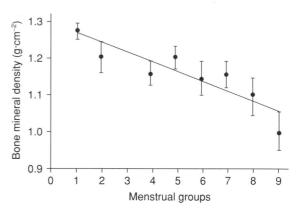

Fig. 7.3 Relationship of menstrual history and BMD in female athletes. From Drinkwater *et al.* (1990).

recent research has demonstrated that low BMD is also seen in the appendicular skeleton, which is less metabolically active cortical bone (Myburgh *et al.* 1993; Wilson *et al.* 1994; Rencken *et al.* 1996). These appendicular sites, however, are also those at risk for the overuse stress fractures that occur in the athletic realm with axial load. Many of these studies have used dual energy X-ray absorptiometry (DEXA) scanning which has become a very exciting new tool for safely assessing BMD as well as body composition (Figs 7.4 and 7.5).

Reversibility of premature bone loss

One of the most significant questions that remain unanswered is whether the bone loss seen as a result of menstrual dysfunction is reversible. The length of time an individual is amenorrheic correlates with lower BMD values. BMD increases with resumption of normal menses, however, it does not appear to return to the levels seen in individuals that have never had menstrual dysfunction (Drinkwater *et al.* 1986). A decrease in training or an increase in caloric intake can also lead to resumption of menses, and these factors should also be assessed. All of these factors underscore the need for early intervention when menstrual dysfunction occurs.

A complete and comprehensive evaluation should take place in an athlete who has menstrual dysfunction. Exercise associated amenorrhea (EAA) and menstrual dysfunction are fairly common, however, they must be evaluated and the assumption should

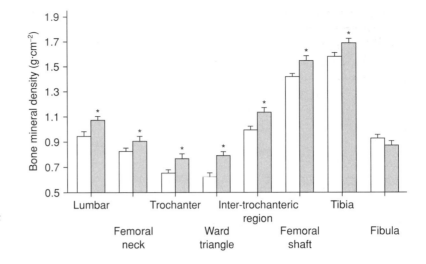

Fig. 7.4 Bone mineral density in amenorrheic (□) and eumenorrheic (▨) athletes. From Rencken *et al.* (1996).

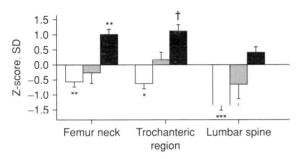

Fig. 7.5 Bone mineral density of proximal femur in amenorrheic (□), oligmenorrheic (▨) and eumenorrheic (■) elite middle distance runners. From Gibson (2000).

not be made that it is "just because they exercise". Evaluation should include a pelvic examination, and laboratory evaluation to include a pregnancy test, FSH, LH, complete blood count, thyroid stimulating hormone, and prolactin levels. Additional laboratory studies may be indicated depending on the athlete's history and physical examination. If the athlete is not sexually active and less than age 16, imaging studies such as an ultrasound can sometimes be used in the place of the pelvic examination to confirm the presence of pelvic organs. Medical problems such as thyroid dysfunction, polycystic ovary disease, prolactinoma, and other adrenal or endocrine abnormalities should be ruled out before assuming that menstrual dysfunction is EAA. An algorithm for the work-up of amenorrhea is shown in Fig. 7.6.

Treatment of menstrual dysfunction

The treatment of menstrual dysfunction must be individualized. When an athlete is evaluated, it is also important to assess for the other entities of the triad: bone health and disordered eating. If laboratory and physical examination confirms EAA, determination of estrogen status is useful. If indicated, treatment for a coexisting eating disorder should be initiated. If there is a history of stress fracture, significant and/or prolonged eating disorder or prolonged menstrual dysfunction, then obtaining a DEXA scan should be considered. This can help to determine treatment options as well as prognosticate the risk for fracture. In the younger athlete, this information may be difficult to interpret. Standards for adolescents and athletes have yet to be determined, and much is still unknown regarding the natural history of bone growth and BMD. Despite these limitations, a DEXA scan can be useful information that provides a baseline that can be used in later years in comparison.

If menstrual dysfunction exists and other medical problems and pregnancy have been ruled out, then consideration for hormone replacement should be made. For athletes older than age 16, many would consider the use of hormonal replacement as a safe and reasonable treatment plan. The ideal situation is for menses to return on its own. If body weight or composition is inadequate, or training is excessive, these factors should be considered. However, given

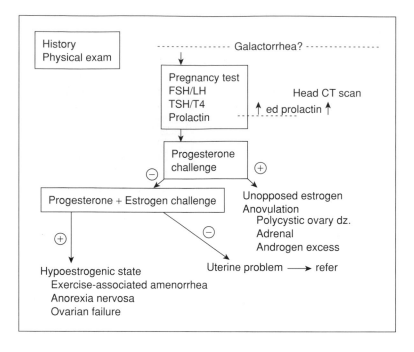

Fig. 7.6 Algorithm for amenorrhea work-up.

the seeming irreversibility of bone loss that occurs with amenorrhea, it is controversial as to how long to wait before initiating treatment. In addition, there is also controversy regarding the optimal form of hormonal replacement. Many have advocated the oral contraceptive pill (OCP), while others have suggested that progesterone alone is enough (Prior *et al.* 1994). Hergenroeder in 1997 found that OCP use for 1 year increased BMD in premenopausal women with hypothalamic amenorrhea compared with no change for those given placebo or medroxyprogesterone alone. Ettinger demonstrated an increase in BMD in runners treated with traditional hormonal replacement (Premarin 0.625 mg or daily 0.5 µg transderm patch along with medroxyprogesterone 10 mg) (Ettinger *et al.* 1987). Only a few well controlled studies have been done with athletes with EAA. However, the data to date suggest that the use of the OCP is protective for BMD, and given that the estrogen levels are higher with OCPs than with traditional HRT, the use of OCPs has remained the mainstay of treatment in the young athlete. For those athletes that are sexually active, the use of the OCP is additionally sensible in order to prevent pregnancy.

Depending on the situation, a progesterone challenge may be indicated. This is a functional test to see if the body's estrogen production is adequate. If an individual with amenorrhea is given progesterone, and there is endogenous estrogen production, then vaginal bleeding will occur. If an individual is given progesterone, and they do not produce estrogen, then no bleeding will occur. This can be a useful test especially if an athlete does not want to consider the OCP. If progesterone alone induces vaginal bleeding, then theoretically the individual can be treated with monthly progesterone.

For those athletes that have osteopenia or osteoporosis, treatment is difficult. All efforts must be made to treat disordered eating, and increase caloric intake if deficient. Ensuring an adequate calcium (1500 mg·day^{-1}) and vitamin D intake, and hormonal replacement, is important. Assessing exercise activity is also important, especially considering the risk for certain sports and risk for collision or contact. Other interventions in this young age group are controversial. Conventional medications used in postmenopausal women, such as the biphosphonates, are contraindicated in younger women given the potential for teratogenic side-effects and unknown long-term effects on bone. There has been limited promise with the use of nasal calcitonin (Drinkwater *et al.* 1993), and the treatment of EAA in the young athlete is an area that needs more research.

Triad conclusions

The female athlete triad remains important in the long-term health of female athletes. Athletes are at a higher risk than nonathletes for developing elements of the triad, and when one component is evident, the health care provider should look for the others. Early detection is useful in avoiding the long-term consequences of premature bone loss, especially given the concern that this bone loss may not be reversible. The best treatment of the female athlete triad is prevention through education.

Pregnancy

One of the special populations to consider is the pregnant athlete. How pregnancy affects exercise, and how basketball play affects pregnancy are important considerations. Determining these effects must be individualized, though guidelines exist that help guide the health care provider in taking care of these athletes (ACOG 2002). The risks of trauma in competitive play may limit participation in basketball. However, exercise and cardiovascular fitness training may be allowed, and the following discussion summarizes the risks of exercise during pregnancy as well as the specific risks of basketball play.

Several changes occur during pregnancy which involve the cardiovascular, respiratory, gastrointestinal, and musculoskeletal systems. The weight gain of pregnancy also incurs effects on balance, coordination and flexibility, that may be important considerations in the basketball player. Cardiac output increases by 30–50% and heart rate will increase by up to 7 and 15 beats per minute in the first and second/third trimesters, respectively (Araujo 1997). Late in pregnancy, cardiac output can decrease if the athlete is in a supine position, thus it is important for the athlete to avoid this position for prolonged periods of time.

Other physiologic changes that occur during pregnancy include an increase in circulating blood volume of 35% to 45%, associated with an increased venous capacitance, keeping blood pressure normalized. A pseudodilutional anemia also occurs with pregnancy due to the increased blood volume. In endurance athletes, an increase in performance ($\dot{V}o_{2max}$) has been noted during pregnancy (Clapp & Capeless 1991), felt due to the effects on the blood volume, and some have considered this a form of "blood doping". After the first trimester, weight gain and other changes can make exercise and competition more difficult, such that the level of performance is more difficult to maintain.

During pregnancy, the nutritional needs of the athlete must be increased. The energy demands include not only those needed for the physical exercise performed, but also the additional demands of pregnancy. During the first and second trimesters, nutritional needs are increased by 150 kcal·day^{-1}, and during the third trimester, these needs increase by 300 kcal·day^{-1} (Araujo 1997). In addition to adding a multivitamin that includes iron on a daily basis, pregnant women should also include folic acid supplementation.

As pregnancy continues, changes in the respiratory system occur due to both a hormonal effect of primarily progesterone, as well as a decrease in the functional residual capacity of the lungs due to the enlarging uterus. An increase in respiratory rate leads to hypocapnia and a mild alkalosis. The effects of progesterone also include a decrease in gastrointestinal motility and relaxation of the lower esophageal sphincter tone, resulting in constipation, and gastric reflux symptoms, respectively.

Fetal tachycardia as well as maternal hyperthermia need to be avoided during pregnancy, though the exact levels of exercise need to be individualized. It is unclear if the fetal tachycardia results from hypocirculation from blood being shunted away from the uterus during exercise, from maternal catecholamine release, or evidence of fetal distress (Morrow *et al.* 1989; Araujo 1997). There has been concern that maternal hyperthermia may be associated with teratogenic defects. Much of this is because of an increased incidence of neural tube defects in women who reported a febrile illness during their pregnancy, along with animal data demonstrating other congenital defects in response to thermogenic stress (Sellers & Perkins-Cole 1987; Shiota 1988; Milunsky *et al.* 1992; Lynberg *et al.* 1994). It is thus important to avoid excessive exercise in the heat or hypovolemia during exercise to avoid fetal tachy-cardia as well as hyperthermia.

Various studies in the athletic population give us some information on the effects of pregnancy on fetal and maternal health. One study of athletes involved in moderate exercise prior to pregnancy and who continued to exercise at either a high or medium intensity exercise program throughout pregnancy until 6 weeks after delivery, found no difference in the duration of labor, birth weight, or 1- and 5-minute Apgar scores (Kardel & Kase 1988). There was a higher maternal weight gain during pregnancy and earlier onset of labor for those women who exercised at the higher intensity of exercise, but only if they gave birth to girls. This was not seen in the group that gave birth to boys. No adverse effects on fetal growth, pregnancy or labor were noted (Kardel & Kase 1988).

In a questionnaire study of 30 Finnish endurance athletes involved in cross-country skiing, running, orienteering, and speed skating, there were no adverse effects on pregnancy, labor or delivery noted (Penttinen & Erkkola 1997). Of these athletes, 53% did not notice a change in performance, whereas 10% thought they were in better condition, and 23% felt they were in worse condition (14% did not answer). Of the 18 athletes that returned to competition, 72% reported performing at a same or better level than before pregnancy, and 28% performed at a lower level. This study supports the individualized effect of pregnancy on athletic performance.

As pregnancy progresses, the developing fetus can compress the vena cava when the woman is in the supine position. This increases as growth occurs and is especially important at the ~20 week mark, when the uterus becomes an intra-abdominal organ. Therefore, it is important to avoid activities such as bench press or other prolonged supine activities after the twentieth week of gestation.

The effects of progesterone on the musculoskeletal system are also important in the athlete. As pregnancy progresses, the center of gravity increases lumbar lordosis and ligamentous and joint laxity increase. With the increase in weight that occurs as pregnancy continues, it becomes more difficult for the pregnant female to participate in high intensity exercise, and the ability to participate in a contact/collision sport also increases. This is due to both physical limitations as well as concerns for the safety of the fetus. Many of these changes are again different from one individual to another, thus making decisions on when it is no longer safe for women to play competitive basketball must be individualized. The biggest risks of participation in basketball during pregnancy are more likely due to the physical limitations that pregnancy incurs, as well as the risk for abdominal trauma that is a significant part of the sport.

Basketball is a sport that entails contact with a resultant risk to the pregnant athlete. Up until the 12–15 week point of gestation, the uterus is protected by the pelvis, and the risk of trauma is decreased. After 20 weeks, however, the uterus becomes more of an abdominal organ, and thus is at risk for trauma. This can potentially cause placental abruption, early labor and preterm labor. Between 15 and 20 weeks of gestation, less is known about the risks to the athlete participating in basketball.

Specific guidelines for exercise during pregnancy are hard to apply in the competitive athlete. The American College of Obstetricians and Gynecologists (ACOG) in 1985 published guidelines that addressed exercise during pregnancy. In these they recommended that the maternal heart rate should remain below 140 beats per minute, maternal core temperature should remain below 38°C, and that exercise should be limited to less than 15 min (ACOG 1985). These recommendations were felt to be reasonable for the general public, however, too conservative for the elite or competitive athlete. In 1994, the ACOG published another set of guidelines which avoided setting specific cut-offs for heart rate and exercise duration, yet still remain somewhat conservative. Despite these limitations, these guidelines are helpful in providing guidance and information to the pregnant athlete (ACOG 1994). In a very recent committee opinion, the ACOG reported that "activities with a high risk of falling or those with a high risk of abdominal trauma should be avoided during pregnancy" (Artal & Sherman 1999; ACOG 2002).

Given these recommendations, it will be important to limit competitive play during pregnancy. However, continued cardiovascular and strength training during pregnancy is safe and healthy given the considerations addressed above. Specific recommendations must be individualized.

Musculoskeletal injuries

Basketball is a sport that requires both anaerobic and aerobic fitness, strength, and agility. It utilizes both the upper and lower extremities, has significant eye–hand coordination demands, and sport-specific skills that require balance, dexterity, and agility. Much of basketball play is short sprints with cutting, pivoting, and jumping activities. Many of the injuries that occur are due to the competitive nature of the sport, and the sport-specific demands placed on the athlete. Although there are no significant differences between the men's and women's game other than the size of the ball, there are differences in injury profiles that are important. At the college level, the relative incidence of injury when compared to other sports is favorable. Table 7.6 shows the incidence of injuries for women's basketball as well as other sports tracked by the NCAA in the 2001–2002 season.

ACL sprains represent one of the most severe injuries that occur and stress fractures, as described earlier, occur more commonly in athletes with menstrual dysfunction and/or disordered eating patterns. Patellofemoral dysfunction (PFD) is the major cause of anterior knee pain, and a common complaint of athletes participating in jumping and running activities such as basketball. Other musculoskeletal problems common in the female athlete include spondylolisthesis, pelvic floor dysfunction, and bunions. The effects of anatomical factors, ligamentous laxity, and the effect of hormonal influences have not been elucidated. In addition, in the pregnant athlete, additional factors may play a role in injury patterns seen in this special population.

In recent years, there has been impressive data demonstrating that female basketball players are at more risk for ACL sprains than their male counter-

Table 7.6 Injury data from NCAA Injury Surveillance System, through 1995–96. From Dick, R. (2001) NCAA data, 2001–2002, Indianapolis, IN, pp. 82–83.

Sport	Game injury rate per 1000 A–E	Practice injury rate per 1000 A–E
Spring football	9.1	
Football	3.8	35.4
Wrestling	4.8	24.1
Women's gymnastics	6.1	13.5
Men's soccer	3.9	18.0
Women's soccer	5.3	17.5
Ice hockey	1.8	12.0
Men's gymnastics		15.7
Men's lacrosse	3.4	
Men's basketball	3.8	9.3
Women's basketball	**5.1**	**9.2**
Field hockey	4.5	7.0
Women's lacrosse	4.2	8.6
Baseball	1.9	6.1
Women's volleyball	4.5	4.2
Women's softball	2.7	4.9

A–E, athlete exposures.

parts (Ireland & Wall 1990; Malone et al. 1992; Arendt & Dick 1995; Arendt et al. 1999). This has been demonstrated at both the college and elite level, and although the exact mechanisms remain unclear, it is likely multifactorial, with several neuroadaptive, biomechanical, and physiological factors playing a role. How female athletes jump, land from jumping, run, pivot and perform skills may differ from males, and these may play a role in the risk for injury. In addition, the strength of muscle groups, as well as the exact firing pattern during these activities may also play a role. Finally, the biomechanical and physiological differences between girls and boys and women and men, may also be factors to consider. Impressive research is underway which will help answer these differences and their role in injury. An excellent review of ACL injuries in women is provided by Arendt (2001). Table 7.7 demonstrates the common mechanisms of ACL injuries, and it is evident that the majority occur as a result of planting and pivoting, landing from a jump, and deceleration; skills often instrumental in basketball play.

ACL injuries occur during basketball play as a player decelerates, plants and pivots, or often when coming down from rebounding or jumping. Often, the player is pushed off balance in the air, or changes direction at the last moment during defensive play. In the female player, noncontact mechanisms predominate. The athlete will often feel or hear a pop, and is most often unable to continue play. Their knee will swell often quite rapidly within the first hour of injury. If these injuries are missed initially, the athlete will often then have recurrent buckling or give-way episodes, demonstrating the importance of the ACL in rotation and deceleration. If seen acutely, an arthrocentesis will often yield blood.

Plain radiographs are important in excluding other bony injury. If a lateral capsular sign or Segond fracture is present, ACL injury has occurred until proven otherwise. Plain radiographs are especially important in the younger athlete, where an ACL avulsion injury may occur and should be recognized prior to undue stress being placed on the knee. A positive Lachman, anterior drawer and/or pivot shift test will confirm the diagnosis, though additional tests may be useful. Complete evaluation of the knee and its associated structures is imperative. The pivot shift test may be difficult to perform in the acute setting. MRI may be useful if there is doubt about the diagnosis or if additional injury to the meniscal or chondral structures is considered.

Treatment of ACL injuries is most often surgical, with complete recovery and return to play often spanning several months to a year. The athlete should be treated acutely with ice, elevation, non-weight bearing, and other measures to decrease pain and swelling. In addition, gentle range of motion and other measures to maintain quadriceps tone are helpful adjuncts to early care. The treatment and rehabilitation of ACL injuries is beyond the scope of this chapter.

An important question to consider is whether these injuries can be prevented. There is again impressive research underway assessing different interventions and how they may play a role in decreasing the incidence of ACL tears in young female athletes. Much of this has been done in basketball, volleyball, and soccer players (Hewett *et al.* 1996, 1999; Griffin *et al.* 2000). It appears that the biomechanics of jumping, as well as the strength and firing pattern of the muscles surrounding the pelvis, as well as the knee may

Table 7.7 Common mechanisms of injury. From Arendt *et al.* (1999).

Mechanism	Frequency	Percentage	Cumulative percentage
Landing from a jump	6	12.2	12.2
Planting/pivoting	28	57.1	69.4
Deceleration	6	12.2	81.6
Going up for a jump	2	4.1	85.7
Hyperextension	6	12.2	98.0
Unsure	1	2.0	100.0
Total	**49**	**100.0**	

be important in preventing these injuries in the future. This is an area where more research is urgently needed.

Stress fractures

Stress fractures occur commonly in the basketball player, and as discussed earlier, athletes with disordered eating patterns or menstrual dysfunction are at significantly greater risk for these overuse injuries. Stress fractures are also common in the female athlete without the entities of the triad, and can be significant time loss injuries. Training factors account for the majority of stress fractures that are not related to the female athlete triad, with an increase in overload the most consistent theme. Athletes will often report a dull ache and occasionally night pain associated with activity, and will give a history of an increase in their volume of training. Other factors to consider include a change in their shoes, additional off the court strength and cardiovascular training, or biomechanical factors.

Most stress fractures in basketball involve the lower extremities with the tibia and metatarsals being the most common sites. Diagnosis should be suspected when the athlete reports increasing pain with activities, with improvement after periods of rest, and worsening with activity. There may be associated swelling and/or night pain, and their area of tenderness is often quite focal. Plain radiographs are often normal, and bone scintigraphy or MRI is often necessary for early detection. Treatment is generally guided by pain, with a period of activity modification to decrease the load on the affected bone. The specific treatment plan will depend on the location of stress fracture, as well as specific issues relating to the athlete.

Early treatment may include modifications of their weight-bearing activity, with continued cardio-vascular training using devices that decrease the load on the bone compared to full basketball play. Examples include using a pool to run in, a bicycle or stairmaster machine, or a treadmill with a harness such that the total body weight is decreased (Zuni). Once the athlete is able to weight bear without pain, progression to allow for sport-specific activities, such as taking free throws or shooting without jumping, can occur. This allows the athlete to return to practice and decreases their time away from sport, as well as improving their confidence and social well-being.

Special considerations in terms of treatment must be made for the fifth metatarsal fracture occurring at the metaphyseal/diaphyseal junction as well as for stress fractures of the tarsal navicular. These fractures often require surgical treatment with internal fixation in the competitive athlete. Stress fractures of the femoral neck are of the utmost importance to identify. If these go on to complete fracture, avascular necrosis of the femoral head can occur due the delicate blood supply to this region of bone.

obliquus (VMO) deficiency, hyperpronation, increased femoral ante-version, patella alta, patellar tendon hypermobility, tight lateral retinacular structures and a shallow patellar groove (Fairbank et al. 1984; Messier et al. 1991; Brukner & Khan 1993; Kannus & Nittymaki 1994; Natri et al. 1998).

Pain in PFD is generally worse after sitting for a prolonged period of time (theater sign) or with climbing or descending stairs. Mild peripatellar swelling is sometimes present and a sympathetic effusion is also not uncommon. Other findings on physical examination include stigmata as mentioned above, peripatellar tenderness, and pain with distal push of the patella during quadriceps contraction. Associated problems often seen with PFD include pes anserine bursitis and tendonitis, patellar tendonitis, and ilio-tibial band friction syndrome.

Treatment often includes modalities and medications to decrease pain and swelling, correction of malalignment and biomechanical factors, strengthening of the VMO structures, and stretching of the lateral structures. Patellar taping techniques have also been utilized (McConnell 1986; Bockrath et al. 1993; Kowall et al. 1996). Surgical treatment is considered if PFD is associated with significant instability, and/or if prolonged conservative treatment is unsuccessful (Fulkerson et al. 1990; Fu 1992). A full review of PFD is presented elsewhere (Fulkerson & Hungerford 1990; Arroll et al. 1997; Baker & Juhn 2000).

Patellofemoral dysfunction

Patellofemoral dysfunction (PFD) is the most common cause of anterior knee pain, and is very common in the female athlete. The athlete will often complain of pain around the patella, and activities such as jumping and running often aggravate their symptoms, thus making this a common complaint in basketball players. Patellofemoral dysfunction is often considered a maltracking of the patella, with or without instability. It is also often considered an overuse problem though not always associated with significant volume of activity. Potential risk factors include an increased Q angle, vastus medialis

Special considerations

It is important that in younger players, the injury profiles include the types of injuries more common in youth. ACL tears and muscle strains are less common, whereas avulsion injuries, apophysitis, and growth plate injuries predominate. It is important when taking care of the younger athlete, to consider these possibilities. It is important to obtain radiographs, and at times additional diagnostic imaging may be necessary. Figure 7.7 demonstrates a Salter II fracture of the distal femur in a 14-year-old girl who sustained a varus injury while playing basketball. This injury was not evident on plain radiographs.

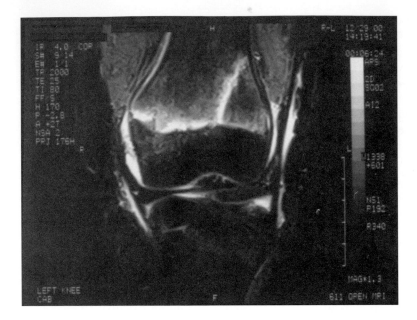

Fig. 7.7 Salter II fracture of the distal femur.

References

ACOG (1985) *Home Exercise Programs: Exercise During Pregnancy, the Postnatal Period.* Washington, D.C.: American College of Obstetricians & Gynecologists.

ACOG (1994) Exercise during pregnancy and the postpartum period. ACOG Technical Bulletin Number 189. *International Journal of Gynaecology and Obstetrics* **45** (1), 65–70.

ACOG Committee on Obstetric Practice (2002) Exercise during pregnancy and the postpartum period. ACOG Committee Opinion Number 267, American College of Obstetricians and Gynecologists. *Obstetrics and Gynecology* **99**, 171–173.

Araujo, D. (1997) Expecting questions about exercise and pregnancy? *Physician and Sportsmedicine* **25** (4).

Arendt, E.A. & Dick, R. (1995) Knee injury patterns among men and women in collegiate basketball and soccer: NCAA data review of literature. *American Journal of Sports Medicine* **23**, 694–701.

Arendt, E.A. (2001) Anterior cruciate injuries. *Current Women's Health Reports* **1**, 211–217.

Arendt, E.A., Agel, J. & Dick, R. (1999) Anterior cruciate ligament injury patterns among collegiate men and women. *Journal of Athletic Training* **34**, 86–92.

Arroll, B., Ellis-Pelger, E., Edwards, A. *et al.* (1997) Patellofemoral pain syndrome: a critical review of the clinical trials on non-operative therapy. *American Journal of Sports Medicine* **25**, 207–212.

Artal, R. & Sherman, C. (1999) Exercise during pregnancy: safe and beneficial for most. *Physical Sports Medicine* **27**, 51–58.

Baker, M.M. & Juhn, M.S. (2000) Patellofemoral pain syndrome in the female athlete. *Clinical Sports Medicine* **19** (2), 315–329.

Bockrath, K., Wooden, C., Worrell, T. *et al.* (1993) Effects of patella taping on patella position and perceived pain. *Medicine and Science in Sports and Exercise* **25**, 989–992.

Brownell, K.D. & Steen, S.N. (1992) Weight cycling in athletes. Effects on behavior, physiology, and health. In: Brownell, K.D., Rodin, J. & Wilmore, J.H. (eds) *Eating, Body Weight and Performance in Athletes: Disorders of Modern Society.* Philadelphia: Lea & Febiger, 159–171.

Brukner, P. & Khan, K. (1993) Anterior knee pain. In: Brukner, P. & Khan, K. (eds) *Clinical Sports Medicine.* Sydney: McGraw-Hill, 372–391.

Cann, C.E., Martin, M.C., Genant, H.K. *et al.* (1984) Decreased spinal mineral content in amenorrheic women. *Journal of the American Medical Association* **251**, 626–629.

Chalip, L., Villige, J. & Duignan, N. (1980) Sex-role identity in a select sample of women field hockey players. *International Journal of Sport Psychology* **11**, 240–248.

Clapp, J.F. III & Capeless, E. (1991) The $\dot{V}o_{2max}$ of recreational athletes before and after pregnancy. *Medicine and Science in Sports and Exercise* **23** (10), 1128–1133.

Colten, M.E. & Gore, S. (1991) *Risk, Resiliency, and Resistance: Current Research on Adolescent Girls*. New York: Ms Foundation.

Drinkwater, B.L., Bruemmer, B. & Chestnut, C.H. (1990) Menstrual history as a determinant of current bone density in young athletes. *Journal of the American Medical Association* **263**, 545.

Drinkwater, B.L., Healy, N.L., Rencken, M.L. *et al.* (1993) Effectiveness of nasal calcitonin in preventing bone loss in young amenorrheic women. *Journal of Bone Mineral Research* **8** (Suppl.), S264.

Drinkwater, B.L., Nilson, K., Chestnut, C.H. *et al.* (1984) Bone mineral content of amenorrheic and eumenorrheic athletes. *New England Journal of Medicine* **311**, 277–281.

Drinkwater, B.L., Nilson, K., Ott, S. *et al.* (1986) Bone mineral density after resumption of menses in amenorrheic athletes. *Journal of the American Medical Association* **256**, 380–382.

Dueck, C.A., Matt, K.S., Manore, M.M. *et al.* (1996) Treatment of athletic amenorrhea with a diet and training intervention program. *International Journal of Sport Nutrition* **6**, 24–40.

Dummer, G.M., Rosen, L.W., Heusner, W.W. *et al.* (1987) Pathogenic weight control behavior of young competitive swimmers. *Physician and Sportsmedicine* **15**, 75–84.

Ettinger, B., Genant, H.K. & Cann, C.E. (1987) Postmenopausal bone loss is prevented by treatment with low-dosage estrogen with calcium. *Annals of Internal Medicine* **106**, 40–45.

Evans, T.A., Putukian, M., Earl, J.E. *et al.* (2000) Frequency of specific entities of female athlete triad among female collegiate athletes at an NCAA Division I institution. *Journal of Athletic Training* **35** (Suppl.), S88.

Fairbank, J.C.T., Pynsent, P.B., Van Poortvliet, J.A. *et al.* (1984) Mechanical factors in the incidence of knee pain in adolescents and young adults. *Journal of Bone and Joint Surgery* **66**, 685–693.

Fulkerson, J.P., Becker, G.J., Meaney, J.A. *et al.* (1990) Anteromedial tibial tubercle transfer without bone graft. *American Journal of Sports Medicine* **18**, 490–497.

Fulkerson, J.P. & Hungerford, D.S. (eds) (1990) *Disorders of the Patellofemoral Joint*, 2nd edn. Baltimore: Williams & Wilkins, 117–119.

Gibson, J. (2000) Osteoporosis. In: Drinkwater, B. (ed.) *Women in Sport*. Oxford: Blackwell Science, 391–406.

Griffin, L.Y., Agel, J., Albohm, M.J. *et al.* (2000) Noncontact anterior curciate ligament injuries: Risk factors and prevention strategies. *Journal of the American Academy of Orthopedic Surgeons* **8**, 141–150.

Harris, S.S., Caspersen, C.J., DeFreise, G.H. *et al.* (1989) Physical activity counseling for healthy adults as a primary preventive intervention in the clinical setting.

Journal of the American Medical Association **261**, 3590–3598.

Hergenroeder, A.C., Smith, E.O., Shypailo, R. *et al.* (1997) Bone mineral changes in young women with hypothalamic amenorrhea treated with oral contraceptives, medroxyprogesterone or placebo over 12 months. *American Journal of Obstetrics and Gynecology* **176**, 1017–1025.

Hewett, T.E., Lindenfeld, T.N., Riccobene, J.V. & Noyes, F.R. (1999) The effect of neuromuscular training on the incidence of knee injury in female athletes: a prospective study. *American Journal of Sports Medicine* **27**, 699–705.

Hewett, T.E., Stroupe, A.L., Nance, T.A. & Noyes, F.R. (1996) Plyometric training in female athletes. Decreased impact forces and increased hamstring torques. *American Journal of Sports Medicine* **24**, 765–773.

Ireland, M.L. & Wall, C. (1990) Epidemiology and comparison of knee injuries in elite male and female United States basketball athletes. *Medicine and Science in Sports and Exercise* **22**, S82.

Kannus, P. & Nittymaki, S. (1994) Which factors predict outcome in the nonoperative treatment of patellofemoral pain syndrome? A prospective follow-up study. *Medicine and Science in Sports and Exercise* **26**, 289–296.

Kardel, K.R. & Kase, T. (1988) Training in pregnant women. Effects on fetal development and birth. *American Journal of Obstet Gynecology* **178** (2), 280–286.

Kowall, M.G., Kolk, G., Nuber, G.W. *et al.* (1996) Patellar taping in the treatment of patellofemoral pain: a prospective randomized study. *American Journal of Sports Medicine* **24**, 61–66.

Leon, A.S., Connett, J. & Jacobs, D.R. *et al.* (1987) Leisure time physical activity levels and risk of coronary heart disease and death: The multiple risk factor intervention trial. *Journal of the American Medical Association* **258**, 2388–2395.

Loucks, A.B. & Horvath, S.M. (1985) Athletic amenorrhea: a review. *Med Sci Sports Exerc* **17**, 56.

Loucks, A.M., Verdun, M. & Heath, E.M. (1998) Low energy availability, not stress of exercise, alters LH pulsatility in exercising women. *Journal of Applied Physiology* **84**, 37–46.

Lynberg, M.C., Khoury, M.J., Lu, X. *et al.* (1994) Maternal flu, fever, and the risk of neural tube defects: a population-based case-control study. *American Journal of Epidemiology* **140** (3), 244–255.

Malone, T.R., Hardaker, W.T. & Garrett, W.E. (1992) Relationship of gender to ACL injuries in intercollegiate basketball players. *Journal of South Orthopedic Association* **2**, 36–39.

McConnell, J.S. (1986) The management of chondromalacia patellae: a long term solution. *Australian Journal of Physiotherapy* **32**, 215–223.

Messier, S.P., Davis, S.E., Curl, W.W. *et al.* (1991) Etiologic factors associated with patellofemoral pain in runners. *Medicine and Science in Sports and Exercise* **23**, 1008–1015.

Milunsky, A., Ulcickas, M., Rothman, K.J. *et al.* (1992) Maternal heat exposure and neural tube defects. *Journal of the American Medical Association* **268** (7), 882–885.

Morrow, R.J., Ritchie, J.W. & Bull, S.B. (1989) Fetal and maternal hemodynamic responses to exercise in pregnancy assessed by Doppler ultrasonography. *American Journal of Obstetrics and Gynecology* **160**, 138–140.

Myburgh, K.H., Bachrach, L.K., Lewis, B. *et al.* (1993) Bone mineral density at axial and appendicular sites in amenorrheic athletes. *Medicine and Science in Sports and Exercise* **25**, 1197–1202.

Natri, A., Kannus, P. & Jarvinen, M. (1998) Which factors predict the long term outcome in chronic patellofemoral pain syndrome? A prospective follow-up study. *Medicine and Science in Sports and Exercise* **30**, 1572–1577.

NCAA (1983–98) *Participation at a Glance*. The National Collegiate Athletic Association, www.NCAA.org.

O'Connor, P.J. & Lewis, R.D. (1995) Kirchner EM. Eating disorder symptoms in female college gymnasts. *Medicine and Science in Sports and Exercise* **27**, 550–555.

Prior, J.C., Vigna, Y.M., Barr, S.I. *et al.* (1994) Cyclic medroxyprogesterone treatment increases bone density; a controlled trial in active women with menstrual cycle disturbances. *American Journal of Medicine* **96**, 521–530.

Rosen, L.W. & Hough, D.O. (1988) Pathogenic weight-control behaviors of female college gymnasts. *Physician and Sports Medicine* **16**, 141–146.

Rosen, L.W., McKeag, D.B., Hough, D.O. *et al.* (1986) Pathogenic weight control behaviors in female athletes. *Physician and Sports Medicine* **14**, 79–86.

Sabo, D.F., Miller, K.E., Farrell, M.P. *et al.* (1999) High school athletic participation, sexual behavior and adolescent pregnancy: a regional study. *Journal of Adolescent Health* **25** (3), 207–216.

Sellers, M.J. & Perkins-Cole, K.J. (1987) Hyperthermia and neural tube defects of the curly-tail mouse. *Journal of Craniofacial Genetics and Developmental Biology* **7** (4), 321–330.

Shiota, K. (1988) Induction of neural tube defects and skeletal malformations in mice following brief hyperthermia in utero. *Biological Neonate* **53** (2), 86–97.

Sundgot-Borgen, J. (1994) Risk and trigger factors for the development of eating disorders in female elite athletes. *Medicine and Science in Sports and Exercise* **26**, 414–419.

Sundgot-Borgen, J. (2000) Eating disorders. In: Drinkwater, B. (ed.) *Women in Sport*. Oxford: Blackwell Science, 364–376.

Sundgot-Borgen, J. & Larsen, S. (1993) Nutrient intake and eating behavior of female elite athletes suffering from anorexia nervosa, anorexia athletica and bulimia nervosa. *International Journal of Sports Nutrition* **3**, 431–442.

Teitz, C.C., Hu, S.S. & Arendt, E.A. (1997) The female athlete: evaluation and treatment of sports-related problems. *Journal of the American Academy of Orthopedic Surgeons* **5**(2), 87–96.

Wilmore, J.H. (1991) Eating and weight disorders in the female athlete. *International Journal of Sports Nutrition* **1**, 104–107.

Yates, A., Shisslak, C., Crago, M. *et al.* (1994) Overcommitment to sport: is there a relationship to the eating disorders? *Clinical Journal of Sports Medicine* **4**, 39–46.

Chapter 8
The special basketball player

Kevin B. Gebke and Douglas B. McKeag

Participation in sports requires the ability to endure physical challenges. Many conditions limit the extent to which people can compete. Basketball players who suffer from medical problems require special attention to minimize the risk of injury or exacerbation of the disease process. This chapter will discuss recommendations for the care of basketball players with diabetes, asthma, and epilepsy as well as the mentally and physically challenged.

Diabetes mellitus

Millions of people worldwide suffer from diabetes mellitus. Various forms of the disease include type 1 (an absolute insulin deficiency), type 2 (relative insulin deficiency usually secondary to insulin resistance), gestational, and secondary diabetes mellitus. The consistent underlying pathophysiologic process is a relative deficiency of insulin resulting in hyperglycemia. Longstanding or poorly controlled diabetes can lead to a wide variety of medical complications from microvascular and macrovascular processes. These include retinopathy, nephropathy, coronary artery disease, cerebrovascular disease and peripheral vascular disease as well as autonomic and peripheral neuropathies. Prior to participation, basketball players with diabetes should be identified and screened for complications of the disease that may place them at increased risk for problems during competition. An understanding of the disease process, the effects of exercise, and the appropriate

treatment adjustments can allow a basketball player to maximize the competitive experience.

Diabetes should be suspected in athletes presenting with complaints of polyuria, polydipsia, polyphagia, or signs of end-organ disease. The diagnosis can be established in an athlete with symptoms suggestive of the disease using the following criteria:
1 Symptoms of diabetes in addition to a random glucose concentration above 200 mg·dL^{-1}
2 Fasting glucose concentration above 126 mg·dL^{-1}.
3 Glucose concentration above 200 mg·dL^{-1} on 2-h glucose tolerance testing.

Diabetes mellitus type 1 is characterized by an absolute deficiency of insulin secretion from the pancreatic beta cells. This form of disease was previously referred to as insulin-dependent or juvenile-onset diabetes. Theoretically, the cause of this form of diabetes is from an autoimmune destruction of the beta cells in genetically predisposed individuals. The disease usually manifests prior to the age of 30, but can occur at any age. Insulin replacement is *required* for control of symptoms and prevention of ketoacidosis. Worldwide, approximately 10% of diabetics are type 1.

Type 2 diabetes is characterized by relative insulin deficiency secondary to insulin resistance. This form of diabetes was previously known as noninsulin-dependent or adult-onset diabetes. Insulin receptors are thought to become blunted leading to ineffective glucose uptake and transport. Obesity is the major predisposing factor to type 2 diabetes and is present in over 80% of newly diagnosed cases. There is a clear genetic predisposition. Type 2 disease accounts for approximately 90% of diabetics and onset is typically after age 40.

Gestational and secondary diabetes are seen infrequently in the athletic population. Gestational diabetes is secondary to insulin resistance during the latter stages of pregnancy. Active participation in basketball and other contact activities are contraindicated in the later stages of pregnancy and should be strongly discouraged. Secondary diabetes occurs as a result of medical diseases (pancreatic disease, Cushing's syndrome), injuries, and drugs (steroids, chlorothiazines). Approach to these conditions should be coordinated with the primary physician caring for the patient.

The effect of exercise on glucose homeostasis is complex. A dynamic interaction between metabolic events and hormonal response is required to maintain an adequate fuel supply in the form of glucose. Exercise inherently facilitates glucose uptake by muscle even in the absence of insulin. Excess insulin can lead to a relative deficiency of available glucose secondary to blood glucose being shifted into tissues and gluconeogenesis being inhibited. For this reason, insulin secretion must be suppressed during exercise to allow the body to efficiently provide glucose through glycogenolysis in muscle, lipolysis in adipose tissue, and gluconeogenesis in the liver.

Diabetic athletes receiving exogenous insulin do not respond to exercise in the way that their healthy counterparts do. Factors that affect blood glucose concentration during exercise include:
1 Hypoglycemic agent prescribed
2 Medication timing
3 Pre-exercise blood glucose concentration
4 Pre-exercise meal
5 Presence of disease complications (nephropathy)
6 Concomitant medication use
7 Duration and intensity of exercise.

Glucose homeostasis is difficult to maintain, especially in the type 1 diabetic. It is impossible for exogenous replacement of insulin to replicate the normal physiologic insulin response and insulin cannot be suppressed once administered. Care must be taken to prevent hypoglycemic episodes during and after exercise.

Exercise is beneficial in people with all forms of diabetes, but is most therapeutic in type 2 diabetics. The mechanism of action is augmentation of the insulin effect through mobilization of glucose across cell membranes. This lowers blood glucose levels and may reduce the medication requirement in type 2 diabetes. Type 1 diabetics do not benefit from this and may actually suffer from the effects of fluctuating glucose levels. Benefits of exercise that are shared among both major forms of diabetes include:
1 Improved lipid profile ($\downarrow$LDL, $\uparrow$HDL)
2 Decreased systolic and diastolic blood pressure (reduced cardiovascular risk)
3 Improved self-esteem
4 Improved socialization.

For these reasons, exercise (including basketball participation) should be encouraged in diabetic athletes.

The diabetic athlete's risk of complication during basketball participation must also be assessed. The systemic involvement of diabetes poses risk to multiple organ systems. The most immediate and frequently occurring complication is hypoglycemia. The warning signs of impending hypoglycemia include palpitations, tremor, anxiety, diaphoresis, hunger, and paresthesias. Exercise-induced hypoglycemia occurs during or immediately after exercise and may be secondary to excessive exogenous insulin usage, location of insulin injection, inadequate caloric intake, or unexpected excessive exercise duration or intensity. Post-exercise (delayed) hypoglycemia may be delayed 8–16 h after strenuous exercise. Delayed hypoglycemia poses a greater risk to basketball players because the symptoms are often nocturnal and severe, including seizures and coma. Post-exercise hypoglycemia is seen when glycogen stores are depleted and inadequately replenished. This is exacerbated by increased post-exercise insulin sensitivity and efficient glucose uptake by glycogen-depleted muscles. Long-standing diabetes can result in impairment of autonomic function. Athletes will lose the ability to sense impending hypoglycemia until blood glucose concentration reaches a dangerously low level. Hypoglycemic basketball players respond well to oral sugar-containing fluids or solids. Other means of therapy such as glucagon or intravenous dextrose may be required if the athlete cannot tolerate oral intake.

Preparticipation evaluation of basketball players is essential in establishing that the athlete is capable of the rigors of competition and is under appropriate medical supervision of care. Evaluation should include a thorough history and physical examination. Key historical information includes duration of disease, previous complications, prescribed medication and dosage, prior participation in sports, and signs or symptoms of diabetic end-organ disease. The physical exam should include evaluation of all organ systems including neurologic testing for evidence of peripheral neuropathy. Longstanding diabetes can result in sensory impairment of the lower extremities. All diabetic athletes must be instructed on proper foot inspection and skin care to reduce the risk of unnoticed lesions developing infection. Fundoscopic evaluation for signs of retinopathy should also be performed. Laboratory testing may be beneficial if recent studies have not been performed. Recommended tests include:

1 Blood urea nitrogen/creatinine
2 Hemoglobin A1c/glycosolated hemoglobin
3 Urine for microalbumin
4 Fasting lipid profile.

Exercise testing recommendations are based on a number of factors that should be identified during the preparticipation evaluation. The American College of Sports Medicine recommends graded exercise testing to screen basketball players for cardiovascular disease in the following situations:

1 Type 1 diabetes and over 30 years of age
2 Type 1 diabetes of over 15 years duration
3 Type 2 diabetes and over 35 years of age
4 Either type 1 or 2 diabetes plus one or more coronary artery disease risk factors
5 Known or suspected coronary artery disease
6 Presence of microvascular or neurologic diabetic complications.

Management of blood glucose during exercise is based on maintaining normoglycemia to provide fuel for exercising muscles. Prevention of hyperglycemia or hypoglycemia is the goal. This is best achieved by establishing a healthy diet with appropriate caloric intake in conjunction with the prescribed pharmacological agent. Medication choice is dependent upon the type of diabetes and any coexisting conditions. Portable glucose monitors should be utilized for establishment of pre-exercise glucose levels and frequent monitoring with changes in the training regimen.

Pre-exercise glucose concentrations can be used to guide participation in insulin-requiring basketball players. This requires an understanding of pregame meal timing (approximately 2 h prior to participation) as well as duration of insulin action (Table 8.1). Three potential scenarios exist. If the athlete is hypoglycemic (blood sugar below 100 mg·dL^{-1}), a snack consisting of 10–20 g of carbohydrate is recommended prior to exercise. Hyperglycemia (blood sugar above 250 mg·dL^{-1}) requires a delay in exercise as well as urine evaluation for ketones and possible insulin administration. Blood glucose in the range of 100–250 mg·dL^{-1} allows for safe participation.

Medication adjustment is dependent upon the duration and intensity of planned activity. For activities of mild to moderate intensity and short duration, no adjustment should be required. More demanding basketball activities should be accompanied by a corresponding decrease in insulin dosage and increase in caloric intake (Table 8.2). Sugar-containing snacks or beverages should be available at activities for consumption if hypoglycemia occurs. Finally, postexercise nutrition should be stressed to allow hepatic and muscular glycogen stores to be replenished. Post-exercise nutrition should be adjusted according to the level of training. Those athletes participating in long duration, high intensity work-outs will require 8–10 g of carbohydrate per kilogram body weight per day (8–10 g CHO·kg^{-1}·day^{-1}). Consumption of 0.7–3.0 g CHO·kg^{-1} is recommended immediately after exercise and every 2 h for a total of 4 h. This practice will prepare the athlete for the next exercise session and help prevent delayed hypoglycemia.

In summary, nutritional assessment, medication adjustment, blood glucose monitoring, and determination of exercise demands are all important factors to consider when predicting exercise response and educating the diabetic basketball player.

Asthma and exercise-induced asthma

Asthma is a common obstructive pulmonary process characterized by reversible bronchospasm, mucus production, inflammation, and edema. Specific triggers have been identified but the profile is unique in each individual case. It is estimated that approximately 90% of asthmatics suffer from exacerbation of symptoms secondary to rigorous physical activity (exercise-induced asthma = EIA). Less frequently,

Table 8.1 ADA insulin table—available types.

Formula	Manufacturer	Dose
Short-acting (Usual onset 0.5–2.0 h; usual duration 3–6 h)		
Human		
Humulin regular	Lilly	U-100
Novolin R (regular)	Novo Nordisk	U-100
Velosulin human (regular)	Novo Nordisk	U-100
Novolin R Penfill (regular)	Novo Nordisk	U-100
Pork		
Iletin II regular	Lilly	U-100, U-500
Purified pork R (regular)	Novo Nordisk	U-100
Regular	Novo Nordisk	U-100
Beef/pork		
Iletin I	Lilly	U-100
Intermediate-acting (usual onset-3–6 h; usual duration 12–20 h)		
Human		
Humulin L (lente)	Lilly	U-100
Humulin N (NPH)	Lilly	U-100
Novolin L (lente)	Novo Nordisk	U-100
Novolin N (NPH)	Novo Nordisk	U-100
Novolin N Penfill (NPH)	Novo Nordisk	U-100
Beef		
NPH	Novo Nordisk	U-100
Lente	Novo Nordisk	U-100
Pork		
Iletin II Lente	Lilly	U-100
Iletin II NPH	Lilly	U-100
Purified pork lente	Novo Nordisk	U-100
Purified porn N (NPH)	Novo Nordisk	U-100
Beef/Pork		
Iletin I Lente	Lilly	U-100
Iletin I NPH	Lilly	U-100
Long-acting (usual onset 6–12 h; usual duration 16–36 h)		
Human		
Humulin U (ultralente)	Lilly	U-100
Beef		
Ultralente	Novo Nordisk	U-100
Premixed combinations		
Human		
Humulin 50/50 (50% NPH, 50% regular)	Lilly	U-100
Humulin 70/30 (70% NPH, 30% regular)	Lilly	U-100
Novolin 70/30 (70% NPH, 30% regular)	Novo Nordisk	U-100
Novolin 70/30 Penfill	Novo Nordisk	U-100
Novolin 70/30 Prefilled	Novo Nordisk	U-100

Table 8.2 American Diabetes Association (ADA) insulin adjustment recommendatons.

Once-daily regimen
Morning exercise lasting >45 min:
Decrease regular insulin by 25% for mild to moderate activity
Decrease regular insulin by 35% for moderate activity
Decrease regular insulin by 50% for strenuous activity (athletes in training)
Afternoon or evening exercise lasting >45 min:
Decrease in NPH/lente by 15% for mild to moderate activity
Decrease NPH/lente by 20% for moderate activity
Decrease NPH/lente by 25% for strenuous activity (athletes in training)

Twice-daily regimen
Morning exercise lasting >45 min:
Decrease morning regular insulin as above
Early afternoon exercise lasting >45 min:
Decrease morning NPH insulin as above
Evening exercise lasting >45 min:
Decrease supper NPH and regular insulin as for once-daily insulin

More than twice-daily injections
Premeal regular insulin can be decreased for exercise occurring postprandially (from 25 to 50% decrements depending on the intensity and duration)
Bedtime or morning NPH or ultralente should be decreased only for very prolonged and intense exercise (tournaments, marathons, etc.) occurring at any time of the day

Continuous subcutaneous insulin infusion
Premeal boluses should be decreased as above for postprandial exercise
For light exercise, the basal rate can be maintained
For moderate or intense exercise, the basal rate should be discontinued for the duration of exercise taking into account that a moderate amount of subcutaneous insulin remaining in the infusion site
(3–5 U) will be absorbed

For unanticipated exercise
Insulin doses cannot be modified, thus hypoglycemia can be prevented by extra food
Mild to moderate exercise = 1 fruit exchange every 30–45 min
Moderate exercise = 1 starch + 1 protein before exercise + 1 fruit every 30–45 min during exercise
Strenuous exercise = 2 starches + 1 protein before exercise + 1–2 fruit(s) every 30–45 min during exercise

Table 8.3 Asthma classification.

Asthma classification	Symptoms	Night symptoms	Lung function
Mild intermittent	(1) Symptoms twice per week or less (2) Asymptomatic with normal peak flow between symptoms (3) Brief exacerbations (few hours to days)	Symptoms no more than twice monthly	(1) FEV1/FVC = 80% or more of predicted (2) Peak flow variability of less than 20%
Mild persistent	(1) Symptoms more than twice weekly (2) Activity alteration required	Symptoms more than twice monthly	(1) FEV1/FVC = 80% or more of predicted (2) Peak flow variability 20–30%
Moderate persistent	(1) Daily symptoms (2) Daily use of short-acting beta agonist medication (3) Exacerbations affect activity (4) Frequent exacerbations lasting days or more	Symptoms more than once per week	(1) FEV1/FVC >60% but <80% of predicted value (2) Peak flow variability >30%
Severe persistent	(1) Continual symptoms (2) Limited activity potential (3) Frequent exacerbations	Frequent symptoms	(1) FEV1/FVC = 60% or less of predicted (2) Peak flow variability >30%

individuals without a history of asthma will develop symptoms of acute airway narrowing with exercise (solitary EIA). Participation in basketball is possible with appropriate management of asthma symptoms.

The exact pathophysiologic mechanism of EIA is unknown, but is thought to be multifactorial. The suspected causes include changes in temperature of air being rapidly inspired and evaporation of water leading to mast cell degranulation. These hypothetical causes are unproven, but supported by the observation of decreased symptom reproduction in warm, moist environments. Individual response in EIA is related to the athlete's airway sensitivity and can be potentiated by other factors such as allergens or upper respiratory infections.

Symptoms associated with EIA are similar to those seen in chronic asthma. Typical symptoms include wheezing, dyspnea, cough, and chest tightness. Other less commonly described symptoms are nausea, stomach discomfort, chest discomfort, fatigue, and deteriorating performance. The usual progression is onset of symptoms after achieving approximately 80% of maximal heart rate with worsening symptoms upon termination of activity. Symptoms typically resolve within 60 min. A refractory period is commonly observed after resolution of symptoms and usually lasts for a minimum of 2 h. Basketball players can actively participate during the refractory period without recurrence of bronchospasm.

Asthma diagnosis is based on symptomatology and objective data derived from spirometry. Asthma is classified as mild intermittent, mild persistent, moderate persistent, or severe persistent (Table 8.3).

Diagnosis of solitary exercise-induced asthma also requires a thorough history and physical examination. Useful historical information includes type of exercise that incites symptoms, timing of symptom onset, environmental conditions responsible (cold and dry), and previous use of pharmacological agents. Identification of symptoms and triggers often uncover EIA during the preparticipation evaluation. Chronic asthma and solitary EIA can typically be distinguished using FEV1, with this value being normal or higher than predicted in EIA and typically less than predicted in chronic asthma. Formal exercise testing may be required to evoke symptoms in some athletes. Diagnosis is confirmed by demonstrating a FEV1 reduction of 15% or decrease in peak flow by 20%. It is acceptable to observe for symptom improvement with a trial of short-acting beta agonists prior to exercise in an athlete with a history suggestive of exercise-induced asthma.

Table 8.4 Asthma treatment recommendations.

Classification	Treatment
Mild intermittent	No daily medication necessary*
Mild persistent	Low-potency inhaled corticosteroid, cromolyn, nedocromil, or leukotriene modifiers *Alternative* = theophylline
Moderate persistent	Low-to-medium-potency inhaled corticosteroid ± long-acting bronchodilator (salmeterol). *Alternative* = theophylline or long-acting beta 2-agonist tablets
Severe persistent	High-potency inhaled corticosteroid + long-acting bronchodilator ± oral corticosteroid
Intermittent symptoms or exacerbations	*All asthma sufferers should maintain a supply of short-acting beta 2-agonist.

Treatment of chronic and exercise-induced asthma begins with education of the athlete. Understanding the symptoms, timing, triggers, and medication action allows for effective basketball participation. Chronic asthma should be approached in such a way as to symptomatically evaluate and treat based on the classification of disease (Table 8.4).

Basketball players with chronic asthma exacerbated by exercise usually respond well to therapy individualized to their asthma profile. In athletes with persistent symptoms or isolated exercise-induced asthma, dosing with short-acting beta 2-agonist inhaler (albuterol, 2–4 puffs) 15 min prior to exercise may provide symptom relief. If symptoms still persist, other pre-exercise regimens can be utilized including cromolyn (4–10 puffs, 15 min prior), nedocromil (2–4 puffs, 15 min prior), salmeterol (2 puffs, at least 30 min prior) or formoterol fumarate inhalation powder (12 µg, 15 min prior). Health care providers must consider therapeutic modalities when recommending therapy. Many substances commonly used in the treatment of asthma are banned. The following drugs are banned by the International Olympic Committee:

1 Clenbuterol
2 Bitolterol
3 Fenoterol
4 Metaproterenol
5 Orciprenaline
6 Pirbuterol
7 Oral, rectal, IM, or IV corticosteroids
8 Oral or injectable beta agonists.

Most inhaled medications require notification of use and medical necessity prior to participation.

Seizure disorder

Seizures are characterized by abnormal neuronal discharge in the brain and are manifest in a variety of patterns. Symptoms directly correlate with the region of the brain involved and may include involuntary muscle movements, sensation or perception impairment, behavioral changes, or alteration of consciousness. People have varying degrees of susceptibility to seizures. Factors have been identified that may lower an individual's seizure threshold including sleep deprivation and electrolyte imbalance.

Seizures are typically seen in an athletic population in one of three situations. (1) Traumatic head injury is a well-documented cause. In basketball, this type of injury can be seen when players collide or when a player strikes his or her head on the floor. (2) A seizure may be precipitated by an underlying metabolic imbalance such as hypoglycemia or hyponatremia. (3) Seizures can be seen in athletes with a history of epilepsy.

Epilepsy is a disorder of recurrent unprovoked seizures with an incidence of approximately 3% in the general population. Seizure frequency varies and long asymptomatic periods between episodes are common. Idiopathic epilepsy can present at any age, but is most commonly seen in the first two decades of life. No underlying abnormality can be identified. Identifiable causes of epilepsy include:

1 Congenital abnormalities
2 Perinatal injury
3 Metabolic diseases
4 Post-traumatic

5 Tumors or space-occupying lesions
6 Vascular disease
7 Degenerative disorders
8 Infection.

The area of the brain that is affected determines seizure classification. Activation limited to one region of the cerebral cortex is termed partial seizure. Electroencephalographic (EEG) evaluation is often utilized for localization of the focus. The location of neuronal activation in partial seizures will dictate the clinical manifestations. Partial seizures can then be subdivided into simple, complex, and complicated. Simple partial seizures involve preservation of consciousness with awareness of symptoms. Consciousness is impaired in complex partial seizures, while progression to generalized tonic, clonic, or tonic-clonic activity is the distinguishing factor in complicated partial seizures.

Generalized seizures involve activation of the entire cerebral cortex simultaneously. Depending on the type and duration of the seizure, significant physiologic manifestations can be seen. Hypoglycemia, hypoxemia, and acidosis are frequently encountered with prolonged tonic-clonic activity of over 30 min duration (status epilepticus). The types of generalized seizures include absence, myoclonic, tonic-clonic, and atonic.

Absence seizures typically manifest during childhood and continue through the first two decades of life. Symptoms may resolve spontaneously or transition into another type of generalized seizure disorder with time. Absence seizures are characterized by sudden lapses of consciousness. Symptoms are usually brief and resolve within a short period of time (usually seconds). Associated clonic, tonic, or atonic components may be seen. Atypical absence seizures differ in that there is frequently a more pronounced change in muscular tone and symptom onset is more gradual. An identifiable underlying structural abnormality is commonly linked to atypical absence seizure disorder.

Myoclonic seizures are characterized by single or repeated muscular contractions. There is an association with metabolic disorders, degenerative conditions of the central nervous system, and anoxic brain injury.

Grand mal seizures may manifest as pure tonic, pure clonic, or tonic-clonic in nature. Tonic-clonic seizures are characterized by a sudden loss of consciousness with an initial tonic component. The tonic phase is manifest by rigidity, arrested respiration, and cyanosis typically lasting less than 60 s. A clonic phase follows which consists of alternating muscular contraction and relaxation seen as jerking movements. This phase can be of long duration, but usually lasts less than 2–3 min. Following a grand mal seizure, a period of unresponsiveness is regularly observed. This postictal period may also include bowel or bladder incontinence, confusion, headache, drowsiness, nausea, and/or myalgia.

Atonic seizures are seen in association with other epileptic syndromes. Symptoms are described as "drop attacks" where an individual will suffer from a brief loss of muscular tone precipitating a fall. Loss of consciousness may be seen, but there are no postictal sequelae. The real hazard is the risk of injury from the fall.

Health care providers must be aware of the exercise response in the basketball player with seizure disorder. The primary concern is precipitation of seizure leading to injury. Relative hypoxia can be seen with maximal exertion and is thought to reduce the seizure threshold. Studies, however, have failed to demonstrate an increase in seizure frequency. Conversely, exercise actually seems to diminish the level of seizure activity without increasing the associated morbidity or mortality. With this knowledge, practitioners should encourage athletes with seizure disorder to participate in regular physical activity.

Studies have shown that exercise training capacity in basketball players with seizure disorder is similar to their healthy counterparts. This determination, of course, depends upon other comorbid factors and limitations. Equivalent improvement in fitness can be achieved in a balanced training program.

In the event of a seizure, the health care providers should be adequately prepared to control the situation. Brief uncomplicated seizures do not warrant hospital evaluation. Observation and support during a brief seizure and throughout the postictal period is appropriate. Return-to-play is possible only if the athlete is fully alert and oriented and without signs of impaired balance or coordination. Status epilepticus represents continuous or repetitive seizure activity and is considered a medical emergency with a mortality rate as high as 20%. Prognosis is directly

Table 8.5 Seizure disorder drugs-of-choice.

Seizure type	Initial drug(s)-of-choice
Absence	Ethosuximide
Partial	Phenytoin or carbamazepine
Generalized convulsive	Phenytoin or valproate

dependent upon duration of the seizure. Treatment of status epilepticus includes airway maintenance, initiation of intravenous dextrose solution, and pharmacotherapy. Diazepam given intravenously is an effective means of aborting seizures. Phenytoin and phenobarbital are also used. Status epilepticus requires a thorough evaluation at a medical facility.

Medication therapy in athletes with seizure disorder is utilized in an attempt to decrease or prevent future attacks. Exercise does not affect anticonvulsive drug metabolism and, as previously mentioned, has not been shown to precipitate seizure. It should be noted, however, that a 10% weight reduction in a basketball player in training might affect the serum level of antiepileptic medications.

Specific drugs-of-choice are identified for each type of seizure and titration of dosage is required (Table 8.5). Typically, dosage is initiated at a safe level and gradually increased until seizures are controlled or a maximal dose has been achieved. If symptoms persist despite maximal drug dosage of the first medication, a second drug can be added. Laboratory monitoring of serum levels is necessary for some antiepileptics and therapeutic concentrations have been established. Anticonvulsant drug use has been associated with hepatotoxicity and aplastic anemia. For this reason, blood cell parameters and hepatic function should be followed as well.

Mentally and physically challenged athletes

Some athletes are faced with obstacles far more difficult to overcome than their able-bodied counterparts. Many physically and/or mentally challenged athletes regularly participate in basketball (Fig. 8.1). The World Health Organization has established

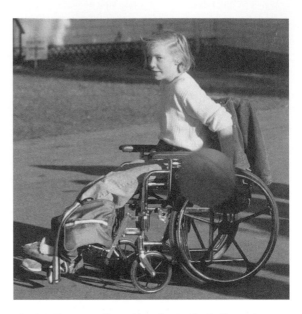

Fig. 8.1 For mentally and/or physically challenged athletes, basketball is an important and popular sport.

specific terminology and definitions to clarify confusion regarding this athletic population. Impairment is defined as any loss or abnormality of psychological, physical, or anatomical structure of function. Disability refers to any restriction or lack of ability to perform an activity in the manner or within the range considered normal for a human being. Handicap implies a disadvantage for a given individual (resulting from an impairment or a disability) that limits or prevents the fulfillment of a role that is normal for that individual based on age, sex, and social and cultural factors.

International competition at elite levels against equally matched disabled persons has become possible over the last half century. The first such international organized games for disabled athletes took place in England at Stoke Mandeville hospital in 1948. This event came to fruition secondary to the determined effort of Sir Ludwig Guttman and was initially intended for paraplegic war veterans of World War II. The Stoke Mandeville games gained popularity as competitions were held every 3 years. Meanwhile, interest mounted throughout the world. In 1960, the first Paraplegic Olympic Games (Paralympics) were held in Rome following the Rome Olympics with participation by 23 countries and over

Table 8.6 Cerebral palsy classification.

Class of cerebral palsy	Description
1	Unable to propel manual wheelchair
2	Able to propel manual wheelchair
3	Able to propel manual wheelchair with near normal function in one extremity
4	Propel chair without limitations
5	Ambulates with assistive device(s)
6	Ambulates without assistive device
7	Involvement of one-half of body
8	Minimal involvement

400 wheelchair athletes. The Paralympics continue to be held every 4 years in conjunction with the Olympic Games. Growth has been constant and over 120 countries now participate.

Many levels of competition for disabled athletes exist and specific groups are represented by organizations based on disability classification (e.g., National Wheelchair Athletic Association). Classification of disability is based on physical involvement and quality and quantity of muscle function required to perform sport-specific activities. Each class is further subdivided based on a medical evaluation and functional assessment of ability. This Functional Classification System (FCS) (4) is a key component to allow for evenly matched competitors. The classification of disability for international competition is as follows:

1 *Visually impaired*: any cause of resultant visual loss.

2 *Cerebral palsy*: includes congenital and early insult; also included in this class are cerebral trauma, cerebrovascular accident, quadriplegia or tetraplegia, and diplegia with spasticity, ataxia, or athetosis (Table 8.6).

3 *Amputation*: any cause of limb loss above or below elbow or knee with prosthesis or orthosis.

4 *Wheelchair athletes*: spinal cord injury or disease with loss of spinal cord nerve function.

5 *Les autres* (French = all others): class includes all conditions that do not fit into other groups such as dwarfism and muscular dystrophy. Functional classification allows for fair competition with athletes from other classifications.

6 *Intellectual disability*: this group has not been included in previous Paralympics, but will be rep-resented in the future and is also well represented in Special Olympics in the United States.

Hearing-impaired athletes are not addressed in the Functional Classification System. Deaf athletes typically have similar motor development and physical fitness levels when compared to their peers. The exception is seen in the hearing-impaired athlete who also has suffered concomitant injury to the semicircular canal system or vestibular apparatus with resultant equilibrium deficits. The major barrier to athletic competition for deaf basketball players is difficulty in communicating with teammates. Various tactics are employed to assist communication using visual rather than auditory cues. The international governing body for deaf athletics is the International Committee of Silent Sports. This committee organizes and hosts the World Games for the Deaf.

Training principles for basketball players with disabilities do not differ significantly from those employed in an able-bodied population. Gains in muscle function and cardiovascular functional performance are attainable goals. Upper body flexibility and strength training should be stressed in wheelchair athletes and can be achieved using a stretching program along with resistance exercise and weight training. Cardiovascular gains are seen as improvements in maximal oxygen consumption with rigorous training.

Certain precautions must be taken during the training process. As in any program, safety is the first lesson and injury prevention must be taught. Athletes with high-level spinal cord injury will fatigue faster and require longer rest periods between training sessions. Also, the heart rate response may not be an accurate measurement to follow for training progression in the spinal cord disabled athlete. Lastly, it is important to educate the athlete on perceived symptoms associated with injury, disease exacerbation, or medication side-effects. As previously mentioned in the seizure disorder discussion, medication adjustments may be necessary if an athlete's body weight decreases by 10% or more during training.

Education and preparation are essential for providers of medical care to the disabled athlete. This requires an understanding of the underlying impairment and the effect on exercise performance.

ABERDEEN COLLEGE

An example of this is the high rate of atlanto-axial instability in athletes afflicted with Down's syndrome. The medical staff must also keep abreast of the continual technological and medical advances related to each individual disability. In addition, understanding the effects of prescribed medications used by basketball players with disabilities is an integral part of assessing the athlete. Problems encountered by disabled athletes can be divided into four types:

1 *Disability-related*: Problems associated with the underlying medical condition (i.e., urinary retention or urinary tract infection in a wheelchair athlete).

2 *Disability-related, exacerbated by competition*: Problems associated with impaired condition, subsequently worsened by competition (i.e., pressure sores in a wheelchair athlete).

3 *Disability-unrelated, competition injury*: acute or chronic sports-related injury.

4 *Incidental*: medical condition encountered unrelated to disability or competition (i.e., upper respiratory infection).

Early diagnosis and intervention by the sports medicine specialist can maximize performance and prevent potentially devastating outcomes.

The musculoskeletal injuries experienced by basketball players with disabilities are similar to those seen in their unaffected counterparts. Overuse injuries are common, especially those involving the upper extremities and shoulders in wheelchair participants. Prevention or minimization of overuse injuries is possible and should be stressed. Means of prevention include stretching and conditioning programs and the use of appropriate protective equipment, taping, and padding. The wheelchair athlete should be fitted with an appropriately sized, efficient chair that minimizes shoulder abduction and rotational movements.

Among the possible overuse syndromes that can be seen is carpal tunnel syndrome. Wheelchair basketball players experience repetitive trauma to the palmar aspect of the hands and can develop an entrapment of the median nerve as it passes through the carpal tunnel. Symptoms are similar to those reported in the general population and include numbness and tingling, pain, and weakness. The use of gloves and a properly sized chair can decrease the likelihood of occurrence.

Wheelchair athletes comprise a high percentage of the total number of disabled athletes that participate in basketball. This group of competitors has attracted a great deal of scientific research and public attention. Although persons with bilateral, above-knee amputations are eligible to compete in this class, the vast majority of these athletes have spinal cord injuries or disease with resultant loss of spinal cord nerve function. Discussion of wheelchair athletes in this text will refer to the group with loss of spinal cord nerve function. Specific topics of discussion include thermoregulatory dysfunction, bladder dysfunction, osteoporosis, pressure sores, and autonomic dysreflexia.

Athletes with spinal cord injury commonly have impairment of autonomic and sensory nervous systems resulting in alteration of the body's normal thermoregulatory function. This dysfunction is secondary to:

1 Reduction in vasomotor and sudomotor responses.

2 Loss of sensory impulses below the level of the spinal cord injury to the hypothalamus causing impaired response to exercise and temperature changes.

3 Reduced venous return from the lower extremities secondary to loss of the skeletal muscle "pump".

Wheelchair athletes experience the most difficulty with extremes of temperature. Hypothermia or hyperthermia can be seen in this group. Preparation is the key to prevention. Recommendations for prevention of hyperthermia and heat injury include minimizing clothing coverage, using damp cloths or cool mist spray (especially for athletes with impaired sweating response), remaining in shaded areas when not competing, and pushing fluid replacement. Dry weight measurements before and after exercise or competition can be used to guide fluid replacement (16 ounces of fluid per pound lost). Signs and symptoms of heat or cold illness should be monitored for and treatment should proceed promptly if suspected.

Bladder dysfunction in the wheelchair basketball player results from neurologic derangement. These athletes are at risk for infection of the bladder, urethra, and kidney. Infection can be associated with significant morbidity and mortality. Bladder rupture is also possible if severe urinary retention occurs. The use of intermittent catheterization and appropriate hydration can decrease occurrence of complications. Antibiotic administration at the first sign of infection is recommended.

Disuse of the paralyzed lower extremities can lead to osteoporosis. Osteoporotic bones are predisposed to fracture from minimal trauma or even muscle spasm. Prevention is best accomplished with liberal padding and good nutritional balance.

Pressure sores are possibly the most common problem encountered by the wheelchair basketball player. Skin breakdown occurs insidiously with prolonged sitting and lack of pressure redistribution. The athlete with spinal cord injury is unable to sense the pain and discomfort usually associated with tissue ischemia and eventually necrosis can occur. Basketball players seem to be at increased risk for pressure sores because of repetitive lateral movements and shifting that creates high sheer forces at the skin–wheelchair interface. The areas most commonly involved are the ischial, sacral, and trochanteric regions. Pressure sore preventive measures include encouragement to frequently redistribute weight, appropriately sized chairs with custom cushions, and moisture-absorbing clothing to decrease frictional force. Early recognition and treatment of pressure sores can minimize lesion progression and reduce the risk of infection.

Wheelchair athletes with a spinal cord lesion above the 6th thoracic vertebrae are predisposed to a condition known as autonomic dysreflexia. This is a commonly encountered condition and health care providers for wheelchair athletes should be familiar with its presentation and treatment. Autonomic dysreflexia manifests with hypertension, tachycardia or reflex bradycardia, headache, anxiety, and profuse sweating. Extreme hypertension can result in hemorrhagic cerebral vascular events. These symptoms are produced by generalized hyperactivity of the sympathetic nervous system. Most commonly, the cause is a distended viscus (bladder or rectum). Other stimuli have been implicated including urinary tract catheterization or infection, sunburn, pressure sores, and tight leg straps. Treatment is based on cessation of activity and removal of the sensory stimuli that provoked the response.

Conclusion

In conclusion, providing care to basketball players with disabilities requires an understanding of the unique impairments and differences in physiologic response. Involvement of multiple disciplines is needed to adequately prepare the athlete for competition. Participation in basketball, and sports in general, has continued to gain popularity over the past several decades. Persons with disabilities will continue to comprise a large percentage of the sports population and sports medicine professionals should be prepared to participate in their care.

Further reading

Albright, A.L. (1997) Diabetes. In: *ACSMs Exercise Management for Persons with Chronic Diseases and Disabilities*, pp. 94–100. Champaign, IL: Human Kinetics.

American Diabetes Association (1997) Report of the Expert Committee on the diagnosis and classification of diabetes mellitus. *Diabetes Care* **20**, 20–35.

American Diabetes Association (2001) Diabetes mellitus and exercise. *Diabetes Care* **24**.

Consult, M. (1998) Consensus statements: medical management of epilepsy. *Neurology* **51**, 39–42.

Cooper, C.B. (1997) Pulmonary disease. In: *ACSMs Exercise Management for Persons with Chronic Diseases and Disabilities*, pp. 74–80. Champaign, IL: Human Kinetics.

Dykens, E.M., Rosner, B.A. & Butterbaugh, G. (1998) Exercise and sports in children and adolescents with developmental disabilities: positive physical and psychosocial effects. *Sports Psychiatry* **7**, 757–771.

Exercise, C. (1990) Diabetes mellitus and exercise. *Diabetes Care* **13**, 804–805.

Fernhall, B. (1997) Mental retardation. In: *ACSMs Exercise Management for Persons with Chronic Diseases and Disabilities*, pp. 221–226. Champaign, IL: Human Kinetics.

Harries, M. (ed.) (1998) *Oxford Textbook of Sports Medicine*, 2nd edn. Oxford: Oxford University Press, p. 957.

Lai, A.M., Stanish, W.D. & Stanish, H.I. (2000) Pediatric and adolescent sports injuries: the young athlete with physical challenges. *Clinics in Sports Medicine* **19**, 793–819.

Lehman, R. *et al.* (1997) Impact of physical activity on cardiovascular risk factors in IDDM. *Diabetes Care* **20**, 1603–1611.

Mellman, M.F. & Podesta, L. (1997) Primary care of the injured athlete. Part II Common medical problems in sports. *Clinics in Sports Medicine* **16**, 635–662.

Moriarity, J. (2000) The diabetic athlete. In: Johnson, R. (ed.) *Sports Medicine in Primary Care.* Philadelphia: W.B. Saunders, pp. 283–302.

Niedfeldt, M. (2000) The asthmatic or allergic athlete. In: Johnson, R. (ed.) *Sports Medicine in Primary Care.* Philadelphia: W.B. Saunders, pp. 278–283.

Niedfeldt, M. (2000) Seizure disorders and athletes. In: Johnson, R. (ed.) *Sports Medicine in Primary Care.* Philadelphia: W.B. Saunders, pp. 311–316.

Palmer-McLean, K. & Wilberger, J.E. (1997) Stroke and head injury. In: *ACSMs Exercise Management for Persons with Chronic Diseases and Disabilities*, pp. 169–174. Champaign, IL: Human Kinetics.

Rice, E.L. (2001) The disabled athlete. Lecture 2/01.

Sallis, R.E. (2001) Exercise-induced asthma. Lecture 2/01.

Spiegel, R.H. & Gates, J.R. (1997) Epilepsy. In: *ACSMs Exercise Management for Persons with Chronic Diseases and Disabilities*, pp. 185–188. Champaign, IL: Human Kinetics.

Wallberg-Henriksson, H., Rincon, J. & Zierath, J. (1998) Exercise in the management of non-insulin-dependent diabetes mellitus. *Sports Medicine*, 25–35.

White, R.D. (2001) Managing the diabetic athlete. Lecture 2/01.

Chapter 9
Psychological issues in basketball

Christopher M. Carr

Introduction

How much of the game of basketball is "mental"? Or more specifically, when one is involved in the game (as a player or coach), how much of the game is related to cognitive (beliefs, attitudes, thoughts) and affective (feelings) components? In many ways, the answer to this question helps to address the psychological aspects of basketball performance. Of course, the answer also addresses the extent to which an athlete or coach incorporates psychological skills to enhance basketball performance. If an athlete or coach docs not believe in these "psychological" components to basketball, there will be little or no teaching of psychological skills to enhance performance. However, when a coach or an athlete recognizes the "mental" skills of basketball performance, and commit themselves to a mental skills training plan, then they are optimizing the opportunities to overcome psychological barriers to performance.

The purpose of this chapter is to highlight some of the psychological components of basketball performance. Specifically, the author will address how a psychological skills program to enhance performance will benefit basketball skills. Issues addressed in performance-enhancement skills will include: (a) effective goal setting skills for basketball; (b) arousal regulation skills for basketball performance; (c) focus and concentration skills (mental imagery) for basketball performance; (d) cognitive-behavioral interventions for optimal basketball performance; and

(e) basketball-specific (e.g., free-throw shooting) mental training skills. These skills can be adapted to enhance performance as a player at any level of competition, although developmental considerations will surely exist. By presenting a general model of psychological skills that enhance cognitive and affective levels of performance, the reader will better understand the "mental" side of the game (Fig. 9.1).

The last section of the book will specifically address the issue of "performance anxiety", which is a general term used to describe an individual's negative performances in the game, in spite of their superior physical talents. Knowing how to differentiate between normal signs of performance anxiety and symptoms of an anxiety disorder is very relevant based on the background of the consulting sport psychologist (who may or may not be a licensed psychologist). The sports medicine professional will also benefit from recognizing differences between an anxiety disorder and typical performance-related anxiety with basketball.

Performance-enhancement techniques in basketball

Basketball combines elements of both team and individual performance; each aspect of performance can be enhanced through the utilization of mental training skills. These skills, which manifest from a cognitive behavioral orientation to human thought,

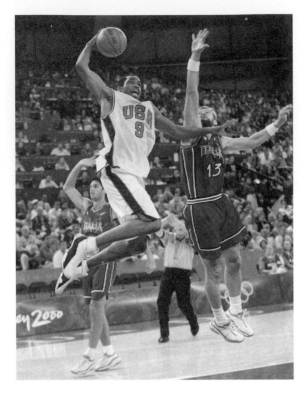

Fig. 9.1 Skills and conditioning are vitally important, but motivation is also essential for high-level performance. Photo © Getty Images/Darren McNamara.

emotions, and behavior, can be learned via repetitive practice. In this brief chapter, the author will highlight the four basic mental training domains, which are: (a) goal setting skills; (b) arousal regulation skills; (c) focus and concentration skills; (d) cognitive–behavioral mental routines; and (e) basketball-specific mental training skills. A basic review of performance-enhancement skills will be presented in each domain. As a sports medicine provider, a basic understanding of performance-enhancement skills may add to your consultation style in the sport of basketball. Basketball players at all levels, whether it is professional, elite amateur, or secondary school, will be seeking ways to enhance their sport-specific skills. This basic review of mental training domains for improving basketball performance will provide the sports medicine professional with helpful information.

Goal setting skills: achieving your best in basketball

As a mental training domain, goal setting represents the very "foundation" of a mental skills program. Goals provide direction, motivation, and feedback in the development of basketball ability. Every basketball team, player, and coach can readily state their "goal" for competing. However, most athletes and coaches do not utilize goal setting in the best manner possible. In fact, a common error observed is for coaches and athletes to state goals as follows: "Win the League Championship"; "Get 15 wins"; or, "Make the playoffs". These outcome goals, although relevant to performance, are only measurable at one point in time: the end of the season. In a league of 15–20 teams, it is a pretty safe bet to think all of the teams have a goal of "winning the league". However, only one will actually accomplish their goal. Thus, the first key to understanding goal setting is to focus on both process and outcome goals.

Outcome goals are results. Scoring averages, assists per game, rebounds per game, and the team's final standing are examples of outcome goals. Of course these goals provide direction for a team, but again are only measurable at the end of competition. Process goals represent the steps that are taken towards the final outcome. For example, an outcome goal of "shooting 85% from the free throw line at the end of season" may be facilitated by such process goals as: "Shoot 75 free throws after each practice"; "Visualize a perfect free throw shot every night"; or, "Make 85% of my free throws in practice". Basketball players and coaches should have a process of setting both process and outcome goals for each player on the team. Again, **outcome** goals reflect the final result, and **process** goals reflect the journey taken on a day-by-day basis. The author often recommends that athletes write their outcome goals on a piece of paper at the beginning of the season, and then place that paper in an envelope to open at the end of the year. Then he recommends that they write 1–2 goals for each practice on a 3″ × 5″ card or piece of paper before each practice. As the achieved process goal cards stack up in his/his locker, internal confidence increases and the player is more likely to play with concentration, confidence, and composure.

Another important element to goal setting as a mental training skill is the ability to state goals that are **specific, challenging, realistic, achieveable**, and **measureable**. Specific goals are clear and relevant to the performance task. For example, an athlete who desires better accuracy in shooting can state a goal as: "Take better shots" (vague), or "Make 60% of my shots within 15 feet of the basket" (specific). Making goals that are specific is often challenging to both the athlete and coach, as it requires a good knowledge of the athlete's present skill level and an ability to specify goals for improving performance.

Challenging goals reflect individual differences. For example, a challenging goal for a 6'11" forward who averaged eight rebounds a game the previous season would be stated as "Average 9 rebounds a game for 15 games". On the other hand, if the same player averaged 60% accuracy in free throw shooting, a goal of 80% may be too challenging. The key to setting challenging goals is to assess the current skill level of the player in the various performance areas (e.g., shooting, rebounding), then set a goal that is just above their current level of performance. A goal that is easily accomplished every practice (nonchallenging) will create boredom and distraction, whereas a goal that is never accomplished in practice (current performance is not close to goal) may create frustration and anxiety in practice. In either situation, boredom or frustration, the player may begin to feel decreased motivation for the game, and the current level of performance will then deteriorate. A goal that is a challenge will maintain intrinsic motivation and focus on the performance-specific task. For example, a college player who plays the point guard averaged eight assists a game in the previous season. After an off-season of training and competition, he has improved his ball-handling skills. In early practices his passes are crisp and he has good court vision. Setting a goal of 10 assists a game may be a challenging goal initially; however, if he starts the first five games with seven assists, the coach may want to adjust the goal to eight assists for the next five games. If, on the other hand, he averages 12 assists in the first five games, the coach may adjust the goal to 13 assists per game for the next five games. All goals must have an ability to be flexible and adjusted, as athletes must clearly redefine goals in certain situations. For example, an athlete who becomes injured must now adjust totally his or her goal-orientation, as the tasks accomplished during rehabilitation are clearly different than those tasks accomplished in full training mode.

Another individual variable to goal setting is the ability to set **realistic** goals. A realistic goal reflects the individual's current level of functioning and skill development. Because of the variety of individual factors, the coach and trainer have the best ability to help the athlete set realistic goals. For example, for a basketball player in the initial stages of ACL reconstruction recovery it would be unrealistic to set a goal of playing full-court basketball in 3 months; the key component is awareness of current functioning/skill, and then adjusting realistic goals for that level.

To maintain motivation and focus, the athlete must be able to set **achievable** goals for performance. By achieving process goals, the sense of satisfaction and confidence from goal-achievement helps to maintain motivation and commitment. The object of process-oriented goals is to achieve them; therefore, the athlete maintains motivation and enthusiasm to set a new and challenging goal to accomplish. As an example, a player sets her goal of 75% from the free throw line for her first three games. After three games, she is shooting 77% from the charity stripe and has a consistent free throw routine that is working for her. She will feel a sense of accomplishment, reward, and confidence, and will also trust her routine and practice it consistently. She can now set a goal of 78% for her next three games, and so on. Her practice free throws will reflect her focus and concentration. Without a goal for this performance skill, she may accept any performance, and thereby limit her own growth in an important facet of the game.

Finally, goals must be **measureable**. That is, both the athlete and coach know if he/she accomplished the goal. A goal that is stated: "Do better today" may be logical, but not very measurable. After all, who knows what "better" is? and is doing "better" accomplished in the athlete's eyes but not in the coach's? A more measurable goal is stated: "Shoot 50 lay-ups after practice". This goal is easy to measure, as the athlete either did or did not shoot 50 lay-ups after practice; they were either successful or unsuccessful in their goal-directed behavior that will improve a basketball-specific skill.

Once a goal-setting process has been established, and the task-relevant goals have been set following the "SCRAM" (specific, challenging, realistic, achievable, measurable) guidelines, the athlete and coach should have clarity regarding the improvement of basketball skills. The author recommends that coaches establish regular goal-setting meetings with each player at the following intervals: preseason; in-season (every week/every other week); and, postseason. Additionally, if a player becomes injured, the coach should consult with the sports medicine staff to set goals related to their rehabilitation compliance and return to play. Coaches can create their own goal-setting handouts to review with each athlete at these meetings; the handouts can be self-developed and typically reflect goals in the sport-specific skill development. For basketball, players may set goals in the following areas: field goal shooting; free throw shooting; ball-handling; rebounding; defensive play; ball movement; movement without the ball (e.g., screens); and other performance domains important to the coach. These can include academics, mental skills preparation, physical conditioning, and off-court behaviors. Although this may appear overwhelming, it does create direction, discipline, and motivation for the athlete if accomplished collaboratively with the coaching staff.

Goal setting therefore becomes the "foundation" for the rest of the athlete's mental skills repertoire. The rest of their mental skills preparation becomes developed and practiced based on the goals the athlete has set regarding his or her mental skills commitment. If the athlete and coach do not create goals for improving performance in the mental skills arena, then the athlete is less likely to engage in the behaviors necessary to master the mental toughness that is required in competition.

Arousal regulation: getting "butterflies" to fly in formation

When an elite basketball player describes his or her optimal basketball performance, they are likely to use words such as "relaxed", "easy", "smooth", and "effortless". In most descriptions of optimal

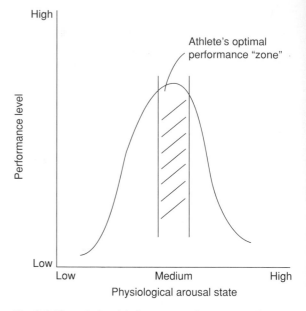

Fig. 9.2 The relationship between performance and physiological arousal state.

performance, the athlete reports a calm and relaxed mental approach to the game. Even when they describe their play as intense and aggressive, they will also report feeling relaxed.

An understanding of the "inverted-U" hypothesis (Landers & Boutcher 1986) best represents (in simplest form) the relationship between physiological arousal and performance (Fig. 9.2). According to the hypothesis of the "inverted-U", performance is highest when the individual has a moderate amount of arousal/activation. When the arousal level (e.g., "nerves", "butterflies") is too high, the athlete's performance decreases. Additionally, if the arousal level is low/flat, the performance is also negatively affected. When the athlete reports a sufficient feeling of arousal (e.g., "energy"), they have increased performance. This model best represents the relationship between arousal states and performance when working with athletes. There will be basketball players who can clearly identify with decreased performance when they were feeling "too nervous", and also when they played "flat, without emotion". Although there are other models and theories (e.g., Zones of Optimal Functioning) that discuss the relationship between arousal states and performance, for purposes of this brief chapter the "inverted-U" hypothesis will be utilized.

The inability to control arousal state in basketball performance creates two significant dilemmas. First, increased arousal may lead to increased muscular tension and biomechanical adjustments. For example, a player who feels nervous at the free throw line may begin to experience the increased arousal state at the moment when the foul is called on the opponent. The athlete begins to worry (cognitive anxiety) and then the body begins to "feel nervous", with resultant increases in muscle tension. If this tension is uncontrolled, and the player steps to the free throw line in a crowded gym with screaming fans (external distractors), the tension may cause biomechanical changes in the execution of the free throw, which may lead to a negative outcome (missing the shot). No wonder then, that athletes who often shoot 25 out of 25 free throws in practice have difficulty shooting even 70% in game situations. The task itself (shooting the free throw) is no different in the games than in practice; however, the athlete's arousal level is higher and uncontrolled, and therefore more likely to be executed incorrectly.

A second problem of uncontrolled arousal states is the attention and concentration changes that occur. Nideffer (1976) has studied extensively the effects of arousal states on attention in athletics. In general, he has found that when athletes increase their arousal, their attention becomes more focused. If the arousal is too high (and uncontrolled), the athlete's focus may be so directed on only one aspect of the performance that they do not concentrate on other relevant cues. For example, when the above player steps to the free throw line, he is aware that he is "really nervous" and "fears" missing the shot and "disappointing my team" (cognitive anxiety). In this high arousal state, he focuses his total attention on the front of the rim, remembering what he has been coached. However, he is unaware that his legs are straight and rigid, and therefore he executes the free throw with an improper base (nonattended task cue).

When the athlete is in "the zone", often used to describe an optimal performance state, he/she is focused only on the cues relevant to the task being performed. The athlete does not attend to the waving fans, the sound of the band, or the fact they have missed their last two free throws (irrelevant to current task). They focus on a deep breath to relax, focus their eyes on the rim, take a few bounces of the ball, bend their knees, and execute the shot with a fluid motion. This optimizes their chance for performance success with that skill (a made free throw). Controlled arousal states can lead therefore to concentration and attention to the relevant tasks for performance.

A common technique used to control arousal states is relaxation training. This form of mental training skill can teach the athlete to control muscular tension and breathing in high-arousal situations. Relaxation techniques must be practiced in order to be effective. There are various forms of techniques, such as progressive muscle relaxation (progressively tensing and then relaxing each of the major muscle groups, accompanied by deep breathing techniques) and autogenic training (focus on kinesthetic feel and association of feelings with relaxation vs. tension). The author has found that athletes, especially at elite levels, are very kinesthetic and body-aware. When given the appropriate tool (e.g., relaxation exercise), they are able to develop mastery of the exercise. Research in areas such as clinical health psychology has praised the benefits of relaxation with pain management, stress management, and cardiac recovery. The author has utilized relaxation techniques in consulting with injured athletes as they progress in rehabilitation.

To utilize relaxation as a mental training skill, the athlete must first set a goal of practicing relaxation training. For example, a basketball player can write a goal of "doing relaxation exercise four evenings a week for 15 min each session". Many of the recommended readings at the end of the chapter have relaxation exercises included; also, individuals can purchase relaxation exercises on audiotape/CD to listen to as an exercise. The following represents a segment of an autogenic relaxation exercise:

(Individual has focused on deep breathing for 2–3 min). . . . "now feel the sensation of warmth flowing from your shoulders into your arms. . . . deep breath in . . . deep breath out . . . feel the warmth flow over and through your biceps and triceps . . . feel the warmth wash away the tension and fatigue in your muscles. . . . feel the warmth flow through your elbows. . . . (continue deep breathing. . . . focus on slowing breaths) . . . feel the warmth flow over and through your forearms. . . . across your wrists. . . . visualize the warmth removing the dark tension in your wrists, hands, and fingers. . . . feel the warmth flow through your hands and through the ends of your fingers as the tension is pushed out of your fingertips . . ." (continue exercise down through the major muscle groups from head to toe) . . .

The above exercise represents a segment of an exercise that requires 10–15 min of quiet focus and concentration. As the athlete practices this skill, a transfer effect occurs on court. When they now step to the free-throw line and receive the ball from the referee, they take a deep breath in and then breathe out. As they breathe out, they feel the sensation of warmth (relaxation) flow from their head to their toes, and the anxiety (tension) leaves their body. They are still activated, but are now "in the zone". Their body feels relaxed, their mind is calm, and they now focus on the successful free throw shot.

Controlling arousal states, which are inevitable in the athletic arena, is essential to maintaining composure (keeping "cool" under pressure). By setting a goal of relaxation practice on a regular basis, the athlete can control his physiological tension in situations where his performance requires fluid

motion (e.g., three-point shot). This control of tension, thus, creates an enhanced sense of self-control and self-confidence. A sample arousal regulation mental training intervention may look like the following:

1 Listen to relaxation CD five nights a week;
2 Do exercise in dorm room with lights off;
3 Develop a "cue" word when relaxed that represents the relaxed state;
4 Record exercise/cue word in mental training journal.

This simple exercise creates a manageable skill for any athlete who desires increased control of arousal states and an ability to manage "butterflies in the stomach". There are, of course, individual differences that are reflected in the interventions of each athlete. A competent sport psychologist will take a careful history of the athlete, including assessment of optimal arousal states. Creating a relaxation CD for the athlete is one positive benefit of the athlete–sport psychologist relationship. Once the athlete has developed a plan for arousal regulation, he/she can more effectively develop concentration and focus mental training skills.

Focus and concentration skills for basketball

As mentioned previously, one of the factors influenced by arousal states is concentration and attentional focus. When arousal states increase, there is a decrease in concentration and focus. When an athlete is in their optimal performance "zone" (comfortable arousal state, Fig. 9.3), they are focused on the relevant task cues. That is, they are paying attention to the elements of performance that represent an optimal performance state. For example, when a point guard is in a "flow" state, he has clear vision of the court and the movements of his teammates. He is aware of his passing lanes and effortlessly handles the ball in pressure without losing his vision and focus. He drives the lanes and either lays the ball in the net or passes to an open post player under the basket. His play is smooth and quick. He is focused on what he needs to pay attention to for each offensive and defensive trip down the court. He does not think about a missed shot or an errant pass; in fact, he has a routine to "let go"

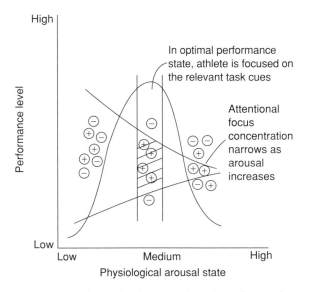

Fig. 9.3 The relationship between physiological arousal state, attentional focus, and relevant task cues for sport.

(cognitively) of these mistakes so he can focus his attention on the relevant cues. Clearly, this is a desired performance state for a basketball athlete.

If the arousal state is too high, then the athlete becomes overly aroused and focused on one aspect of performance, while not attending to other relevant cues. After a bad pass, for example, a player gets frustrated (high arousal state) and then loses concentration long enough for his opponent to break-off of a screen and score an easy basket. Because the player was already frustrated, the coach starts to yell, he gets more frustrated, and now he is in an anxiety-stress spiral. The risk of unmanaged frustration and arousal is that it creates a negative cognitive distraction, which subsequently increases the arousal state to a higher level.

The key to focus and concentration skills (in the sport of basketball) is to gain awareness of what are the important task cues to execute the requisite skills. When the athlete is in an optimal performance state, she is focused on only the relevant cues (Fig. 9.3). Therefore, the key to effective mental skills preparation is to recognize and teach/learn those relevant task cues. How can an athlete create this concentration and focus prior to competition? Imagery is now introduced as a focus and concentration mental skill.

Imagery: "seeing" is believing!

Imagery is a cognitive-behavioral intervention that athletes use to imagine their actual performance in a quiet, uninterrupted environment. "Seeing through the mind's eye" represents the technique of imagery. Successful imagery utilizes multiple senses, and can be conducted as either an **external** or **internal** imagery exercise. External imagery represents an observational view; that is, the athlete (with eyes closed) watches himself execute a successful three-point shot from the top of the key. The best way to describe external imagery is to see it as when you watch videotape; however, individualized external imagery is more of an external "close-up" (e.g., a basketball player visualizing himself making a perfect free throw; watching himself make the smooth mechanical release).

Internal imagery, however, is a more kinesthetic intervention. In this type of exercise, the athlete incorporates feeling, vision, tactile senses, auditory senses, and in-the-moment reflection as she sees "from her own eyes" herself steal the ball from her opponent and throw a perfect outlet pass to start a fast break. With internal imagery, since the athlete is practicing the performance from within her own mind, she incorporates the sense of touch and movement. An athlete who reports the following: "I watched myself take the outlet pass, dribble past the half-court line and thread a pass in the lane to my center for an easy lay-up" is describing external imagery. If the athlete used the following description: "I felt the ball come into my hands off the backboard . . . when I landed on my feet, I turned my head and saw the two guard break open to the right. . . . I started my dribble and didn't look at the ball . . . after six dribbles I looked to my left and released a quick pass to my right, where the two set-up for a wide-open three . . . I felt the bodies bang into mine as I got in position for the rebound. . . . I felt fast, quick, and strong", she would be describing an internal imagery exercise.

Keys to using imagery in basketball

In order to use imagery effectively as a mental training skill, there are some important variables to consider. First of all, internal imagery has been found to be more effective in the mastery of skills, whereas external imagery may be more effective in the initial learning stages of a specific skill. For example, a coach would recommend that his perimeter players "feel" the shots from the perimeter, especially the feel of successful shots. On the other hand, a middle school (11–13 year olds) basketball coach may show a video of crossover dribbles before taking the players on the court for drill work. Secondly, relaxation training enhances imagery practice. When the author develops a performance tape/CD for an athlete, a 10–15 minute autogenic relaxation exercise is followed by a brief guided (internal) imagery exercise. Again, understanding individual athlete skill levels is imperative to guiding mental skills interventions.

Third, imagery skills will develop over time. It is unrealistic for an athlete to expect an instant response. The author recommends that imagery practice focuses on brief elements of skills until mastery develops. For example, a player can visualize the successful completion of two free throws rather than visualizing all of the attempts they may expect in a game (e.g., 15 shots). Create a basic set of skills (remember to go back to the relevant task cues for each skill) and practice internal imagery. A coach may observe his players doing a fast-break drill very well; at that point the coach may stop the drill, have the players close their eyes, reflect on the feeling they have at that moment, and then replay the movement in their minds. This reinforces the "feeling" state of optimal basketball performance, which creates subconscious confidence. Fourth, utilize positive images of performance. Simply put, visualize "how to do it" rather than "how NOT to do it". Words can inappropriately guide our images. If a coach yells out to a player on the court "Don't let your man drive past you", what image is created? Usually the player would visualize his opponent driving past him for two points. However, the coach may instead yell out "Maintain good balance and guard the lane". By changing his words to a positive focus, the player can now visualize the feeling of a good defensive posture and incorporate positive execution of the performance.

Finally, imagery skills can be developed only with repetition and practice. Although the athlete may experience some immediate feelings of confidence and focus, the skills must be practiced regularly for optimal results. Practice, practice, practice, and most importantly, create vividness and control in imagery. From the past 12 years of applied sport psychology work with athletes, the author has found that very few successful elite athletes visualize the outcome (e.g., medal ceremony). In fact, elite athletes can recall vivid details of performance surroundings and replicate the "feeling" of optimal performance (e.g., the feeling of a perfect jump shot).

Cognitive-behavioral interventions: developing mental routines

Once the athlete has established goals for performance, and has begun to practice relaxation training and imagery exercises to gain composure and concentration skills, the mental skills program can be individualized. Cognitive-behavioral interventions are targeted to enhance the cognitive (thoughts/thinking/attitudes) and behavioral (plans/behaviors/rituals) aspects of performance. This orientation to performance enhancement posits the belief that once the athlete has committed to a mental skills routine, the plan becomes an integral component in the state of "mental readiness". Some of the interventions that can be used to enhance basketball performance include: self-talk/self-confidence strategies; mental training journals; premental rituals; and, the use of "cues" in performance focus.

Self-talk and self-confidence are complimentary to each other. The dialogue that an individual generates in their own mind (self-talk) often represents the degree of confidence they have in themselves. Sport psychologists have defined confidence as "the belief that you can successfully perform a desired behavior" (Weinberg & Gould 1995). Beliefs represent a cognitive paradigm. Although it is expected that many athletes may verbalize "I'm confident in my shooting skills", how many of them actually *believe* this at an internal (self-talk) level. Perhaps they may state their confidence externally (e.g., "Coach, I can make this shot"), when in reality, they have doubt in their internal self-talk (e.g., "Don't miss it . . . coach is counting on me"). Athletes are often limited by their own negative self-talk and lack of self-confidence. In the history of sport this has been true. For years before 1954, no runner had run the mile in under 4 : 00 min. When Roger Bannister believed, then accomplished the feat, running the mile under 4 minutes, within one year more than a dozen runners broke the 4-minute mark. Why? Perhaps because those competitive runners now *believed* it could be done, so they visualized themselves being fast enough.

A basketball athlete may incorporate self-talk strategies to enhance confidence and focus in his or her performance. The use of positive self-statements ("I am a confident defender" or "I am strong in the paint") on a series of 3×5 cards or in a mental training journal that can be viewed daily will enhance confidence. The techniques are not overly complicated; rather, they are a simple set of replicable and positive self-statements that can be utilized to enhance confidence. By associating positive self-statements with preparation for competition, an athlete can build confidence and positive performance. False confidence represents an external perception of performance with little intrinsic belief.

The use of a mental training journal (logbook, diary) can be a cognitive process that allows the athlete to reflect not only on positive outcomes, but to "let go" of negative performances. For example, a college basketball player discusses his journal use:

> "The journal allows me to revisit my game. . . . If I had a good performance, I can write about how I felt, what I was focused on, my use of cue words. . . . it creates a positive picture in my mind. If I had a bad game, I can write down my mistakes . . . acknowledge my being human, and then tear out that page and throw it away. . . . Surprisingly, I even have good plays in the games I thought I played horrible. My journal helps me to become aware. . . . now I use it to read before every game, because when I read about my good games I start to get that excited feeling . . ."

The use of a mental training journal does not have to follow a rigid pattern. In fact, the author encourages individualism in journaling. The key is to do it! The author often challenges athletes this way: If doing something different for 5 minutes a day (writing in journal) will help you improve your game by one assist, or two points, or two more rebounds, is it worth it? The answer is self-determined. A journal may also contain the athlete's pregame mental routine, which can then be a "checklist" for mental preparation and confidence.

A fourth cognitive-behavioral intervention is the development of a premental routine. For example, in basketball a player may have a preshot, prefree-throw, pregame, and during-game (refocus) mental routine. The bottom line to any preparation mental routine is to achieve the optimal performance state for that task. For example, a prefree throw mental routine should be developed first from the player's optimal performance. The player would write down her best free-throw performance, then identify the relevant tasks and cues for that performance. If a player discovers that their optimal performance at the free-throw line is enhanced when they feel relaxed, easy, and smooth ("cues"), then their prefree-throw routine will incorporate those cues into the preparation of executing the shot. Again, the individual variables are extensive and must be assessed to help the athlete develop the "best fit" for

a mental routine. "One size fits all" mental training routines are not especially helpful.

Finally, "cue" words represent an associative phenomenon. For example, when the player sees the shot clock go to "02" seconds, they automatically respond with a move towards a shot. The cue is the clock, and more specifically, the time on the clock. When an athlete incorporates cue words into his or her mental preparation plan, the cues are best associated with optimal performance. For example, if a power forward has used the word "strong" in many of his journal entries to describe his feeling when he is productive around the basket, then he may write the word "strong" on his wrist or top of his shoes. Thus, when he begins to feel distracted or doubtful regarding his performance, he can look at his "cue", close his eyes, take a deep breath, and create the image of being "strong" around the basket. It refocuses his attention and recreates a confident (vs. doubting) feeling. In working with collegiate basketball players, the author has encouraged them to have their "cue" words visible; the sight of the word can create a subconscious connection to performance that may be missed if the athlete only "thinks" about the cue word. Creativity and utilization of these cognitive-behavioral strategies becomes more effective as the athlete commits to a mental skills plan and uses the interventions to "weave" together the goals, feelings, and focus (concentration) of optimal athletic performance.

Basketball-specific mental training tools

Every sport has dynamics that are unique. The author has experience not only with collegiate and elite-level basketball players, but has worked with professional/world class alpine skiers, baseball players, race car drivers, and soccer players (among others). In understanding each sport, there are unique components of the game that are relevant to mental training skills. Even though the components of mental training skills development (goal setting, arousal regulation, focus/concentration, and cognitive-behavioral skills) remain constant among sports, there are some unique components of basketball that will be briefly discussed. Included are: free throw shooting mental routines; regaining focus

---

Free throws: creating a mental routine

What's the difference? Nothing, really. The mechanics of shooting a free throw are the same in practice and in games. Only the EXTERNAL dynamics are different; the crowd, the noise, the game situation, and the players on the court. The ability to "mentally" focus on shooting free throws has to do with your practicing the "mental" aspects of the performance. When you are "focused" on the free throw, chances are you will make it most of the time. Here are a few mental "tips" to creating a positive mental free throw routine:

(1) Practice RELAXATION . . . When you teach your body how to relax, you will be able to relax it during a game when the situation creates more anxiety. You will be able to achieve the relaxation feeling often with just one deep breath.

(2) VISUALIZE successful free throw shooting in a game situation. At least once a day, you can practice visualizing yourself making the front end of a one-and-one in a tight game situation. The better you can feel it, see it, hear it, and make it . . . the more likely it will happen in reality.

(3) Practice SIMULATION. When you are shooting in practice, create "scenarios" that may occur in a game. Close your eyes and visualize the arena, hear the crowd, then execute your routine.

(4) Create CUE WORDS that represent the "state of mind" you are in when you are making your free throws. If you go 10 for 10 in a stretch of practice, close your eyes and think of a word that reminds you of that feeling (in that moment). Then write the word down and use it during your pre-game routine so that the feeling of successful free throw shooting is AUTOMATIC.

(5) CREATE A PRE-SHOT ROUTINE. A sample routine would include the following:

> *1–3 deep breaths (to create relaxation) before stepping to line*
> *1–3 deep breaths after getting ball from official*
> *Positive "cue" word to focus on during routine*
> *Consistent actions during routine (dribbles, spins, etc.)*
> *Feeling relaxed, Focused on rim, Smooth and fluid release*
> *Positive self-talk after shot, even if miss, Stay consistent!*

I hope these "tips" help in your mental preparation for free throw shooting. Remember to stay consistent, relaxed, and positive. . . . Good Luck!!

Fig. 9.4 Mental training skills.

after substitution; and, dealing with sport-specific distractions.

Figure 9.4 is a free-throw mental training handout that the author used while at The Ohio State University as the Psychologist for the Athletic Department. After observing the college basketball game and environment, it was apparent that free throw shooting was the one performance area that players had the most trouble adjusting to from practice to the game. It was common for players to shoot 70%, 80%, even 90% in practice, but struggle to shoot 60% in games. An observation of the author was the lack of a structured mental routine to prepare for the execution of the free throw. The figure represents guidelines that were given to players to use a mental training "tool" to develop their concentration and confidence at the charity stripe.

Another aspect of basketball performance that can create mental "barriers" is the ability to refocus

and regain confidence after spending time on the bench. This can be observed from the scenario of a role player coming off the bench 15 min in the game, or the scenario of a starter committing unforced errors, being substituted out, then re-entering the game later. In both instances, the player may utilize a structured focus/refocus routine. For example, a small forward is usually the second frontline player off the bench. He will come out and go through warm-ups, then sit on the bench until his name is called. He may feel that he needs "a few minutes" to get in the flow of the game. In fact, that creates a self-limitation, as his total playing time may only equate to "a few minutes". Therefore, he benefits from having a "cue" word that he can look at when he is called off the bench. This cue word represents the feeling of being in flow . . . being aggressive . . . being focused. . . . being comfortable handling the ball . . . and so on. By having a routine, he becomes more self-determined (focused on what he controls) rather that situation-determined (focused on distractions). He thus optimizes his chance for optimal play during his brief time on court.

In the other situation, a point guard commits two unforced turnovers, has the ball stolen from her, and then commits a "silly" second foul when she reacts out of frustration. The coach substitutes her out, and may or may not talk with her on the bench. If the player does not "let go" of the mistakes (turnovers, fouls), she may re-enter the game thinking "Don't throw the ball away". If she has a refocus mental routine, she may come off the court, sit down, get the feedback from the coach, then as she wipes away sweat from her forehead say to herself "I am wiping away my mistakes". A drink of water may be followed by the self-statement "I feel the water refuel my engine . . . I am quick and focused". She may then glance at a cue word on her wrist or shoes, close her eyes, take a deep breath, and "let go" of the mistakes and then see herself (external imagery) on the court making a great assist. By recreating her focus with a routine, she is less situation-dependent (extrinsically motivated) and more self-dependent (intrinsically motivated).

Finally, the game of basketball is filled with numerous external distractions including (but not limited to) rowdy fans, loud arenas, officiating (both positive and negative), media, and travel. Each of these distractions can impact player performance negatively if the player does not utilize a coping mechanism (e.g., mental preparation routine). In research with Olympic athletes, the most successful of competitors have the most detailed plans and strategies of what they want to do. They also have alternative plans for distractions (Gould *et al.* 1992). The author recommends that athletes create a mental routine for dealing with distractions associated with basketball. As an example, a player will have a cue word they use whenever they feel an official's call was incorrect. Once the call is made, the game continues. Therefore, the player will choose if they want to continue "in the flow", or by playing distracted. If they recognize that they feel frustrated, then perhaps the snap of a rubber band around their wrist will refocus their attention (as an example). Again, the individual variation of athletes comes into relevance here. A well-planned coping routine

will always create a better result than attempting to correct "in the moment" (due to the anxiety-stress spiral). As soon as the player regains focus on themselves, they can regain the composure and confidence necessary for optimal performance. If they are unable to "let go" of distractions, they will create a heightened awareness of the distraction and become even more distracted. . . . and further away from their optimal performance state.

Putting it together: a mental training "recipe"

Using the metaphor related to cooking, an athlete should see the development of a mental skills plan as making a recipe (for optimal performance on the court). Each ingredient is necessary for the final product to be satisfying. Not every attempt will turn out the same, but with practice and repetition, the recipe becomes more ingrained and focused. After significant practice, the athlete doesn't have to look at the recipe to get the ingredients. Everything "comes together" and the end product is very good! The following represents a general and basic mental training "recipe" for enhancing performance as a basketball player:

1 Get a notebook for a mental training journal. Start with one entry a day.

2 In your journal, write down 2–3 goals for your next practice. Further back in the journal, write down the goals that you desire, but can only be measured at the end of the season. . . . don't go back to that page very often, focus more on the daily goals.

3 Begin a relaxation exercise for 4–5 days each week. Find a script in a sport psychology book or buy a relaxation tape from a record/book store. Record in your journal how the exercise feels and if you have "cue" words you associate with relaxation. Stay with it.

4 At the end of each relaxation exercise, visualize yourself executing 2–3 plays (e.g., free-throw shot, rebound) exactly how you want them to happen. If you can do it while seeing it through your own eyes (internal), start there. If that is difficult, watch a videotape of your practice and then recreate that positive play in your mind (external). While at practice, close your eyes and see if you can recreate (in that moment) the feelings/images associated with

positive play. Record your imagery exercises in your journal.

5 Develop a pregame and prefree throw mental routine. Start by writing about your "best game" you've ever played in basketball (then best shot, free throw, etc.) in your journal. Create a simple, 2–3-step routine that you control and creates the positive feelings associated with optimal performance.

6 Record your self-talk in your journal and challenge negative thinking and self-talk. Reframe your negative thoughts into positive challenges and reflect in your journal.

By following this basic "recipe" an individual athlete can begin the framework of an individualized performance-enhancement program.

Performance anxiety in basketball

Anxiety is a multidimensional concept within the field of sport psychology. When discussing anxiety in a performance context, one can focus on cognitive anxiety (thoughts, worry) or on somatic anxiety (physiological responses) (Weinberg & Gould 1995). Performance anxiety in sport can be manifested in the form of an athlete's exaggerated movements in the locker room 10 minutes before tip-off to the excessive perspiration of a teammate under minimal exertion.

For the sports medicine professional that provides care for basketball athletes, it is important to "know" your athletes. In this sense, you have awareness of how the athlete responds to practice and game situations. By establishing an observed baseline of behavior, the sports medicine professional/coach/sport psychologist can become sensitive to changes, both subtle and drastic, in the behavior of an athlete prior to competition. The obvious risks of performance anxiety responses are that they are generalized to other performance areas (e.g., academics), or they "trigger" symptoms of an anxiety disorder. The following disorders are classified as anxiety disorders and are found in the *Diagnostic and Statistical Manual of Mental Health Disorders* (DSM-IV): panic attack; agoraphobia; panic disorder without agoraphobia; specific phobia; social phobia; obsessive-compulsive disorder; post-traumatic stress disorder; acute stress disorder; generalized anxiety disorder; anxiety disorder due to a general medical condition; substance-induced anxiety disorder; and, anxiety disorder not otherwise specified (American Psychiatric Association 1994). An overview of each anxiety disorder is not necessary for the context of this chapter; however, a general discussion of symptoms of anxiety conditions is warranted to differentially diagnose between an actual anxiety disorder and "performance" anxiety.

Whereas anxiety disorders such as post-traumatic stress disorder and acute stress disorder can have immediate onset of symptoms, most clinical anxiety disorders (e.g., generalized anxiety disorder) may have a 6-week to 6-month period where symptoms can manifest. When there is a concern that an athlete may be exhibiting atypical anxiety symptoms, a prompt intervention and referral would be warranted. In this instance, the referring source (e.g., team physician) should have clear knowledge of the referral source's training. If the individual is listed as a "sport psychologist", make sure to inquire about licensure as a practicing psychologist. If they are licensed, then question the amount of training/experience they have in working with an athletic population. The author, who has worked with athletes as a psychologist for the past 15 years, has often observed various behavioral and cognitive symptoms that may meet DSM-IV criteria for an anxiety disorder, when in fact, they are typical responses to the competitive athletic environment (for example, feelings of accelerated heart rate, sweating, shaking, and shortness of breath may indeed be symptoms of a panic attack; however, when about to take the court in the NCAA Final Four Basketball Tournament these symptoms may be experienced by everyone on the team).

In brief summary of differentiating between performance anxiety and anxiety disorders, there is a general rule one can follow. Because the world of sport and competition generates significant situational stress (e.g., crowd noise, performing in front of large crowds), there will be some physiological (e.g., elevated heart rate) and cognitive (e.g., worry about performance) symptoms that are not reported in other situations. However, if those symptoms (e.g., excessive worry) cause a significant disruption in the athlete's day-to-day functioning, an underlying anxiety disorder may be occurring. Using one's best clinical judgement and use of appropriate referral sources (e.g., sport psychologist) is recommended.

The sports medicine professional will be able to observe cognitive, affective, and behavioral changes in athletes based upon knowledge of baseline data (individual athlete responses) and deviations in these observed baselines. At this point, a gentle intervention of dialogue can help promote referral or the acceptance of a referral. If a sport psychologist (licensed psychologist) is available, a sports medicine professional can consult on the case without disclosing athlete information. In the treatment of anxiety disorders, cognitive-behavioral interventions have been found to be most effective, with some pharmacological interventions also helpful (dependent upon diagnosis/type of anxiety disorder). Proper knowledge of symptoms, knowledge of athletes, and knowledge/availability of competent sport psychologists is necessary in the care of athletes who struggle with anxiety related to competition.

Conclusion

The game of basketball requires confidence, focus, goal-direction, and composure to be successful. The utilization of cognitive-behavioral interventions has been shown to be effective in enhancing performance in sport. There is no "magic", no "motivational stories", no "quick fixes" to developing a solid mental skills routine to enhance athletic performance. However, a commitment to goals and a commitment to activities discussed in this chapter can help the basketball athlete to gain control of arousal states, develop enhanced concentration for performance, and create a sense of confidence and focus in his or her basketball abilities. Understanding that the game of basketball creates energy and anxiety is important in providing athletes with clear guidance as to differentiating between typical responses and atypical anxiety responses, which may inhibit performance.

References

American Psychiatric Association (1994) *Diagnostic and Statistical Manual of Mental Disorders*, 4th edn. Washington, DC: American Psychiatric Association,

Gould, D., Ecklund, R.C. & Jackson, S.A. (1992) 1988 U.S. Olympic wrestling excellence. I. Mental preparation, precompetitive cognition, and affect. *Sport Psychologist* 6, 358–382.

Landers, D.M. & Boutcher, S.H. (1986) Arousal-performance relationships. In: J.M. Williams (ed.) *Applied Sport Psychology: Personal Growth to Peak Performance*, pp. 163–84. Palo Alto: Mayfield.

Nideffer, R.M. (1976) *The Inner Athlete*. New York: Crowell.

Weinberg, R.S. & Gould, D. (1995) *Foundations of Sport and Exercise Psychology*. Champaign, IL: Human Kinetics.

Further reading

Csikzentmihalyi, M. (1990) *Flow: the Psychology of Optimal Experience*. New York: Harper & Row.

Jackson, S.A. & Csikzentmihalyi, M. (1998) *Flow in Sports*. Champaign, IL: Human Kinetics.

Martens, R., Vealey, R.S. & Burton, D. (1990) *Competitive Anxiety in Sport*. Champaign, IL: Human Kinetics.

Orlick, T. (1986) *Psyching for Sport: Mental Training for Athletes*. Champaign, IL: Leisure Press.

Orlick, T. (1990) *In Pursuit of Excellence*. Champaign, IL: Human Kinetics.

Chapter 10
Basketball injuries: head and face considerations

William F. Micheo and Enrique Amy

Introduction

Basketball, once considered a noncontact sport, has evolved into a game of speed, strength, and aggressive play. These factors, along with the increasing popularity of the sport, have resulted in an increase in the number of injuries associated with playing the sport (Kunkel 1994). At the present time, basketball is considered a contact-collision sport with significant risk of injury to head, facial, and oral structures (American Academy of Pediatrics Committee on Sports Medicine and Fitness 1994) (Fig. 10.1). Unlike other sports like football, in which mandatory use of facial protective equipment has resulted in a decrease in injuries, basketball has no universal regulations regarding the use of this equipment for the prevention of facial and oral injuries.

The prevalence of tooth injuries in children and adolescents has been described in the past in different studies. One survey of the dental literature indicates that the incidence of reported injury ranges from 4% to 14% of the patients examined with males two to three times more likely to suffer some sort of trauma than females. It is interesting to note how the incidence of dental trauma has increased in the last 50 years. The age in which these injuries are more frequent is between 8 and 15 years. The majority of the cases of trauma are in the anterior maxillary area or the upper anterior teeth, especially the two central incisors and the superior lip (Amy 1996). In a study conducted by Olvera in the United States between 1988 and 1989 in data reported by

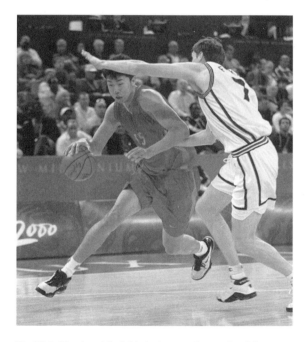

Fig 10.1 Head and facial injuries are the result of the contact-collision nature of contemporary basketball. Photo © Getty Images/Darren McNamara.

the National Federation of High Schools, it was revealed that of a total of 254 956 cases evaluated in the sport of basketball, the majority of injuries were to the anterior area of the face (Olvera 1990). Gomez *et al.* (1996) reported 14% incidence of dental injuries in a study of girls participating in high school basketball. Another site of significant incidence of injury in basketball players is that of the eye. In a study conducted to evaluate the epidemiology of eye injuries in professional basketball players 50% of the injuries were lacerations to the eyelid, 28% contusions to the periorbital region and 12% were corneal abrasions (Zagelbaum *et al.* 1995).

Management of injury to the head and face requires knowledge of the most common conditions associated with the sport of basketball. Members of the sports medicine team should have basic knowledge in the management of these conditions. Oral health professionals should be an integral part of the medical team with additional consultants available for the management of complicated head and face lesions (Chapman 1989). The dentist, together with other professionals in the field, should emphasize oral and visual health as elements of general health in all sports and, because of its particular relevance, in contact-collision sports. Problems of the head and face are frequent and many times they are the principal cause of a poor performance by an athlete or of his/her retirement from competition. In this chapter we want to emphasize the importance of appropiate diagnosis, management, and referral in the treatment of the injured basketball player. However, in this particular type of injury, prevention strategies are of utmost importance given the fact that the use of appropriate equipment such as protective eyewear and mouthguards may result in a significant reduction of injury (Kerr 1986; Zagelbaum *et al.* 1995).

Head injuries

Recognition of a severe head injury is relatively easy particularly if the athlete has a complete loss of consciousness. However, mild head injuries are much more frequent in contact-collision sports. In these injuries, there is no loss of consciousness but rather only a transient loss of alertness or a brief period of post-traumatic amnesia that may be difficult to recognize. More than 90% of all cerebral concussions fall into this mild category (Cantu 1996).

The majority of these mild traumatic brain injuries result in a transient neurologic syndrome without structural damage to the brain. Concussion is defined as a clinical syndrome characterized by the immediate and transient post-traumatic impairment of neural function such as alteration of consciousness, disturbance of vision or equilibrium due to brainstem involvement (Sonzogni & Gross 1993; Johnston *et al.* 2001). In basketball, injury may occur secondary to a direct blow to the face from an elbow or a fall in which the player strikes their head against the floor.

Damage to the brain associated with acceleration forces applied to the head can be the result of compression, tensile, or shear forces. The mechanisms of traumatic brain injury include coup/countercoup in which a forceful blow to the resting head produces injury beneath the point of impact (coup), as well as damage to the opposite side of cranial impact because of movement of brain structures inside the skull (countercoup). Other mechanisms of brain damage are direct compressive forces associated with a skull fracture and the application of external forces to the head when the neck muscles are weak or in a relaxed state (Cantu 1996).

The acute symptoms of concussion have been described in detail in many published studies. Signs and symptoms include amnesia, loss of consciousness, headache, dizziness, blurred vision, attention deficit, and nausea. In addition, there are a wide variety of subjective findings that may be encountered in concussed athletes. These include descriptions of vacant stare, irritability, emotional lability, impaired coordination, sleep disturbance, noise/light intolerance, lethargy, behavioral disturbance, and altered sense of taste/smell. The time to resolution of these signs and symptoms is extremely variable (Torg & Gennarelli 1994; Johnston *et al.* 2001).

When evaluating an athlete with a brain injury who is unconscious, it must be assumed that they have suffered a neck fracture, and the neck must be immobilized. In assessing an athlete with a head injury who is conscious, the level of consciousness or alertness is the most sensitive criteria for both establishing the nature of the head injury and subsequently following the athlete. Orientation to person, place, and time should be ascertained. The presence or absence of post-traumatic amnesia, and the ability to retain new information such as the ability to repeat words immediately or after 15 min, as well as the ability to repeat one's assignments on certain plays in the contest should be determined (Grindel *et al.* 2001) (Table 10.1). It is also important

Table 10.1 Sideline tests of memory.

Immediate recall of three words
Recall of three words after 15 min
Recent memory items (game score, period quarter, who scored last/won, describe last play, field location)
Months in reverse order
Orientation (name, date of birth, age, year)

Modified from Grindel *et al.* (2001).

to do a complete neurologic examination and to establish the presence, absence, and severity of neurologic symptoms such as headache, lightheadedness, difficulty with balance, coordination, and sensory or motor function.

Injury severity can be classified based on the presence or absence of loss of consciousness and post-traumatic amnesia. Multiple classification scales exist which attempt to establish the severity of concussion. Dr Robert Cantu and the American College of Sports Medicine, the Colorado Medical Society, and the American Medical Society for Sports Medicine among others have published scales of severity classifying the injuries into mild, moderate, and severe categories (Johnston *et al.* 2001) (Table 10.2).

The two most serious sequelae to mild traumatic brain injury (i.e., concussion) are irreversible and crippling cognitive deficits, and death due to second impact syndrome. Return to play before the brain can recover from an injury may lead to either of these serious complications, though prolonged cognitive deficits can be seen after a single initial insult. Second impact syndrome can lead to death within minutes and may occur if a second mild traumatic brain injury follows an initial unresolved brain injury in young athletes (Torg & Gennarelli 1994; Cantu 1996).

A less serious, yet potentially debilitating result of a concussion is postconcussion syndrome. Postconcussion syndrome involves prolonged, disabling, and sometimes permanent symptoms such as headache, dizziness, nausea, tinnitus, depression, irritability, slowed mental processing, impaired attention, and deficits in memory. Multiple concussions, particularly within a short period of time, have been shown to lead to long-term and sometimes permanent cognitive deficits as well as increasing one's risk of postconcussion syndrome (Johnston *et al.* 2001).

After a diagnosis of concussion has been made, there are many factors that may influence the return-to-play decision. These include injury severity, past history of the athlete, demands of the chosen sport, the presence of postconcussive symptoms, and the speed of resolution of the acute symptoms. While scientifically validated return-to-play guidelines do not yet exist, the consensus of experts in this field would suggest that complete resolution of concussion symptoms (both at rest and with exercise) would be mandatory prior to the resumption of training or playing. An example of guidelines to return to competition after concussion endorsed by the American College Sports of Medicine is shown in Table 10.3 (Cantu 1996).

Rare but severe brain injury associated with basketball includes second impact syndrome or malignant brain edema, hematomas, and intracranial hemor-

Table 10.2 Severity of concussion.

Grade	Cantu (1986)	Colorado (1991)	AMSSM
Mild	No LOC PTA <30 min	No LOC No PTA confusion	No LOC Symptoms <5 min
Moderate	LOC <5 min PTA >30 min	No LOC PTA confusion	LOC <1 min Symptoms 5 min–24 h
Severe	LOC >5 min PTA >24 h	LOC	LOC >1 min Symptoms >24 h

LOC, Loss of consciousness; PTA, Post-traumatic amnesia.
Modified from Johnston *et al.* (2001).

Table 10.3 Guidelines for return to play after concussion.

	First concussion	Second concussion	Third concussion
Grade 1 (Mild)	Return if symptom free for 1 week	Return in 2 weeks if symptom free for 1 week	Terminate season, return next season if symptom free
Grade 2 (Moderate)	Return if symptom free for 1 week	Return in 1 month if symptom free for 1 week Consider terminating season	Terminate season, return next season if symptom free
Grade 3 (Severe)	After 1 month return if symptom free for 1 week	Terminate season, return next season if symptom free	

From Cantu (1996).

rhages. As previously mentioned, the second impact syndrome may occur when an athlete is still symptomatic from an initial head injury and sustains a second head injury. Usually within seconds to minutes of the second impact, the initially conscious but stunned athlete precipitously collapses, with rapidly dilating pupils, loss of eye movement, and evidence of respiratory failure. Epidural hematomas are characterized by head injury, mild symptoms such as headache, and deterioration of consciousness 15–30 min after the initial injury. This lesion typically occurs with a temporal skull fracture from a blow received in the temporal area and is associated with a tear in the middle meningeal artery. In these patients death may result from the mass effect of the rapidly expanding blood causing brain herniation. Subdural hematomas, which are the most common cause of death in athletic head injury, are usually associated with immediate loss of consciousness that does not get better. Intracerebral hematomas usually occur deep within the brain and are associated with an extremely severe acceleration injury to the head. Typically consciousness is not regained unless this lesion is extremely small (Torg & Gennarelli 1994).

The management of severe brain injury in an athlete who has collapsed includes protection of the cervical spine, cardiopulmonary resuscitation, and prompt transportation to a medical facility with the capability to perform computed tomography or magnetic resonance imaging of the brain. Other techniques of management may include hyperventilation, intravenous steroids, and intravenous osmotic diuretic administration.

Ocular and orbital injuries

In some areas of the world basketball is the most common cause of sports-related ocular trauma. Basketball players are therefore placed in the "high risk" category for sustaining eye injuries by the International Federation of Sports Medicine (Guyette 1993). A wide range of injuries to the eye can occur ranging from eyelid injury, corneal abrasion, periorbital contusion, hyphema, or orbital fracture. The majority of injuries occur in the act of rebounding and are caused by fingers or elbows in athletes not wearing protective eyewear.

Significant ocular injury can occur that may be missed on superficial examination. Therefore, if a player presents with decreased vision, persistent pain, diplopia, or any question as to the location or extent of the injury, prompt ophthalmologic consultation should be obtained.

A common injury found in basketball players is corneal abrasion or laceration. The player will usually present with pain, epiphora, and photophobia. The diagnosis is made by topical fluorescein staining and examining the eye under ophthalmoscopic magnification. Minor injuries can be treated with topical medication and patching of the eye.

The globe is protected from penetration by objects by strong bones of the orbital rim. When there is an anterior blow to the orbital region by a nonpenetrating object, such as a ball, fist, or elbow, the orbital contents are forced backward into the narrow portion of the bony orbit. The sudden increase in intraorbital pressure by the noncompressible soft tissues of the eye can result in fracture and displacement of the thin bones of the medial wall and floor of the orbit. If the orbital rim and other facial bones remain intact, the fracture is termed a "pure" orbital blow-out fracture (Guyette 1993). In some cases this injury can result in enophthalmos, infraorbital paresthesia, and diplopia.

There is considerable controversy regarding the treatment of these injuries including the indications for and timing of surgical intervention. In the patient with an orbital fracture without symptoms such as diplopia, conservative treatment may be attempted. Many surgeons feel that surgical repair is indicated when there is a combination of radiographic or computed tomographic evidence of extensive fracture, limitation of forced rotation of the eye, and significant positional change of the globe (Guyette 1993).

Because of the significant risk of ocular injury the use of eye protectors should be considered for basketball players. Glass lenses, lenseless eye guards, and ordinary plastic lenses do not provide adequate protection and, in many situations, can increase the risk and severity of eye injury. The ideal eye protector should prevent injury to the eye by dissipating force onto the glabella and supraorbital ridges, protective eye wear should be light, comfortable, and should not increase the chance of injury by limiting vision. The lenses should be constructed of polycarbonate because of its superior impact resistance (Zagelbaum *et al.* 1995).

Facial and dental injuries

Facial and dental trauma occur more frequently than is generally believed. Evaluation of oro-facial trauma is, in great part, an art. It requires experience, finesse, knowledge, patience, agility and a very creative, intuitive and quick mind to make the correct decisions in a tense situation.

Dental trauma should always be considered an emergency and should be treated immediately (Amy 1996). It is very important to obtain the most complete information from the history and the examination given that it can help the clinician to make decisions about clinical management. The exam or evaluation should be conducted in a systematic and organized manner. The dentist or clinician should look for facial asymmetry, injuries of soft intraoral and extraoral tissue. Also, the dentist should look for subcutaneous hematomas and possible bone fracture, especially under the tongue. If bleeding is present, the origin of this should be determined and then controlled. In many cases, this helps determine whether there is bone fracture. The clinician should also determine whether there is an anomaly of the occlusion or bite of the patient and whether the patient can close the mouth easily. Many times, the bite can be crossed or deviated toward one side. This can indicate the possibility of fracture or dislocation of the jaw. It is important to palpate the alveolar process (bone), the temporomandibular joint and the soft tissue, as well as the tongue and intraoral mucosa.

When dental trauma occurs in primary dentition (deciduous), it usually results in tooth displacement instead of alveolar or bone fracture. In permanent teeth, damage depends on the angle, strength and direction of the impact. Frequently, the root or crown of the tooth fractures. Displacements, such as intrusion, extrusion, lateral displacement or complete avulsion can also occur. When dental trauma occurs, movement of the tooth and change in tooth color can be detected.

When impact is toward the lips, it can result in contusion, subluxation, lateral luxation (i.e., dislocation) or intrusions of teeth, together with laceration of the lips. Indirect impacts can result in intrusion with or without laceration of the lip. In a case where the athlete receives an impact on the jaw during competition, that energy will be absorbed by the condyles and the symphysis which could cause a tooth fracture. In some instances, tooth fragments that are not palpable can be impregnated in the soft tissue and noted radiographically. These fragments can cause acute or chronic infection and disfiguring fibrosis (scar). The purpose of performing radiographic studies is to evaluate the maturation stage of the root and to identify trauma to the bone structures. The radiographic views utilized more frequently are the periapicals and the occlusal but other studies that can be taken include the panoramic, Towne's or

Water's view as well as a chest radiograph to detect a swallowed tooth or tooth particles (Amy 1996).

Injuries in soft tissue

The soft tissues that are usually involved are the lips, gingival tissue, alveolar mucosa, and tongue. The lips are the ones affected the most in contact sports. The treatment will depend on the location and extent of the injury. The oral cavity is characterized by great vascularity and when an intraoral laceration occurs, bleeding is abundant. It is necessary to control the hemorrhage first to decide on the most adequate way to correct the problem. An airway should be kept open at all times.

Lacerations in the oral cavity can be classified into four types:

1 Simple laceration—it produces an open cut in the gingiva or oral mucosa as a result of a hit or contact with an object with edges.

2 Combined laceration—results from a hit or contact with a nonedged object and is accompanied by a hematoma of the mucosa.

3 Erosion or scraping—injury that results as a consequence of a fall. It is characterized by loss of skin and exposure of subcutaneous tissue with bleeding.

4 Multiple lacerations—various lacerations occur with luxation, dental avulsion or bone fracture.

The resulting lacerations from trauma can be clean or contaminated. Clean injuries do not generally need antibiotic therapy and heal in less than 48 h. Contaminated injuries are those that have been invaded by pathogenic bacteria of the oral flora, saliva or pharynx. These should always be treated with antibiotics, preferably penicillin or third generation cephalosporins, if the patient is not allergic to them. If the patient is allergic, erythromycin, tetracycline or clyndamycin can be used. Tetanus prophylaxis and a booster of tetanus toxoid is recommended as well.

Lacerations can generally be managed with local anesthesia given by way of an anesthetic injection with or without vasoconstrictor. In some cases where alveolar fractures occur, it is necessary to administer general anesthesia in a center where the patient can be hospitalized. The suture material mainly used in the oral cavity is 3–0 or 4–0 silk. For the subepithelial tissue, catgut collagen or catgut chromic is re-commended. This material is removed after 5–7 days (Amy 1996).

Soft tissue injury to the face includes abrasions, contusions, and lacerations. Most lacerations occur over a bony prominence of the facial skeleton. Because of the excellent blood supply in the facial region, wounds usually heal quickly with minimal scar formation. The wound should be thoroughly irrigated and should be closed in layers with absorbable sutures in deeper tissues and a subcuticular closure of buried absorbable sutures. This allows for adhesive paper strips or small caliber inert sutures to be placed for closure of skin without tension. Cutaneus sutures should be removed in 5–7 days to avoid permanent suture marks (Guyette 1993).

In summary, recommendations for management of soft tissue lacerations of the mouth include:
- Appropriate antibiotic coverage and analgesia.
- Treatment for teeth trauma, after controlling the bleeding. It is recommended to suture soft tissue after the tooth and bone trauma have been corrected.
- Take radiographs of the area to determine whether a bone fracture exists.
- Keep the tissue wet (sterile saline water).
- Keep the injury as clean as possible.
- Consultation with an oral and maxillofacial surgeon in the case of severe or combined lesions.

Tooth displacement

When a tooth displacement occurs, time is the most critical factor and the tooth should be repositioned as soon as possible. It is desirable to have a dental evaluation within the first 2 hours after the trauma and to make a splint or fix the tooth with wire or resin for 7–10 days.

The following are the various types of tooth luxations that exist:
- Contusion—it is described as trauma that occurs to the structures that hold the tooth in place without abnormal displacement taking place. The tooth may be sensitive to percussion.
- Subluxation—it is described as trauma to the structures that hold the tooth in place, with displacement. This displacement is not easy to detect clinically or radiographically. The tooth retains its

position in the arch; there can be hemorrhage in the gingivae, which indicates periodontal damage.

• Extrusion—it is an avulsion or partial displacement of the alveolar bone; it will have the appearance of an elongated tooth.

• Lateral luxation—it is an eccentric displacement of the tooth towards the tongue. In many instances, it is associated with a fracture of the alveolar wall.

• Intrusion—it occurs when a tooth penetrates the alveolar bone; and it can be accompanied by a comminuted fracture of the bone. When the area is examined, it is easily noticed that the tooth is very firm inside the bone. This is a rare type of trauma associated with falls or direct facial trauma in contact sports.

After the facial trauma it is convenient to examine carefully the affected area and to make sure that the exact placement of the tooth is known. Endodontic treatment is recommended when the displacement is more than 15 mm, depending on the degree of maturity of the root of the tooth. When displacement is less than 15 mm, the tooth should be evaluated periodically to make sure that it is still vital. If the tooth cannot be seen, the tooth may be completely in the bone or in the nasal cavity. It is very possible that these teeth will not respond normally to vitality tests for a few months.

Avulsed tooth

An avulsion can be described as complete displacement of a tooth (Fig. 10.2). It occurs when a tooth comes out of the bone and falls to the floor or competition field. Tooth avulsions generally occur during car accidents or participation in contact sports. An avulsed tooth should be reimplanted as soon as possible. It is recommended to recover the tooth and place it in a sterile isotonic solution such as Hank's or Eagle solutions, or milk. Because of the possibility of bacterial contamination it is not recommended to put it in the patient's mouth unless there is no other option. The tooth should be examined carefully, cleaning it gently with tap water or Ringer's solution to remove dirt or debris. It should not be rubbed vigorously with gauzes filled with solutions that contain chemicals. For a tooth to be reimplanted it should be free of advanced periodontal disease or extensive fractures. It is desirable to have

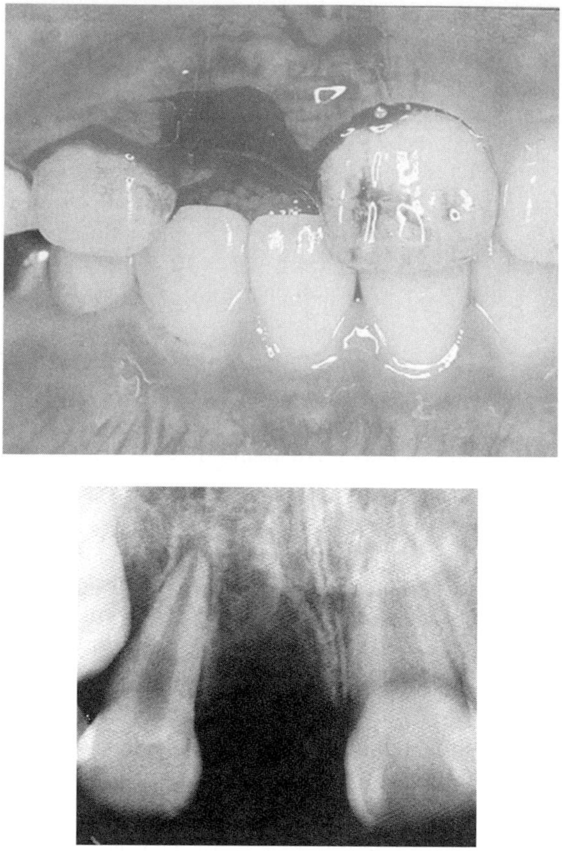

Fig. 10.2 Avulsed tooth (maxillary right central incisor).

a dentist reimplant the tooth; but in case that there is no dentist when the accident occurs, the clinician should conduct the reimplantation (Table 10.4).

After a referral to the dentist if an endodontic treatment is needed, it is recommended to wait one week prior to treatment. If the apex is immature, the recommendation is to wait one to two weeks after the reimplantation has occurred to begin endodontic therapy. If evidence of pulp pathology is detected, the tooth canal is thoroughly cleaned and filled with calcium hydroxide. The patient should be followed up every 6 to 8 weeks. In many cases, liquid fluoride is applied to avoid reabsorption of the root (Amy 1996). Survival of avulsed teeth varies and many last up to 20 years.

When a tooth is to be reimplanted, it is always recommended to irrigate it with water to clean the

Table 10.4 Steps for tooth reimplantation.

• Gently wash the tooth with water or Ringer's solution and eliminate any dirt or debris.
• Place the tooth between your fingers using the index finger and thumb. With both fingers insert the tooth holding it by the crown. Make sure that the convex or curved part of the tooth is towards the lip or facing outside.
• Slowly take the tooth toward the bone or the space where it came out of and push it until you see that it is in place. Compare the position with the adjacent teeth.
• If the patient was using a mouth protector, place the protector in his/her mouth after reimplanting the tooth. Antibiotics and analgesics can be prescribed at that moment.
• Take the patient to the dentist as soon as possible. Success of the reimplantation improves if it is done in the first hour after the trauma.

debris. The alveolus in the bone should also be cleaned to remove the contaminated clot. As is well known, the blood clot plays a very important role in the revascularization process and if the clot is contaminated, the reimplantation process could be affected. Some authors recommend the tooth to be submerged in tetracycline solution for 15 min and the alveolus to be irrigated as well.

When an avulsion takes place, the periodontal ligament is affected and the blood vessels break, and this increases the likelihood of pulp infection. If reimplantation occurs within the first 6 hours, there is probability of success, however, reimplantation within the first hour gives the best results. Following the reimplantation infection should be controlled. Despite appropriate treatment one of the most com-

mon consequences of tooth avulsion is reabsorption of the root (Kehoe 1986).

Root fracture

When a root fracture occurs, time is critical and the patient should be seen as soon as possible. The affected tooth should be splinted with a wire splint and resin temporarily and pain should be be treated adequately. The location of the fracture will determine the treatment which could include tooth extraction, surgical exposure of the fractured surface, orthodontic treatment, or surgical extraction of the root. The final treatment could be instituted several days after the trauma.

Fracture of anterior teeth

When a dental fracture that involves the enamel and dentine occurs and the pulp is not involved, it should be covered with calcium hydroxide and splinted with resin and wire (Fig. 10.3). It should finally be restored at 6–12 weeks. When the fracture involves the nerve of the tooth with an open apex, after the first 3 hours of the injury, calcium hydroxide should be applied. When the pulp exposure is massive and more than 3 hours have passed since the trauma, a pulpotomy should be performed to maintain vitality and maturation of the root. Afterwards, an endodontic treatment such as root canal could be performed. Once the root canal is performed, the tooth can be restored with the appropriate method.

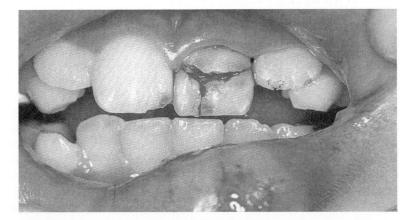

Fig. 10.3 Tooth fracture and labial contusion.

Nasal fracture

The external nose is a pyramidal structure with a central septum. The framework is composed of bone in the upper third and cartilage in the lower two-thirds. The prominent position and projection of the nose make it a common site of injury during team sports such as basketball. The paired nasal bones are thick and narrow superiorly and rarely fractured but the lower portion of the nasal bones are broad, thin, and subject to fracture. Direct frontal force to the nasal dorsum usually results in fracture of the lower half of the nasal bones. Lateral impact accounts for most nasal fractures and can produce a wide variety of injuries. Fractures and dislocations of the anterior (cartilaginous) septum often accompany nasal fractures.

In examining a player with a nasal fracture, crepitance and mobility of the fractured segments are found. External nasal deviation may be present but in many instances it can be masked by edema. The intranasal structures should be thoroughly examined and shrinkage of the mucosa with a vasoconstrictor may be required. A complication that should not be missed is a hematoma of the septum because it can lead to collapse of the nasal structures secondary to loss of septal cartilage associated with abscess formation or pressure necrosis (Guyette 1993).

The treatment of nasal fractures is similar in children and adults. Under intravenous sedation or general anesthesia, the nasal bones should be realigned. In some cases an osteotomy may be required to improve facial symmetry. After treatment of a nasal fracture approximately 6 weeks is required for the nasal bones to heal.

Fracture of the mandible

Fracture of the mandible or the lower jaw inferior maxilla is relatively frequent in sport because of its shape. Mandibular fractures are classified according to anatomic location with the most common sites being the condyle, mandibular angle, and the alveolar process. Of all the bone fractures, 50% involve teeth in the line of the fracture. The location in which fractures of the mandible occur more frequently is in the area of third molars, canines and premolars. In many occasions, periodontal defects and defects in the bone are related to the position of the line of fracture (Amy 1996).

The common signs and symptoms include changes in occlusion, mobility of mandibular segments, pain, inability to chew or open the mouth widely, numbness or paresthesia of the lower lip, ecchymosis of the gums or the floor of the mouth, and deviation of the lower jaw on opening. On examination careful palpation is recommended to verify changes in the contour of the bone and crepitation in the joint. Bimanual manipulation helps to detect mobility between the fragments.

Initial management includes securing the airway, immobilization of the lower jaw, and transportation to a facility with consultants in maxillofacial surgery for definite treatment. As a general rule radiographs should be taken for diagnosis and to determine the extent of the fractures. Some of the commonly used views include panoramic, lateral oblique, posterior-anterior, occlusal, periapical and reverse Towne's.

Fractures of the maxilla

Maxillary fractures which involve the upper jaw and associated bony structure are classified by location and severity into: Le Fort I, Le Fort II and Le Fort III. In Le Fort I fractures, the palate and alveolar process are separated from the maxilla by a fracture line above the antral floor and the floor of the nose (Schultz *et al.* 1987; Guyette 1993). The clinical signs of this type of fracture are edema, hematoma, malocclusion, open bite, mobility of the alveolar process, epistaxis and paresthesia. Emergency treatment should include temporary immobilization and referral to an oral and maxillofacial surgeon.

In Le Fort II fractures, the line of fracture goes through the lateral and anterior walls of the maxillary sinus and continues through the infraorbital borders to unite with the bridge of the nose. This fracture is commonly known as a "floating fracture". The signs and symptoms of this fracture are bilateral infraorbital paresthesias, diplopia and abnormal sensation. Treatment for this type of fracture should include transporting the patient directly to the emergency room of a hospital and referral to a maxillofacial surgeon.

Le Fort III fractures are similar to Le Fort II except that the patient presents with loss of cerebral spinal fluid through the nose. The patient may present other features of traumatic brain injury and managed with protection of the cervical spine.

Fractures of the zygoma

Fractures of the zygoma or cheek bone occur frequently because of its prominent lateral position in the facial structure. These fractures occur in basketball with lateral impacts to the face such as that from a fall, elbow, or fist. Signs and symptoms of this fracture include periorbital ecchymosis, edema, molar prominence, orbital margin deformity, epistaxis, crepitation, diplopia, and difficulty with opening or closing of the mouth. The zygomatic bone should be palpated feeling for flatness of the cheek or steps in the orbital rim.

Treatment may vary and depends on the extension of the fracture but includes transportation to a hospital and maxillofacial surgery consultation. In many cases, this fracture will require surgical treatment with reduction under general anesthesia.

Temporomandibular joint

The temporomandibular joint is found in both sides of the face, immediately under the ear, close to the hearing canal. This joint unites the mandible or inferior maxilla to the cranium and it is formed by joint disk and a mandibular condyle. There are also two ligaments that are important in the function of this joint, which are the sphenomandibular and the stylomandibular ligaments.

The disk or meniscus is one of the most important structures of the joint; since it absorbs functional stress and facilitates a smooth slide of the condyle. The meniscus is made up of collagen tissue. The posterior insertion of the disk is highly vascular and is innervated by the auriculotemporal branch of the fifth cranial nerve, the trigeminal. The lateral head of the pterygoid muscle provides the anterior insertion. Normally, the disk should maintain a position that covers most of the surface between the osseous contact points, the condyle and the temporal bone.

Trauma is the etiologic factor of the majority of the disorders of the temporomandibular joint (Schultz *et al.* 1987; Amy 1996). There is a higher probability of trauma to this joint in athletes who participate in contact-collision sports. Many of these athletes who suffer acute trauma with direct or indirect blows or hits to the joint may in the long run present with chronic symptoms that are very difficult to correct.

Injury to the temporomandibular joint may result in hemarthrosis, capsulitis, internal derangement, subluxation, dislocation, or fracture. Clinical evaluation may reveal swelling in the joint area, limitation of oral opening, deviation of the mouth toward the affected side, open bite in the opposite side of the trauma, and localized pain to palpation. In the case of condylar fracture blood may be present in the external auditory canal.

Initial management includes immobilization of the mandible, analgesics, and referral for definite diagnosis and treatment. Minor injuries to the joint may be treated with a soft diet, moist heat, and anti-inflammatory medications.

Chronic symptoms associated with temporomandibular joint disorders include pain, inflammation of the masticatory muscles and ligaments, as well as referred pain to the cervical region and in some cases, the arm. Chronic symptoms of the joint can be seen associated with psychological problems such as anxiety and depression.

Custom-built mouth protectors

Mouth protectors are used to protect various structures in the oral cavity during athletic events, usually in contact sports and their construction is an important service provided by sports dentistry. It can be said that mouth protectors are essential in the practice of contact sports (Chaconas 1985; Amy 1996).

Mouth protectors are removable appliances that usually cover the maxillary teeth (upper teeth) but there are mouth protectors that cover both arches, maxilla and mandible. These protectors are made up of a flexible material that is constructed from a plaster model of the patient's teeth. Custom-made mouth protectors are preferred and they should be fabricated by a trained dentist (Fig. 10.4).

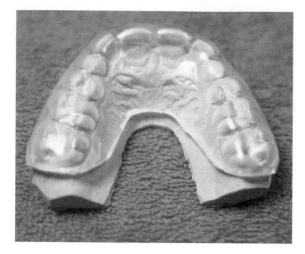

Fig. 10.4 Custom-made mouth protector.

The main functions of mouth protectors are:
• To protect oral soft tissues and the lips from teeth to avoid lacerations with contact.
• To help cushion and distribute the force of direct punches to the jaw, preventing fractures of the teeth, and minimizing the possibility of a fracture to the angle of the jaw or fracture of the condyles.
• To help prevent trauma to the temporomandibular joint.
• To serve as a splint, keeping teeth in their place when a strong hit is received.

Types of mouth protectors

There are three types or basic categories of mouth protectors, which are:
• Off the shelf mouth protectors which are found in department or sporting goods stores. They come in a universal size and are placed over the upper teeth.
• Mouth-formed protectors which can be thermo-set or chemo-set. The thermo-set type is found in sporting goods stores and is softened in hot water, tempered in cold water and adapted directly over the teeth. The chemo-set type is adapted through the use of soft autopolymerized resin. It can be said that the majority of athletes use this type of mouth protectors.
• Custom-built protectors which are fabricated on a stone model of the athlete's denture. This type

is preferred because it is more adaptable to the oral tissues, its comfortable and interferes minimally with breathing and speech. They are fabricated by a dentist or a dental technician. During the fabrication process, the specific anatomical structures are considered so that the protector adapts better. The material used is polyvinyl acetate (plastic vinyl). They are available in different colors, though athletes prefer them transparent. They are more durable than the other protectors and are the only ones that really guarantee maximal protection to the intraoral structures. They can be vacuum formed or pressure laminated (Chaconas 1985; Amy 1996).

As it has been previously mentioned, the use of a custom-built mouth protector is highly recommended, given that they have proven to be a great help in preventing injury since trauma to the oral cavity can occur in many types of sports. The American Dental Association has included a list of 23 sports or sporting activities which includes basketball in which the use of a mouth protector is recommended. In our experience the custom-built mouth protector is very well accepted by competitive athletes.

In summary a well constructed mouth protector should have the following properties:
• Custom-made for the specific patient
• Constructed with fine and smooth edges
• Built with enough retention to avoid its coming out of place during competition
• Strong enough so that teeth cannot penetrate it
• Resistant in order to last approximately 2 years
• Temperature resistant, so that it can be sterilized
• Priced at a reasonable cost for the athletes.

References

American Academy of Pediatrics Committee on Sports Medicine and Fitness (1994) Medical Conditions Affecting Sports Participation. *Pediatrics* **94** (5), 757–760.
Amy, E. (1996) *Oral Health in Sports*. San Juan: Ediciones Mitológicas.
Cantu, R.C. (1996) Head and Neck Injuries. In: W.B. Kibler, (ed.) *ACSM's Handbook for the Team Physician*, pp. 188–204. Williams & Wilkins, Baltimore.
Chaconas, S.J. (1985) A Comparison of Athletic Mouth-Guard Materials. *Am J Sport Med* **13** (3), 193–197.

Chapman, P.J. (1989) Mouth-Guards and the Role of Sporting Team Dentist. *Aust Dental J* **34** (1), 36–43.

Gomez, E., DeLee, J.C. & Farney, W.C. (1996) Incidence of Injury in Texas Girl's High School Basketball. *Am J Sports Med* **24** (5), 684–687.

Grindel, S.H., Lovell, M.R. & Collins, M.W. (2001) The Assessment of Sport-Related Concussion: The Evidence Behind Neuropsychological Testing and Management. *Clin J Sport Med* **11**, 134–143.

Guyette, R.F. (1993) Facial Injuries in Basketball Players. *Clin Sports Med* **12**, 247–264.

Johnston, K.M., McCrory, P., Mohtadi, N.G. & Meeuwisse, W. (2001) Evidence-Based Review of Sport-Related Concussion: Clinical Science. *Clin J Sport Med* **11**, 150–159.

Kehoe, J.C. (1986) Splinting and Replantation after Traumatic Avulsion. *J Am Dental Assoc* **112**, 224–230.

Kerr, I.L. (1986) Mouth-Guards for the Prevention of Injuries in Contact Sports. *Sports Med* **3** (6), 415–427.

Kunkel, S.S. (1994) Basketball Injuries and Rehabilitation. In: R.M. Bushbacher & R.L. Braddom (eds) *Sports Medicine and Rehabilitation: a Sport Specific Approach*, pp. 95–109. Philadelphia: Hanley & Belfus.

Olvera, N. (1990) *Newsletter Academy for Sports Dentistry*, January Issue, pp. 4–7.

Schultz, R. *et al.* (1987) Athletic Facial Injuries. *J Am Dental Assoc* **252** (24), 3395–3398.

Sonzogni, J.J. & Gross, M.L. (1993) Assessment and Treatment of Basketball Injuries. *Clin Sports Med* **12**, 221–237.

Torg, J.S. & Gennarelli, T.M. (1994). Head and Cervical Spine Injuries. In: J.C. Delee & D. Drez (eds) *Orthopaedic Sports Medicine*, pp. 417–462. Philadelphia: W.B. Saunders.

Zagelbaum, B.M., Starkey, C., Hersh, P.S. *et al.* (1995) The National Basketball Association Eye Injury Study. *Arch Ophthalmol* **113** (6), 749–752.

Chapter 11
Cardiovascular considerations in basketball

Andrew L. Pipe

Introduction

The physiological adaptations to exercise are nowhere as complex, or as fascinating, as the changes in cardiac and cardiovascular function that occur in the athlete. The heart responds in a specific and characteristic way to the exercise load upon it by the practice of a particular sport. Those who care for basketball players must appreciate the cardiovascular changes that occur in association with the practice of this sport.

There is an unfortunate tendency to regard the practice of sport medicine as a discipline dominated by considerations of the musculoskeletal system or sports trauma. But fractures heal and ligaments can be repaired. There are a variety of situations in which the health, and the life, of the athlete may be jeopardized by disorders of other organ systems. Athletes, or would-be athletes, can have significant underlying cardiovascular disease; disease that if unrecognized can be fatal.

It is important for every sport medicine professional to be familiar with the syndromes or conditions that may predispose an athlete to cardiovascular collapse or sudden cardiac death (SCD). Rare those conditions may be, the death of a young athlete is a tragic event. The identification of such conditions is a fundamental challenge, and responsibility, for the sport medicine practitioner in order that appropriate action may be taken—usually the disqualification from further participation in sport—before a tragedy occurs. In North America a number of highly publicized deaths in basketball have drawn attention to this phenomenon and the misperception has grown that such events are more common in basketball than in other sports. There is no epidemiological evidence to support this contention (the incidence is the same in American football—the two most popular games on that continent.) Nevertheless, a principal feature of Marfan syndrome (a syndrome associated with SCD) is tall stature; such individuals may, understandably, be drawn to basketball but are at high risk of cardiovascular complications as a consequence of the features of this condition. The practitioner caring for basketball players must be critically aware of the importance of identifying, to the extent possible, all athletes who may be at risk of a cardiovascular complication or incident.

Two fundamental considerations must not be ignored: First, the conditions predisposing to a cardiovascular event or sudden death are often inherited; the importance of knowing an athlete's family history cannot be overemphasized. Secondly, a cardiovascular catastrophe may be preceded by exercise-associated syncope. A syncopal attack in an athlete *must* be very carefully evaluated if there is *any* question about such an event being cardiac in origin. An understanding of the athlete's personal history in sport is paramount.

Remember the left and right ventricles—not the anterior cruciate ligaments!—are the most important structures in an athlete.

Cardiovascular adaptations in basketball players

For many years it was thought (and sometimes taught!) that intense training would produce changes in the heart that were harmful to the athlete—the term *athlete's heart* took on an inappropriate and sinister meaning! We now understand that training will produce specific, predictable and completely physiological changes in the size and function of the cardiac structures. The most marked changes often occur in the left ventricle.

It is important to appreciate that the type and intensity of any form of exercise training will determine the nature of the cardiovascular response: the size and function of the weightlifter's left ventricle will be very different from that of an endurance athlete. Perhaps the most common adaptation to dynamic exercise training is a lowered heart rate. As an athlete's fitness increases so the mitochondria of the muscles become more adept at extracting and utilizing oxygen and the heart does not have to beat as frequently, at any given work load, to deliver oxygen. The volume of blood ejected with each cardiac contraction also increases in response to dynamic training, further reducing the demands on the heart at any given level of exercise. Athletes respond to the increased cardiovascular requirements of sport by increasing their heart rate and stroke volume—the heart rate may triple and the stoke volume will typically double.

Basketball has been described as a "dynamic sport of moderate intensity" (Fig. 11.1). Dynamic exercise produces changes in muscle length with very little change in tension. Static exercise, on the other hand, produces little change in muscle length but a marked increase in tension. (It will be useful for purposes of this discussion to view cross-country skiers or distance runners as representing the most dynamic sports and weightlifting as the most static.) The hearts of athletes exposed to dynamic training (e.g., running), experience a *volume overload*—such training produces an increase in plasma volume and the increased demands of exercise are met by increasing the stroke volume (the amount of blood ejected with each cardiac contraction) as well as by increasing

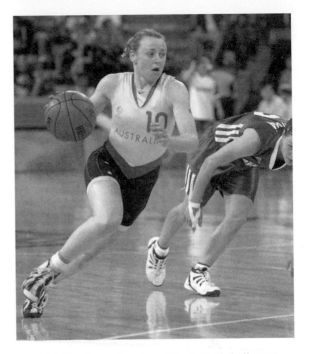

Fig. 11.1 The dynamic nature of basketball challenges the cardiovascular system. Photo © Getty Images/Robert Cianflone.

the heart rate. The demands of basketball training, and the nature of the game are such that the capacity of the left ventricle can be expected to enlarge somewhat and the thickness of the ventricular wall will also increase to a moderate degree (a condition referred to as *eccentric hypertrophy*).

Basketball players also experience *pressure overloads* both in training and during game situations as a result of the static exercise loads to which they are exposed—whether weightlifting in training, or powering to the basket following a rebound with an opponent on one's shoulder! The characteristic response to a pressure overload is for the ventricular wall to thicken without any associated change in the size of the ventricular capacity (a condition referred to as *concentric hypertrophy*). The demands of basketball are such that both eccentric and concentric hypertrophy may occur in well-trained players.

The hallmark of a well-trained individual is an increase in the capacity to deliver and utilize oxygen, a trait referred to as the *maximal oxygen uptake* or the $\dot{V}O_{2max}$. Typically basketball players have a $\dot{V}O_{2max}$ of approximately 50–55 mL·kg^{-1}·min^{-1}. The frequency, intensity and duration of exercise will influence the degree of cardiovascular adaptation. An athlete's heart rate is a good indicator of the training intensity—and a heart rate of between 130 and 150 beats per minute is generally felt to be necessary for a training response to occur; exercise sessions should take place at least three to four times a week for a period of at least 30–60 min if a significant training effect is expected.

Basketball players therefore will have a lowered resting heart rate, an increased stroke volume and a degree of ventricular wall thickening as a consequence of the unique training and competition demands of their sport. The changes in wall thickness and ventricular cavity enlargement may be small but can lead to a significant elevation of overall left ventricular mass. These changes are remarkably consistent within a particular sport discipline, reflecting the specificity of the response to a unique exercise load, and will normally be evident on an echocardiogram or reflected in an electrocardiogram (ECG) tracing (Table 11.1). They may develop rapidly in response to training, and most importantly, may regress quickly in the absence of continued training. (It is impossible to predict, however, that an individual athlete will always demonstrate these changes given the influence of genetics and environment on an individual's physiological response.)

Table 11.1 Common findings in basketball players.

Physiological adaptations
Increased left ventricular cavity size
Increased left ventricular wall thickness
Increased cardiac output at any given work load

Physical examination
Bradycardia
Soft systolic murmurs
Third heart sound (S3)

Electrocardiogram
Sinus bradycardia
Sinus arrhythmia
First degree AV block
Voltage changes of left and right ventricular hypertrophy
ST segment changes (elevation, depression)
Incomplete RBBB

The sport medicine professional must be able to differentiate the normal adaptations of training from the abnormalities that are indicative of underlying cardiac disease. Echocardiographic examinations are particularly helpful in this respect. At times, however, such distinctions may not be easy and require sophisticated or specialized expertise and investigations.

The physical examination of the athlete

A comprehensive approach to the preparticipation evaluation of a basketball athlete is found elsewhere in this volume. As noted in Chapter 5, it is essential that any such evaluation include a carefully conducted family and personal history designed to explore any suggestion of cardiovascular disorder and, more specifically, those associated with exercise-related death (Table 11.2). A history of exertional chest pain, syncopal episodes (especially if associated with exercise), unexpected degrees of shortness of breath or unanticipated fatigue should sensitize the examiner to the need for further, careful examination and investigation. The importance of obtaining a careful family history cannot be overemphasized; any incident of sudden or early cardiac death in the family must be deemed significant and pursued appropriately.

At the time of physical examination a careful inspection for any evidence of the stigmata of Marfan syndrome must be automatic (see below). The blood pressure should be measured in both arms. The presence of hypertension, or borderline hypertension, is an important finding in a young athlete; one should be sensitive to this issue, particularly when examining black athletes. Careful palpation of the carotid pulse, the femoral pulses, examination of the jugular venous wave and precordial palpation can be performed quickly and easily. Auscultation should be performed in a quiet setting while the athlete is supine, seated and standing. The athlete can be asked to carry out simple exercises, or to perform a Valsalva maneuver in order to assist in detecting and identifying murmurs. Systolic murmurs are not uncommon in athletes

Table 11.2 History taking, physical examination and basketball players.

Personal and family history
Always ask:
1 Have you ever collapsed or fainted in association with exercise?
2 Have you ever experienced chest pain or an unanticipated degree of breathlessness in association with exercise?
3 Have you ever experienced a rapid heartbeat, with or without a feeling of lightheadedness?
4 Has anyone in your family (parents, grandparents, uncles, aunts, brothers, sisters) ever died suddenly? Died at a young age?
5 Does anyone in your family have any form of heart disease?
6 Has anyone in your family been diagnosed with Marfan syndrome?
7 Has anyone in your family been diagnosed with hypertrophic cardiomyopathy?
8 Is there a history of inherited deafness in your family?*

Physical examination
Always check:
1 Body height
2 Pubic ramus to floor/height ratio
3 Arm span measurement
4 Evidence of myopia or dislocated lens
5 Chest wall abnormalities (pectus carinatum or excavatum)
6 Blood pressure in both arms
7 Femoral pulses
8 Abdominal bruits? Enlarged abdominal aorta?
9 Careful auscultation of the heart—supine, seated and standing (Listen for murmurs of aortic regurgitation, mitral valve prolapse)

* The long QT syndrome, a rare cause of sudden death, is an inherited condition associated with congenital neural deafness

and generally reflect a hyperdynamic state. Diastolic murmurs are never benign and require further evaluation.

It must also be recognized that many conditions that place the athlete at risk may be incompletely developed or manifest in youth; the importance of repeating history taking and physical examinations on a regular basis should be noted.

Questions frequently arise about athletes with heart murmurs. It must be recognized that there are many circumstances where athletes do not have ready access to specialized care or investigations. In these situations, it may be reasonable to consider that an athlete with a soft grade I–II systolic murmur, who has been active without incident for all their life, who has no personal or family history of cardiovascular disease or collapse, has a completely normal chest X-ray and electrocardiogram, and a completely normal physical examination, be permitted to participate in sport. In communities where there is a high incidence of rheumatic valve disease very careful consideration needs to be given to the investigation and follow-up of any athlete with a heart murmur particularly when the mitral valve is thought to be involved.

Mitral valve prolapse (MVP) is a common finding, present in 4–7% of the population, and is more common in females. It is frequently identified by the presence of a mid-systolic click and, except when associated with Marfan syndrome (see below) is usually a benign condition. There is scant evidence to support the contention that sudden death is exercise related in MVP. Athletes with MVP and no evidence of Marfan syndrome or mitral regurgitation should have no limits placed on their activities. Athletes with MVP and syncope, chest pain, significant mitral regurgitation or a family history of sudden death should be removed from strenuous physical activities.

It follows that any athlete with a positive personal or family history, or any evidence of cardiovascular disease on physical examination should receive a 12-lead electrocardiogram and consideration should be given to further investigations. Sir William Osler once noted that physicians should "listen to your patients; they are telling you their diagnosis!" The importance of a focused and carefully taken history cannot be repeated enough!

The electrocardiogram and the athlete

An athlete's electrocardiogram has been said to "reflect the extremes of normality more than any other test used in a cardiovascular examination." The ECG of an athlete very commonly demonstrates "abnormalities" that are suggestive of heart disease (see Table 11.1). It is essential that these changes not be misinterpreted. Almost characteristically an athlete's ECG will demonstrate sinus bradycardia; a sinus arrhythmia is also frequently present at rest. Such changes reflect the influence of training and its influence on the athlete's autonomic state. Other disorders of rhythm are not unusual in athletes: first degree (and sometimes second degree) atrioventricular block is common and reverses with exercise; junctional rhythms are often noted on ambulatory recordings in association with sinus bradycardia; ectopic ventricular beats and arrhythmias have also been reported in athletes during exercise and the immediate postexercise period. Left ventricular hypertrophy (LVH) as judged by voltage criteria is frequently present in athletes and changes of the T wave, including inversions, are not uncommon but usually normalize with exercise. It is important to be aware of the likelihood of such changes in an athletic individual and to interpret them as part of an overall evaluation, which includes particular attention to family and personal history and a careful physical examination.

The 26th Bethesda Conference

At the conclusion of this chapter are found a number of recommended publications for those who wish to read further about cardiovascular concerns in the athlete. Most important among them, perhaps, are the proceedings of the 26th Bethesda Conference, which provide particular guidance for assessing eligibility for participation in sport for athletes with cardiovascular abnormalities. Reference is made to this document throughout this chapter; the author would recommend it to anyone involved in the care of basketball players.

Sudden cardiac death

The death of an athlete is always a tragedy; if such an event occurs during the practice of sport the anguish is compounded. Sport is quite properly regarded as being health and life enhancing and deaths in sport, though exceedingly rare, are devastating for the family and perplexing to the public. A number of high profile cases involving basketball players have drawn attention to this phenomenon in our sport. Black athletes seem to be disproportionately represented in series of cases of sudden cardiac death (SCD); the phenomenon seems to be more common in males. All health professionals associated with the care of basketball players must be vigilant in ensuring that the athletes entrusted to their care are appropriately screened and examined for the conditions that could place them at risk.

Table 11.3 The causes of sudden cardiac death in 158 athletes. Adapted from Maron *et al.* (1996).

1 Hypertrophic cardiomyopathy (HCM)	36%
2 Coronary artery anomalies	19%
3 Cardiac changes consistent with HCM?	10%
4 Ruptured aorta	5%
5 "Tunneled" LAD coronary artery	5%
6 Aortic stenosis	4%
7 Myocarditis	3%
8 Dilated cardiomyopathy	3%
9 ARVD, MVP, CAD & other	13%

ARVD, arrhythmogenic right ventricular dysplasia; CAD, coronary artery disease; LAD, left anterior descending; Tunneled LAD, LAD buried in the left ventricular muscle; MVP, mitral valve prolapse.

The overall death rate in sport among US high school and college athletes has been noted to be 0.75 and 0.13 per 100 000 athletes for men and women, respectively. Trauma is the most common cause of death among young adults; heat-related deaths, rhabdomyolysis in those with sickle cell trait, asthma and gastrointestinal hemorrhage are the major noncardiac causes of deaths in an athletic population.

In recent years our understanding of the conditions and causes most likely to result in sudden cardiac death has grown considerably. The sport medicine community owes a particular debt to Dr Barry J. Maron whose work in this area has been seminal. As a consequence of his contributions we know that the most common causes of exercise-associated SCD in individuals below the age of 35 years are hypertrophic cardiomyopathy (HCM), which is found in 36% of such incidents, and coronary artery anomalies which are noted in 19% of these deaths. The remainder are due to a variety of 20 or more primarily congenital cardiovascular diseases, which underscores again the importance of proper history taking when examining athletes (Table 11.3). The most common cause of exercise-associated death in those over the age of 35 is coronary artery disease.

From time to time the suggestion is made that intensive screening strategies should be employed in athletes to detect the lesions that might lead to a sudden cardiac death. Such approaches are unrealistic both because of their expense and their very low "yield". It has been calculated that it would be necessary, for instance, to perform 200 000 echo-cardiograms to identify one individual *at risk* of a sudden cardiac death. At the same time it must be realized that there are inherent limitations in an approach utilizing only a standard history and physical examination—such interventions lack the power to reliably identify many of the potentially lethal abnormalities.

Hypertrophic cardiomyopathy

The most common cause of death among young (less than 35 years of age) athletes is hypertrophic cardiomyopathy (HCM), a genetically transmitted disorder with diverse expression that may result in the development of an enlarged ventricle character-ized by the presence of abnormal and disordered myofibrils. The nature of the enlargement may vary considerably; enlargement may encroach on the left ventricular outflow tract and thus limit cardiac output during exercise in some patients (producing the syncopal symptoms sometimes associated with this disorder). But the nonobstructive forms of HCM are more common. The tangled, abnormal myofib-rils of the enlarged ventricle are the origin of the ventricular arrhythmias that are the usual cause of death in this condition. It is an uncommon abnorm-ality and is calculated to occur in about 0.2% of the population (1 in 500). HCM is more common in males and seems to be more frequently associated in the USA with death during exercise among black athletes; black patients with HCM are far less fre-quently identified in US hospital populations, which may be reflective of limited access to specialized care rather than a differing incidence rate.

It is the hypertrophy of the left ventricle, associ-ated with a normal sized ventricular cavity that is considered the gross anatomic and diagnostic marker of this condition. Such enlargement is infrequently detected on clinical examination because the clinical features associated with the condition (history of syncope, family history of cardiovascular collapse or the presence of a loud systolic murmur) are relat-ively uncommon. The diagnosis is usually con-firmed following echocardiographic examination when there is clear-cut evidence of abnormality. Such a distinction may be difficult to make, how-ever, as there may be considerable overlap with the

echocardiographic findings that may occur com-monly in athletes reflecting the left ventricular hypertrophy that occurs in response to training. Thus there may be considerable challenge in mak-ing the diagnosis of this disorder in some athletes—a challenge that is best left to those with experience in echocardiography and an understanding of the changes in cardiac size that normally occur in athletes. A period of detraining may be particularly helpful in resolving diagnostic dilemmas given that the adaptive changes in ventricular wall size that follow athletic training regress with rest; no such changes occur in the individual with HCM. The clearest evidence of HCM may be the demonstration of the characteristic echocardiographic features in a relative.

It is recommended that individuals with HCM should be excluded from participation in intense competitive sport—basketball would be absolutely contraindicated. Aggressive treatment is recom-mended for those considered to be at significant risk of sudden death; at present this often consists of treatment with maintenance doses of amiodarone or consideration of the use of an implantable defibrillator.

Coronary artery anomalies

Abnormalities of the coronary arteries are the second most common cause of exercise-associated sudden death in individuals less than 35 years of age. These anatomical abnormalities may take multiple forms many of which produce significant obstruction of coronary artery blood flow and are incompatible with exercise or sport activity. Others are unlikely to produce ischemia or symptoms.

The most common anomaly noted in young athletes who have died during sport activity is that of the left coronary artery arising from the anterior sinus of Valsalva. The unusual coronary artery there-fore lies between the aorta and the pulmonary artery. Such an anomaly is likely to result in the formation of a "slit-like" coronary ostium that may be subject to compression, by expansion of the aorta and the pulmonary artery in association with exercise, leading to ischemia and perhaps sudden death. It has also been suggested that in some cases spasm of such arteries may be the principal factor in the development of ischemia and resulting death. The obstruction or spasm is undoubtedly intermittent and probably occurs episodically given the fact that most with these lesions have exercised uneventfully and to a significant degree countless times before a catastrophic event occurred. Many in the basketball community will be familiar with the sudden death of "Pistol Pete" Maravich, an accomplished professional player who died in a pick-up game at age 40 and in his retirement, who was found to have this abnormality.

It is important to realize that most patients with such lesions are asymptomatic. Their abnormalities come to light only at the time of coronary arteriography. On occasion an incidental echocardiogram may identify such an anomaly. While most patients report no symptoms, some (as many as a third in some series) have described chest pain or syncope. The tendency of athletes or regular exercisers to minimize the development or presence of symptoms must be appreciated by any who care for such individuals. Once again, careful and sensitive history taking can be seen to be of obvious importance in screening athletes.

The presence of such lesions must be suspected in any individuals who have chest pain or syncope during or immediately following exercise. Exercise stress testing, and possibly coronary angiography, are recommended for such individuals. Transesophageal echocardiography may permit the identification of the origin of the coronary vessels in some cases. When abnormal origins of the coronary arteries are detected in young individuals coronary bypass surgery is often recommended.

The remaining causes of SCD occur infrequently; some additional clinical syndromes are of particular relevance to those involved in basketball. They are discussed below.

Myocarditis

Athletes are susceptible to the same range of illnesses as the general public. The incidence of myocarditis varies among different communities—Chagas' disease is the most common cause of inflammatory cardiac illness in many regions and is widespread in Central and South America—but approximately 5% of individuals with a viral infection will experience mild myocardial inflammation. (This is of more than passing interest to sport medicine practitioners who see viral illnesses very commonly among their athletic patients.) Myocarditis has been noted to be the fourth most common cause of death in exercising individuals. It has been the leading cause of sudden cardiac death in studies of military recruits who share barrack accommodations. The incidence of myocarditis may wax and wane in association with changing rates of prevalence and virulence of infecting agents in any particular community. A variety of organisms are associated with myocarditis; the most common infectious agents are felt to be the coxsackie B viruses. Viral infection is said to cause myocardial cell destruction, produce a secondary immune reaction and finally to produce endothelial injury and microvascular spasm. Some patients may be extremely ill during the acute phase of an episode of myocarditis but most will have only minimal, flu-like symptoms. Myocarditis is felt to be the precipitating factor in many, if not most, cases of dilated cardiomyopathy (DCM). Deaths that occur in individuals with myocarditis are felt to follow episodes of ventricular tachyarrhythmia.

The most relevant questions concerning myocarditis and sport relate to the management of presumed or actual cases. Given the likelihood of myocardial involvement in a small, but significant, number of viral illnesses it would seem prudent to preclude from competition and training any athlete with a fever or other systemic signs of viral infection. Some authors have suggested that any athlete with a viral illness with symptoms "below the neck" (e.g., chest congestion, chest-wall pain, generalized myalgias, productive cough, etc.) should not participate or practice until there has been resolution of the illness. This simple approach seems, intuitively, to be a useful one to follow though there is no objective evidence to support it.

Any athlete with suspected myocarditis should be removed from sport to allow further evaluation. There is evidence from animal studies that continued training during an acute episode may lead to increased rates of viral replication, more myocardial damage and increased risk of serious complications. Treatment of those with established myocarditis is aimed at preventing the development of DCM in the event that there is any evidence of ventricular dysfunction and usually consists of the use of after-load reducing agents like the ACE inhibitors. The most recent Bethesda Conference on athletes and cardiovascular disorders identified the risk of sudden death in athletes with this disorder and was clear in its recommendation that athletes with myocarditis should be removed from sport for a period of 6 months following the onset of symptoms. It is sobering to consider that the 5-year mortality rate is approximately 50% following an episode of myocarditis and that the persistence of ventricular arrhythmias, after the resolution of the illness, has been noted in children and young adults.

Marfan syndrome

Marfan syndrome is a congenital disease of connective tissue that expresses itself through abnormalities in a number of organ systems. In its "classic" form, patients are very tall, with long limbs and fingers, there are often deformities of the chest and sternum, dislocation of the lens is sometimes present and there may be a high, narrow arched palate. The fundamental disorder is reflected in the production of defective elastic tissue as the result of abnormalities in the genes that code for the production of *fibrillin*. Elastic tissues are found abundantly in the cardiovascular system (heart valves, blood vessel walls, chordal structures of the heart), in the eye fibrillin is a principal component of the ligaments which support the lens, in the musculoskeletal system fibrillin is to be found in cartilage and tendons and is present in the elastic structures of the skin. The prevalence of Marfan syndrome is felt to be much higher among individuals who participate in sports in which tall stature and long limbs are seen as being advantageous; basketball is the prime example! This genetic disorder is relatively common (1 in 10 000) and is found in all races and genetic groups and men and women equally. Those caring for basketball players must become familiar with the features of this syndrome and develop a high index of suspicion for its presence.

The detection of Marfan syndrome patients is an important goal of any screening process in sport, particularly in basketball. The diagnosis of Marfan syndrome can be made on the basis of three of the following four criteria: (a) a positive family history;

Table 11.4 The features of Marfan syndrome.

The diagnosis is based on the presence of findings from any *three* of the following four groups of criteria:
1 Family history

2 Cardiac findings
(a) Dilated ascending aorta
(b) Aortic regurgitation
(c) Mitral valve prolapse
(d) Abdominal aortic aneurysm

3 Musculoskeletal findings
(a) Tall stature
(b) Chest deformities (pectus carinatum or excavatum)
(c) Long limbs
(d) Altered length of body segments
(e) "Spider" fingers
(f) High arched palate
(g) Malocclusion
(h) Hypermobile joints
(i) Skin laxity and striae

4 Ocular findings
(a) Dislocated lens
(b) Elongated globe
(c) Myopia
(d) Flattened cornea
(e) Retinal detachments

Note: The clinical findings in Marfan syndrome can vary enormously; it is unusual for all features to be present. Those caring for basketball players must have a very high index of suspicion for the presence of the syndrome. Adapted from: Gibbons, G. (1999) The Marfan syndrome: implications for athletes, In: A. Williams (ed.) *The Athlete and Heart Disease* pp. 69–78. Philadelphia: Lippincott Williams & Wilkins.

(b) the presence of any of the cardiovascular features of Marfan syndrome; (c) the presence of any of the musculoskeletal features of Marfan syndrome; and (d) the presence of any of the ocular features typical of Marfan syndrome (Table 11.4). It has been estimated that 20–30% of cases occur as a result of a spontaneous mutation and thus have no family history; in addition, the features of the syndrome may develop over time—some changes may not be evident until after adolescence.

Cardiovascular complications are the most common cause of death in patients with this syndrome. They typically include aortic dissection, aortic regurgitation and heart failure secondary to valvular heart disease. It is the defects in the elastic tissues of the vessels and valves, particularly those of the aortic root, that lead to the cardiovascular features of this syndrome. In association with the mechanical stresses imposed on such tissues the abnormalities cause an insidious process of dilatation and enlargement eventually leading to aortic valve regurgitation and aortic enlargement. Mitral valve prolapse is very common in Marfan syndrome and has a more ominous course in such patients.

The musculoskeletal features of the syndrome may be quite obvious. The increased height of the patient is combined with very long limbs, "spider" fingers, a reduced upper to lower body ratio (measure the lower segment—top of pubic ramus to the floor—and divide into the height) and joint laxity. (The ability to overlap the distal phalanges of the thumb and fifth fingers when wrapped around the wrist of the opposite hand and the tendency of the thumb to protrude beyond the ulnar border of a clenched fist are often cited as simple screening tests for the presence of Marfan features.) Pectus deformities of the chest are common and may be associated with a degree of scoliosis; a high arched palate may be accompanied by malocclusion and, in general, such patients have poorly developed muscle mass.

A slit-lamp examination permits the identification of the characteristic ocular features; lens dislocation (present in 50%) may be accompanied by an elongated globe and a flattened cornea. Marfan patients are at increased risk of retinal detachment and are frequently myopic.

In addition to the "classical" features of the syndrome, Marfan patients may have increased laxity and striae of the skin, and a tendency to develop pneumothorax and hernias. All of which are reflective of the abnormal elastic tissue that is the basis of this syndrome.

The most important element in facilitating the diagnosis of Marfan syndrome is a high index of suspicion. Any family history of sudden death, aortic aneurysm, dissection or rupture should stimulate a very careful and systematic examination. Similarly, any suggestion of the musculoskeletal features of this syndrome, the identification of the murmur of aortic insufficiency or mitral regurgitation or the signs of mitral valve prolapse should trigger a thorough investigation for the presence of the syndrome. A careful history and a comprehensive physical examination should permit the identification of the majority of individuals with this syndrome who are at high risk of sudden death. The recommendations of the 26th Bethesda Conference are quite clear in advising that those with Marfan syndrome should not be permitted to participate in basketball with its associated cardiovascular demands and risk of frequent bodily collision.

Drug use, sport and sudden death

It is an unfortunate reality of sport that there will be those who seek to enhance their athletic performance pharmacologically, or who use "social" drugs for reasons of their own. Both forms of drug use carry with them the risk of significant cardiovascular complications.

Anabolic-androgenic steroids (AAS) have been associated with a variety of cardiovascular problems including premature myocardial infarction, sudden cardiac death, cerebrovascular accidents, and the development of cardiomyopathy. There are numerous case reports of such occurrences in the literature although the absolute risk of such events is probably low. Anabolic steroid use is associated with a distortion of lipid profiles, changes in the coagulation status and hypertension.

The sympathomimetics (ephedrine and related compounds) are found in a variety of common, over-the-counter medications and are present in an extraordinarily large array of nutritional "supplements", dietary products and "natural" health products. Their use has been directly implicated in a significant number of deaths as a consequence of their ability to provoke significant coronary artery spasm and to alter the threshold for arrhythmia development. In sports where endurance capacity is prized, the abuse of recombinant erythropoietin (rEPO) has been implicated in many deaths. Such deaths are believed to be related to the development of a state of hyperviscosity caused by an increased red blood cell mass.

The use of cocaine has been associated with countless cardiac disasters, and, sadly several cardiac deaths among basketball players. Cocaine's ability to produce marked coronary artery spasm and increase the likelihood of arrhythmia, while increasing the heart rate and blood pressure make it capable of inducing a cardiac catastrophe in a totally normal heart. The increased sympathetic activity that accompanies exercise might be expected to accentuate the cardiovascular effects of cocaine.

Those involved in sport have a responsibility to counsel their athletic patients about the hazards associated with the use of performance-enhancing drugs. Specific advice about the use of nutritional "supplements" will not only ensure athlete safety but also, in all likelihood, enhance the quality of the dietary practices of the athlete.

Commotio cordis

The recognition that a sudden blow to the chest can induce a fatal arrhythmia has important implications for those who provide care at basketball events. It is known that the application of a critical force to the anterior chest wall at a precise point in the cardiac cycle is capable of inducing a fatal arrhythmia (ventricular fibrillation). To the author's knowledge there has been only one documented incident of this phenomenon in basketball. Cases have been reported in ice hockey, soccer, and baseball; they typically follow a blow with a ball or other object, or a collision with another athlete. This syndrome is seen almost exclusively in children and young adults, perhaps as a consequence of the increased elasticity of the chest wall in the young. Sadly, it has been suggested that victims of commotio cordis may be strangely resistant to attempts at resuscitation. It is entirely conceivable that the force delivered by a rapidly thrown basketball striking an athlete in the sternum could induce a potentially fatal arrhythmia. Clearly there is no way to anticipate, or perhaps even prevent, such an incident in basketball; it is important that sport physicians and others be aware of this condition and are prepared to respond rapidly with appropriate resuscitation efforts.

Coronary artery disease

So far in this discussion we have focused our attention on the needs of athletes who, typically, are considered to be young players. The most common cause of sudden death in those over the age of 35 is coronary artery disease. There are many involved

in the sport of basketball who continue to be active in the game beyond this age as players or officials. Thus it is appropriate to consider issues surrounding the cardiac health of these older individuals.

In reviewing the reports of sudden death that have occurred in older individuals it is striking how many have premonitory symptoms; the tendency to deny such symptoms would seem to be common particularly among those who are particularly dedicated to sport or unusually competitive. The presence of cardiac risk factors is likely to be lower in those with a history of life-long physical activity; hypertension, hyperlipidemia and cigarette smoking are much less frequent among such individuals. Exercise stress testing is much less reliable in those in whom the pretest likelihood of coronary disease is low. It is also important to recognize that sudden cardiac events usually follow plaque rupture and thrombosis at a previously unobstructed site in a coronary vessel—stress testing usually produces a positive result in the presence of a pre-existing, obstructive lesion. Given the unique physiological and emotional demands associated with refereeing, consideration might be given to conducting exercise stress tests in individuals over the age of 40, or with more than one major risk factor or known cardiac disease. It is important to ensure that ex-athletes and officials understand common approaches to the prevention of cardiac disease, especially the importance of smoking cessation. Physicians and other health professionals need to be sensitive to the complaints or questions of older athletes or officials, which may reflect the presence of cardiac symptoms. Attempts should be made to introduce a discussion of cardiac health and the prevention of coronary artery disease at meetings of basketball coaches and officials.

Resuscitation skills and equipment in basketball

It has been observed that basketball has a high frequency of cardiac events and sudden cardiac death among players; most emergencies of this kind occur during training sessions; and cardiac emergencies among spectators are not uncommon. In many communities a sophisticated approach to the management of cardiac emergencies is in place and includes training in cardiopulmonary resuscitation (CPR) of the general public, access to emergency medical personnel trained in CPR and defibrillation and who provide rapid transportation to advanced life support facilities. The advent of automatic external defibrillators (AEDs) means that prompt access to what may be definitive resuscitative care is now potentially available at any site where athletic training and competition take place. These devices require minimal training before use, sense an unusual cardiac rhythm and, when appropriate and with a high degree of accuracy, deliver a defibrillating electric current.

Sadly, there have been examples in basketball where the resources for early defibrillation and resuscitation have been available but were inappropriately or belatedly applied with fatal results. It would seem a minimal requirement that all involved in the care of basketball players receive basic training in CPR, and where appropriate and available, training in the use of an AED. It is essential that a simple protocol for the management of sudden collapse or a cardiac emergency be developed for the medical staff of every basketball team. Similarly, it would seem reasonable for AEDs to be made available, and for specific protocols to be applied for the management of cardiac emergencies at the sites of tournaments and major competitions.

Conclusion

The health professional providing care to those involved in basketball should be familiar with the cardiovascular adaptations that occur in such athletes, sensitive to the reality that basketball has been frequently associated with sudden cardiac death, and specifically aware of the conditions and circumstances that predispose to such tragedies. It is important that all basketball players receive an appropriate preparticipation examination and undergo careful questioning regarding their personal and family medical history. A carefully taken history (with a special emphasis on symptoms or episodes of syncope occurring in association with exercise, and/or any family history of sudden, premature cardiac death or exercise-related collapse) must be followed by a vigilant physical examination supplemented, when appropriate, with special investigations (of which the echocardiogram is perhaps the most useful). It is important that officials and older athletes learn about the major risk factors for coronary artery disease and its common symptoms. The tendency of those active in sport to deny cardiac symptoms must be appreciated. Health professionals involved in any sport must be capable of providing cardiopulmonary resuscitation and develop a site- or event-specific protocol for the management of cardiovascular collapse in an athlete, official or spectator.

"Success" it has been noted "consists of doing ordinary things, extraordinarily well". An appropriate and apt observation when applied to the challenge of detecting and managing cardiovascular abnormalities in the basketball athlete.

Further reading

Estes, N., Salem, D. & Wang, P. (eds) (1998) *Sudden Cardiac Death in the Athlete.* Futura Publishing, Armonk.

Maron, B. (ed.) (1997) The Athlete's Heart and Cardiovascular Disease. *Cardiology Clinics 3.* Philadelphia: W.B. Saunders.

Maron, B. & Mitchell, J. (1994) 26th Bethesda Conference: Revised eligibility recommendations for competitive athletes with cardiovascular abnormalities. *Journal of the American College of Cardiology* **24**, 845–899.

Maron, B., Shirani, J., Poliac, L. *et al.* (1996) Sudden death in young competitive athletes: clinical, demographic and pathological profiles. *Journal of the American Medical Association* **276**, 199–204.

Maron, B., Thompson, P. & Puffer, J. (1996) Cardiovascular preparticipation screening of competitive athletes. *Circulation* **94**, 850–856.

Williams, R.A. (1999) *The Athlete and Heart Disease: Diagnosis, Evaluation and Management.* Philadelphia: Lippincott Williams & Wilkins.

Chapter 12
Medical illness

Margot Putukian

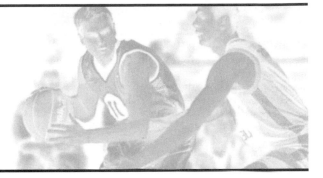

Introduction

Basketball is a sport that entails both aerobic and anaerobic conditioning, strength, and agility. It is a collision sport where contact occurs and fairly significant injuries can occur. Certain medical problems, such as reactive airway disease, skin diseases, infectious mononucleosis, and concussions occur commonly in the basketball player and require proper identification and treatment. Other medical issues that are important to consider are those that put the athlete or their opponents at risk during play, such as infectious diseases, and the potential for transmission of blood-borne pathogens. Medical problems that may limit participation include gastrointestinal diseases, genitourinary problems, cramps, and environmental exposures. Many of these issues have been discussed in detail elsewhere in this book. This chapter will briefly discuss those medical illnesses not discussed previously as they pertain to the basketball player (Fig. 12.1).

At the professional level in the United States, the medical conditions that occur in the male basketball player were assessed over a 3-year period by the National Basketball Association (NBA) Trainer's Association (Steingard 1993). They reported a total of 3260 reports (93% response rate) with 844 (25.9%)

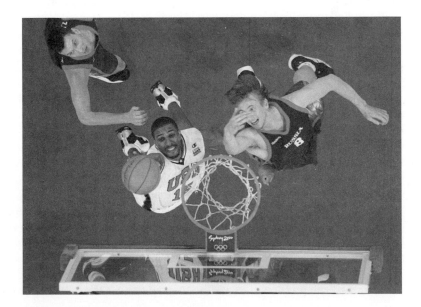

Fig. 12.1 Successful play depends upon the prevention of medical problems. Photo © Getty Images/ Jed Jacobsohn.

Table 12.1 Frequency of illness during a basketball season (adapted from Steingard 1993; with permission).

Illness	Frequency
Dermatitis	11
Sinusitis	16
General illness	25
Gastritis/upset stomach	42
Diarrhea	74
Cold	113
Influenza	118
Upper respiratory tract infection	140
Sore throat	159

considered nonsport injuries. These were defined as those conditions which involved: (1) time loss from practice or competition; (2) physician intervention; (3) prescription medication necessary; or (4) extraordinary care necessary. A total of 859 practice or game days were lost due to nonsport illness, accounting for 3% of the total time lost over the 3-year time frame assessed. The most common medical problems encountered are shown in Table 12.1.

One must be careful in interpreting these data in that these represent many problems which overlap in presentation, and also only those injuries reported to the sports trainer. It may miss several other important medical problems such as sexually transmitted diseases, depression, anxiety, and other problems that athletes most likely underreport. However, it does present useful information in terms of the types of problems encountered in the United States professional player who participates in almost full-year training and competition.

The initial interaction that many health care providers have with the basketball player is during the preparticipation examination (PPPE). During this evaluation, separating out conditions that put the athlete at risk for illness or injury is important. Certain conditions, such as hypertension, exercise-induced asthma, and musculoskeletal abnormalities, are often detected during the PPPE. Other medical problems such as single organs, history of significant head injury, or medical problems such as infectious mononucleosis may also be detected during the PPPE. The PPPE is an important opportunity to address chronic medical problems, as well as to identify acute medical problems that preclude participation until they resolve. Immunizations for measles, mumps, rubella and tetanus should be reviewed, and in the basketball player, hepatitis B immunization should be encouraged. For the adolescent and college age athlete, meningitis immunization should also be discussed. The PPPE is discussed in greater detail in Chapter 5, though certain conditions that preclude participation will be discussed below.

Athlete's heart is a syndrome of findings that are physiologic adaptations to exercise. These are normal alterations that occur as a result of physical training, and include an increase in the chamber size, muscle wall thickness, with resultant increase in stroke volume. These alterations are often associated with changes in the electrocardiogram, chest X-ray, and echocardiogram, and importantly are rarely symptomatic. Differentiating athlete's heart from the abnormalities associated with sudden cardiac death is often challenging. This is one of the most important medical system to consider in the PPPE and is discussed in further detail in Chapter 11.

Hypertension

Hypertension in the athlete is not uncommon, and in the young athlete, secondary causes should be sought (Working Group Report 1996; Kaplan 2001; Glover, in press). These include renal artery stenosis, adrenal hyperplasia, coarctation, renal parenchymal disease, medications or supplement use. In adults, normal blood pressure is defined as systolic pressure (SP) <130, and diastolic pressure (DP) <85, with high normal blood pressure being SP 130–139, and DP 85–90. Hypertension is then divided into stages; stage I (SP 140–159, DP 90–99), stage II (SP 160–179, DP 100–109), and stage III (SP >180, DP >110). Blood pressures are different for athletes of varying ages, and are also dependent on height and gender. In children, blood pressure is considered normal if it is below the 90th percentile. Blood pressures between the 90th and 94th percentile are considered "high normal" blood pressure. Hypertension is blood pressures between the 95th and 99th percentile, and severe hypertension is above the 99th percentile (Bartosh & Aronson 1999).

Hypertension is also differentiated by whether additional risk factors and end organ damage is present. Risk factors include family history of coronary artery disease (CAD) in men <55 years or women <65 years, smoking, hypercholesterolemia, diabetes, and age >60 years in men or postmenopausal in women. End organ damage can be expressed as retinopathy, coronary artery disease, left ventricular hypertrophy, heart failure, nephropathy, peripheral and cerebral vascular disease. Testing often includes complete blood count, renal function, urinalysis, electrocardiogram, echocardiogram, and exercise treadmill testing.

In the basketball player with hypertension, it is important to exclude medication or supplement use as the cause or aggravating factor of their elevated blood pressure. These agents include medications (nonsteroidal anti-inflammatory drugs, oral contraceptives, decongestants), illicit drugs (amphetamines, cocaine, alcohol in excess), and ergogenic aids (steroids, growth hormone, ephedrine, amphetamines, erythropoietin, phentermine). A careful history is important in excluding these medications and agents in the athlete that may or may not be aware of their hypertensive side-effects.

Return to play with hypertension

The earliest stage of hypertension is labile hypertension, where high normal blood pressures exist. This can be associated with high serum renin levels, catecholamine levels and renal blood flow. Identifying the hypertensive athlete is important, and if after evaluation, no secondary cause is identified, then treatment should be initiated. The Bethesda Conference provides guidelines for participation in exercise with hypertension (Kaplan *et al.* 1994; Mitchell *et al.* 1994). Before participation in exercise such as basketball, blood pressure should be controlled (American Academy of Pediatrics 1997). If this occurs, basketball play is not contraindicated, and can be part of the treatment. In stage III hypertension where diastolic dysfunction is present and left ventricular hypertrophy exists, exercise is contraindicated unless well controlled. The treatment of the athlete with hypertension should be individualized, with promising data using dietary approaches (Appel *et al.* 1997; Sacks *et al.* 2001) as

well as several medication options which have a negligible effect on performance (Swain & Kaplan 1997; Sachtleben *et al.* 2002).

Gastrointestinal conditions

Conditions that most commonly affect the gastrointestinal (GI) system can range from gastritis, gastroenteritis, to inflammatory bowel disease. In addition, gastrointestinal symptoms may be the presentation for systemic disease such as thyroid, endocrine, neoplasm, irritable bowel disease or vascular compromise. Gastrointestinal symptoms can also occur as a result of fluid and solid foods, as well as medications. Both upper and lower GI tract should be considered. The most common entities to consider will be discussed briefly below.

Upper GI tract symptoms include dyspepsia, gastric and peptic ulcer disease, and gastritis. The most common cause of upper GI symptoms is gastroesophageal reflux (GER). The exact etiology of GER in athletes is unclear but symptoms are often made worse during intense exercise. It is important to exclude cardiac and respiratory disease in the evaluation of these athletes, especially in the older individual. Additional testing may be indicated, and a thorough evaluation should be performed to rule out ulcer disease or other treatable causes of upper GI disease.

Some GI disorders present with both upper and lower GI symptoms. Acute gastroenteritis is common in the young athlete, with viral causes being the most likely etiology. The viral causes of gastroenteritis include rotavirus, enterovirus and most commonly Norwalk virus. Bacterial causes include *Salmonella, Shigella, Campylobacter, Escherichia,* and *Yersinia.* Other causes to consider include the protozoans *Giardia, Cryptosporodium,* and *Entamoeba.* Symptoms include abdominal pain, nausea, vomiting, and watery or bloody diarrhea. In general, viral infections are self-limited, with prevention of dehydration and other supportive measures the only treatment necessary.

Salmonella, Shigella, Campylobacter and *Yersinia* should be considered when there is evidence of acute illness after eating foods that have not been washed such as meats, poultry or vegetables. These illnesses are often accompanied by a bloody diarrhea as well as fever, and laboratory tests should include cultures for these organisms as well as fecal white blood cells. Treatment otherwise includes supportive care, fluids, and antibiotics only when appropriate.

Traveler's diarrhea

Enterotoxic *Escherichia coli* is the most common cause of traveler's diarrhea, although the other bacterial or protozoan sources can also be causative, and often the etiology is unknown. Treatment of traveler's diarrhea includes either trimethoprim/sulfamethoxazole or doxycycline. Prevention should be considered in those situations where travel into an endemic region will occur, or where elite competition is going to occur. Prophylaxis should also be considered for athletes with underlying gastrointestinal disease or high risk situations. The most common prophylactic medications used include ciprofloxacin (500 mg), ofloxacin (400 mg) or norfloxacin (400 mg) due to their side-effect profile and once daily dose (Statement on Traveler's Diarrhea 1995). Anti-diarrheal agents are not recommended unless the diarrhea is severe. Antispasmodics can help alleviate cramping, but must be given carefully if competition is to be considered.

Other considerations

When evaluating the athlete with gastrointestinal symptoms consistent with gastroenteritis, it is important to consider those entities requiring antibiotics, but also to consider both inflammatory bowel disease (IBD) and an acute appendicitis. If the abdomen is tender, symptoms are persistent, or if the clinical history is otherwise suspicious, obtaining a complete white blood cell count with a differential can be very important. If the white blood cell count is elevated, or if fever is present, then both bacterial infections and appendicitis should be considered. If on examination the abdomen is tender or significant guarding or rebound is present, surgical consultation is indicated.

The athlete with bloody diarrhea, or with symptoms of previous episodes of gastrointestinal bleeding, apthous ulcers, or a family history of IBD should prompt the physician to consider IBD as a possibility. Appropriate testing may include gastric endoscopy or colonoscopy or both. Consultation with a gastroenterologist is helpful in determining appropriate testing and further treatment. Other causes of bloody diarrhea include hemorrhagic gastritis, medication induced gastritis, peptic ulcer disease, polyps, and hemorrhoids. Hemorrhoids are the most common cause of lower GI bleeding in young adults and can often be diagnosed by physical examination including anoscopy. Further management of these disorders depends on thorough evaluation, proper diagnosis, and individualized treatment. (Schwartz *et al.* 1990; Green 1992; Putukian 1997; Butcher 1999).

Return to play considerations

For the athlete with gastroenteritis, or with any form of bloody diarrhea once identified, return to play decisions should be made only after the athlete is hemodynamically stable, and able to exercise without significant compromise. If the hematocrit is stable, the athlete is afebrile and can tolerate fluids, and has no evidence for dehydration, return to play can be considered. Measurement of orthostatic blood pressure and pulse is an important adjunct to measuring vital signs for accurately determining blood volume and hemodynamic stability. Whether participation will adversely effect the illness, or whether the illness will compromise performance, should be considered when making return to play decisions.

Cramps can occur during basketball, and can be caused by gastrointestinal cramping as a result of upper gastrointestinal distress or related to gastroenteritis. In addition, general muscle cramping can also occur and involve several muscle groups, most commonly the gastrocnemius–soleus complex, or other leg muscles. In the former, treatment should be aimed at ruling out upper GI disease, and should consider H_2 blockers if there are significant GER symptoms. The timing of fluid and food intake prior to activity should also be discussed and modified as necessary. For muscle cramps that occur in the late stages of activity, improper hydration is often the source, and assessing the athlete's diet, hydration, and ensuring electrolyte balance is important. Assessment for hyponatremia, hypomagnesemia or other electrolyte abnormalities should be considered, with careful history, examination, and appropriate laboratory testing as a guide to evaluation.

Genitourinary problems

Genitourinary problems can occur in the basketball player, and can be a result of trauma, or represent conditions that are not specific to the sport. Examples of the latter include proteinuria and hematuria, epididymitis, inguinal hernia, varicocele or hydrocele, nephrolithiasis or testicular tumor. Examples of those injuries that can occur as a result of trauma that can occur during basketball play include testicular torsion or rupture, or renal contusion, laceration or renal fracture. Some of these problems are briefly discussed below.

Proteinuria is not uncommon, and has been reported in 5–85% of screening urinalysis and 70% of athletes (Burroughs & Hilts 2002). In most instances, proteinuria in athletes is benign, but evaluation for persistent proteinuria should be thorough and complete (Carroll & Tenite 2000). Evaluation should include repeat testing, and history should include assessment of renal disease, hypertension, anemia and diabetes as well as infections (streptococcus), medications (antibiotics or nonsteroidal anti-inflammatories), or supplements. If repeat morning testing demonstrates persistent proteinuria, additional testing that includes complete blood count (CBC), fasting glucose, and a 24-h urine measuring protein, creatinine and creatinine clearance should be obtained.

Hematuria is similarly common in athletes, and can be benign or represent more serious underlying medical problems. Hematuria can be related to trauma, either from a direct blow to the kidney or bladder, or indirect trauma from recurrent jumping or running. Hematuria can also be due to renal pathology, infection, nephrolithiasis, malignancy, urinary tract infection, rhabdomyolysis, sickle cell disease, or coagulopathy. It can also occur as a result of certain medications, polycystic kidney disease or arteriovenous malformations. If repeat testing confirms hematuria, additional testing including blood urea nitrogen, CBC, electrolytes, creatinine, and renal ultrasound as well as intravenous pyelogram should be considered. In individuals older than 40, if the above tests are normal and hematuria is persistent, cystoscopy should also be considered to assess for urethral and/or bladder lesions. Hematuria related to exercise is a diagnosis of exclusion, and a complete work-up must be done before making this diagnosis, especially in older athletes (Abarbanel et al. 1990).

In the young athlete, assessment of scrotal or testicular masses is important and should be complete. Although the incidence of benign lesions such as varicoceles and hydroceles is high, the possibility of testicular malignancy should always be considered in the male athlete. Testicular cancer remains the most common cancer in young men, and during the PPPE, not only should the athlete be assessed for an inguinal hernia, but also discussion of the self-testicular exam should take place. Any suspicious masses should be assessed further with ultrasonography.

During basketball play, blows to the kidneys, bladder, or genitals can occur. In general, the amount of trauma is minimal and thus renal lacerations or fractures are not common. If significant trauma and bleeding occur, a blood count and orthostatic blood pressure should be obtained to rule out significant vascular compromise. For less severe trauma, an intravenous pyelogram can demonstrate cortical laceration where extravasation of dye occurs. Computed tomography may be needed for more significant injuries and can localize injury.

Direct trauma to the genital area can cause contusions in both genders, but in male athletes, testicular or epididymal fracture can occur and can be a medical emergency. Symptoms will include pain, swelling, nausea and anxiety. Evaluation should be complete with attempt to identify intact testes and epididymis structures. Early treatment includes ice and elevation. Hematuria should be aggressively followed and urethral injury should be ruled out. For the athlete with acute trauma with symptoms, testicular ultrasound should be obtained to rule out fracture of the testes or epididymis as well as testicular torsion (Galeis & Kass 1999).

Return to play

Return to play after genitourinary problems depends on the nature of the problem, and will differ depending on the individual. For both hematuria and proteinuria in the absence of trauma, the athlete can be allowed to participate as long as they are hemodynamically stable, and acute infection is controlled. For the entities related to trauma, exercise should be limited until definitive diagnosis has been made. Further decisions should be individualized depending on the specific medical problem and the level of play considered.

Skin conditions

Conditions affecting the skin are common in basketball, as in all sports. These can be divided into simple abrasions and lacerations, and infectious diseases. Abrasions and lacerations occur commonly during basketball play, the former from contact with the playing surface, and the latter from contact with an opponent, the playing surface or the basketball rim or surroundings.

A common mechanism for a laceration to the face is an elbow being thrown during rebounding. The timely care of abrasions and lacerations is important, and as discussed later, universal precautions should be used in taking care of the bloody athlete. The first thing that must occur when taking care of abrasions or lacerations is to control any active bleeding, and assess for associated injuries. If the laceration involves the head or face, caution should be taken such that mild traumatic brain injury (mTBI) is not missed. Depending on the location, underlying fracture or joint involvement should also be considered.

Once the bleeding is controlled, an assessment for the severity of injury should be made. The area should be cleansed and cleaned, and compression applied. If the laceration is deep enough to warrant suturing, but can be controlled with steri strips or some other form of coverage, this will allow the player to return to activity with minimal time loss. These lacerations can then be addressed properly after the game. Blood must be cleaned from the court surface and clothing before the athlete can return to play.

Other skin conditions include those that are at risk for transmission to others, and those that are not. Contact dermatitis, acne vulgaris, tinea versicolor and tinea cruris ("jock itch") are examples of skin conditions that pose minimal risk to others that occur in the basketball player. Skin conditions that are at risk for transmission on the basketball court include herpes gladiatorum, tinea corporis, erysipelas, and impetigo. Contact dermatitis can occur in response to knee sleeves or other sports equipment, or can occur from exposure to plants such as poison ivy if the athlete is playing outside. Treatment generally includes avoidance and proper cleansing of braces, topical corticosteroids, and on occasion, a short course of oral corticosteroids (prednisone), as well as antipruritic agents.

Acne vulgaris is common in all athletes, irrespective of gender and sport, often exacerbated by the perspiration and resultant increased bacteria present on the skin. Topical agents, such as tretinoin gel, can be used if not severe, though many athletes prefer to use an oral antibiotic, such as erythromycin or tetracycline. Treatment should also include education regarding general hygiene and proper skin cleansing. If these measures are not satisfactory, referral to a dermatologist should be considered.

Tinea infections can occur in several areas of the body, and are named according to the body part involved. Tinea cruris (groin area) and tinea pedis (feet) are generally not in contact with opponents during basketball play, though they can be transmitted via common areas such as shower facilities. Tinea corporis (body) and tinea capitis (scalp) are other examples of tinea. Tinea cruris ("jock itch") appears as erythematous lesions which are sharply demarcated, irregular and scaly. It can appear in the groin, perineum and perianal area, is more common in men, and generally does not occur on the genitalia because of the scrotal sebum which has an antifungal effect (Basler 2002). In "jock itch" prevention includes keeping the groin area dry, using antiperspirant powders, and using absorbent undergarments which breath (boxers instead of briefs) when not practicing or playing. Tinea pedis ("athlete's foot") appears as irregular, scaly patches with erythema and if severe, maceration and erosions can occur. Diagnosis of tinea infections is often made by history and physical examination, though definitive diagnosis can be made by evaluating scrapings in potassium hydroxide under a microscope. Treatment of fungal infections includes topical antifungal agents, and oral antifungal agents can be used in severe or widespread infections. Terfenadine (250 mg·day^{-1}), itraconazole (200 mg·day^{-1}), or fluconazole (150 mg·day^{-1}) are all examples of appropriate oral medications used for treatment of these disorders. Areas that are exposed must be covered with an impermeable bandage such that transmission is avoided.

Tinea versicolor is more correctly called pityriasis versicolor in that it is caused by a commensal yeast (vs. tinea which is a "cutaneous infection by a dermatophyte agent") (Helm & Bergfeld 2001). Pityriasis versicolor is a common skin disease in all athletes, and is often more obvious in African American athletes because it shows up as hypopigmented scaly patches seen over the trunk and torso. This skin infection is generally benign and self-limited, and only occasionally will these lesions be pruritic. Athletes often seek treatment because they are cosmetically obvious. Treatment can include selenium sulfide 1% lotion applied for 10–15 minutes then washed off daily for 2 weeks, topical antifungal creams, or oral antifungal agents, and treatment should be individualized. In general, oral agents should only be used if the other treatments fail, given the potential for hepatotoxicity of oral antifungals. Pityriasis versicolor often recurs, and if this occurs, prophylactic treatment on a monthly basis can be considered.

Herpes gladiatorum is another skin infection that, although more commonly associated with wrestlers, can occur in the basketball player, and must be treated. These infections can limit participation if they cannot be covered. Primary herpes infection is associated with high fever, myalgias, malaise, headache and lymphadenopathy. After 1–2 days, these systemic symptoms are followed by a group of vesicles that are often associated with burning and itching. In secondary infections, the systemic symptoms are not present and the grouped vesicles occur generally in the same dermatome with tingling and burning predating the onset of the rash.

Herpes infection is again often treated emperically with diagnosis made by history and physical examination, though definitive diagnosis requires viral culture. Herpes is often difficult to culture, thus cultures may be falsely negative, and emperic treatment with antivirals is often indicated if clinical suspicion is high. Treatment with aciclovir, famiciclovir or valacyclovir should be initiated and lesions should be treated for five to 10 days. Herpes is contagious for the day before and the four days after the rash is present, and is less contagious when the lesions are dry. Some authors have recommended unroofing these lesions and applying benzoin or injecting dilute triamcinolone into the lesions (Basler 2002). These lesions must be adequately covered, and if this is not possible, the athlete cannot participate until the lesions have crusted over, which generally takes a minimum of 72 h after treatment is initiated.

Impetigo and erysipelas are bacterial skin infections caused by staphylococcus and streptococcus bacteria that must be treated and covered. These infections are contagious and also pose a risk to the athlete if left untreated. Toxic shock syndrome, bacterial myositis, scarlet fever, pyomyositis and glomerulonephritis can all occur as a complication to bacterial infection. Diagnosis is often made by culture, and treatment with systemic antibiotics that treats both staphylococcus and streptococcus should be initiated empirically once cultures have been obtained. Further treatment should be continued based on culture results and sensitivities. These lesions must also be covered to prevent transmission.

Exercise-induced bronchospasm

Exercise-induced bronchospasm (EIB) is a common medical problem in all sports, including basketball. It is classically described as shortness of breath, coughing, chest tightness and/or wheezing which typically occurs after 8–10 min of moderate exercise. It is associated with a decline in pulmonary function tests; >15% drop in forced expiratory volume in 1 second (FEV1), >35% decrease in forced expiratory flow rate, >10% decrease in peak expiratory flow rate, and an increase in both residual lung volume and total lung capacity (Kobayashi & Kobayashi 2002). EIB in basketball can be precipitated by playing in the cold weather, or by allergens that are present when playing outdoors. Other precipitants include viral infections, air pollution, or dry air. Because basketball involves strenuous activity with intermittent sprinting and prolonged play, it carries a higher risk for EIB than sports such as swimming or baseball. Several mechanisms for EIB have been described, though the current thinking is that it is due to water loss in combination with release of cholinergic or inflammatory mediators.

Diagnosis can often be made by the clinical presentation, and in these situations, emperic treatment with a bronchodilator prior to activity can be considered. If the diagnosis is questionable, or if a therapeutic challenge is not useful in alleviating symptoms, further standardized testing should be performed. This can include bedside spirometry performed before and after an exercise challenge. FEV1, FEF (forced expiratory flow), and PEFR (peak expiratory flow rate) should be measured prior to exercise, and then again after exercise every 5 min for 30 min. An exercise test in the setting that the athlete is symptomatic is often preferable in that it reproduces the environmental and sport-specific demands the athlete is accustomed to. Other options include formal pulmonary function tests with or without methacholine. In both standardized tests, whether there is improvement both clinically as well as objectively after a bronchodilator has been given is also useful.

Non-pharmacologic treatment can include proper warm-up, avoidance of triggers, and cardiovascular training. An initial exercise trigger will induce a drop in FEV1 and then a refractory period, such that if a second exercise trigger is presented during this refractory period, the second exercise trigger is followed by a smaller drop in FEV1. This has been termed "running through your asthma" and entails either hard sprints, or 10–15 min of exercise at 75–80% $\dot{V}_{O_{2max}}$; it can be very useful in lessening the symptoms of exercise-induced bronchospasm in the competitive athlete. The athlete should also be encouraged to increase their cardiorespiratory fitness in that if the athlete is trained, a more intense exercise challenge is required for a bronchoconstrictive response to occur.

Pharmacologic treatment often starts with a beta-agonist used prior to exercise. If this fails, the next step is to add either cromolyn sodium or nedocromil sodium prior to exercise. Other medication options include inhaled corticosteroids, antihistamines, and leukotriene modifiers. Theophylline has fallen out of favor due to its side-effects and drug interactions, though can still be used as an adjunct. The treatment of EIB should be individualized and the physician should ensure that the medications being used are not banned by the appropriate governing bodies (National Asthma Education Program 1991; Rupp *et al.* 1993; Drazen *et al.* 1999; Kobayashi & Kobayashi 2002).

Upper respiratory illness

Otitis, pharyngitis, sinusitis and other upper respiratory infections are common in basketball players, as well as all athletes. These are most commonly caused by viruses (adenovirus, rhinovirus, Ebstein–Barr virus (EBV) coxsackievirus A, influenza, or cytomegalovirus), bacteria (streptococcus, groups A, B, C and G), or atypicals (*Chlamydia twar*, *Mycoplasma*). The majority of these should be diagnosed by either clinical presentation with supporting culture and laboratory tests as indicated, and are not discussed in further detail here. There is no basketball-specific concerns for these illnesses though EBV and group A β-hemolytic streptococcus (GABHS) deserve special mention, and are discussed below.

Return to play after upper respiratory illness

In general, an athlete that has a fever greater than 100.5°F, no matter the cause, should not be allowed to participate in any type of exercise. This is due to the potential for developing myocarditis and the hypermetabolic state induced by fever. If an athlete has a high fever, or other signs of infection, a full evaluation should be performed to identify the source. This often requires further laboratory and diagnostic testing. In addition, the febrile athlete should be assessed to ensure that concomitant dehydration is not present. Orthostatic measurements of blood pressure and heart rate should be performed to make this assessment. Dehydration can be a predisposing factor for the development of heat related illness.

Participation during an illness can have an effect on the course of the illness, leading to a prolonged clinical course for diseases such as viral meningitis and Ebstein–Barr virus. Exercise can change the levels of lymphocytes, both T and B cells, IgA, interferon, and interleukin-1 (Martin 2002). To what extent these changes will affect the clinical course of illnesses, as well as how exercise affects illness or how illness affects exercise, remains unclear.

Group A β-hemolytic streptococcus

The classic presentation of GABHS is fever, headache, malaise, and exudative pharyngeal and tonsillar erythema with associated tender cervical adenopathy, anorexia, nausea, vomiting and abdominal pain, or scarlet fever (Vukmir 1992; Kiselica 1994). Unfortunately, most patients do not present with classic symptoms, and differentiating GABHS from viral illness is often challenging. It is important to

diagnose and treat these individuals quickly to limit their infectivity and the possibility of developing complications such as peritonsillar abscess and acute rheumatic fever and acute glomerulonephritis. Effective diagnosis and treatment remains controversial, with some advocating emperic treatment depending on clinical presentation, rapid strep tests with back-up throat cultures, or just culture data (Pichechero 1995; Perkins 1997; McIsaac et al. 1998; Wald et al. 1998; Miser 1999). Two scoring systems are presented in Table 12.2.

Return to play after GABHS

Once treatment is initiated, individuals are no longer effective within 24 h and generally can return to basketball play as long as they feel well, are hemodynamically stable, and do not have an elevated temperature. It is important to monitor these individuals, and it may be prudent to limit activity if they are unable to eat or drink enough to sustain recovery as well as exercise.

Table 12.2 Streptococcal scoring systems.

McIssac *et al.*		Wald *et al.*	
Criteria	*Points*	*Criteria*	*Points*
Temperature > 38°C	1	Temperature ≥38.3°C	1
No cough	1	No upper respiratory symptoms	1
Tender anterior cervical nodes	1	Tender or enlarged cervical nodes	1
Tonsillar swelling or exudate	1	Erythema, swelling, or exudate of pharynx or tonsils	1
Age 3–14 years	1	Age 5–15 years	1
Age 15–44 years	–0	Season (Nov–May)	1
Age >45 years	–1		
Total score ____		**Total score** ____	

Management based on streptococcal score			Positive predictive value of streptococcal score	
Total score	*Chance of GAS infection (%)*	*Suggested management*	*Score*	*PPV for positive throat culture*
0	2–3	No culture or antibiotic required	1	N/A
1	4–6		2	24%
2	10–12	Culture all: treat only if culture is positive	3	22%
3	27–28		4	41%
4	38–63	Culture all: treat with antibiotics on clinical grounds	5	59%
			6	75%

From McIsaac WJ, White D, Tannenbaum D, Low DE: A clinical score to reduce unnecessary antibiotic use in patients with sore throat. *Can Med Assoc J* **158**: 75–83, 1998, with permission © 1998 Canadian Medical Association; and Wald ER, Green MD, Schwartz B, Barbadora K: A streptococcal score card revisited. *Pediatr Emerg Care* **14**: 109–111, 1998, with permission.

Infectious mononucleosis

One important infection to assess for in the basketball player is infectious mononucleosis. Infectious mononucleosis is caused by the Ebstein–Barr virus (EBV), and is important in that it is common in the adolescent and young adult, presents with common symptoms, and is associated with hepatosplenomegaly. In general, the earlier the infection occurs, the more likely that it will be asymptomatic. EBV is very common in adolescence and early adulthood, with 70% of college freshman having had previous EBV disease. Acute infectious mononucleosis occurs in 1–3% of college students (Miser 1999). EBV is transmitted by extensive mucous membrane contact, and can be spread by sharing food and drinks. The presenting symptoms and signs include a prodrome of fatigue, malaise, myalgias, headache, and occasionally anorexia and nausea. This is soon followed by fever, chills, sore throat, and tender posterior cervical lymphadenopathy. The athlete will often have fever, an exudative pharyngitis, swollen eyelids and palatal petechiae. Jaundice and a morbilliform rash is seen in up to 10% (Miser 1999). Superinfection with streptococcus, group A, occurs in roughly 30%, and if the athlete is given amoxicillin or ampicillin, a maculopapular rash can also occur.

Diagnosis of EBV disease can be confirmed with laboratory testing, immunoglobulin testing being the most specific. The complete blood count will demonstrate a lymphocytosis, with atypical lymphocytes predominating. Neutropenia and thrombocytopenia can occur in the second week of illness, whereas anemia is not common and should heighten the possibility of splenic rupture. Mild elevations of liver function tests can be seen in the third week in up to 90% of EBV disease, though these generally return to normal by the fifth week. Superinfection with group A beta hemolytic strep occurs commonly and should be cultured for and treated, though avoiding ampicillin and amoxicillin, for the possibility of inducing a rash. Otherwise, treatment is generally supportive with rest, acetominophen or codeine for analgesia, and other supportive measures. Rarely, corticosteroids are required for obstruction of the airways due to severe tonsillitis. Most athletes will feel better after the second week of illness, with a majority feeling 100%

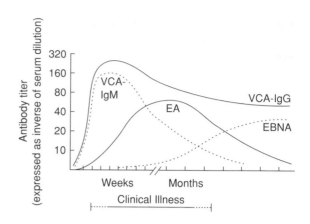

Fig. 12.2 Typical human serologic response to Epstein–Barr virus infection. At clinical presentation (usually 4–7 weeks after exposure), antiviral capsid antigen (anti-VCA) response may consist of IgM and IgG antibodies, anti-early antigen (anti-EA) response is often present, and anti-EBV nuclear antigen (anti-EBNA) is commonly negative. IgM anti-VCA response usually subsides within 2–4 months, and anti-EA response usually disappears within 2–6 months. Chronically infected, asymptomatic persons maintain measurable IgG anti-VCA and anti-EBNA titers for life. (Modified from Andiman *et al.* 1981.)

by 8 weeks. Complications of splenic rupture, autoimmune hemolytic anemia, granulocytopenia, and upper airway obstruction are rare.

The monospot test is a heterophile test that is positive in roughly 90% by the third week of illness in those with acute EBV disease. In some individuals with acute disease, however, the monospot test remains negative, making the use of specific antibody tests more useful if high clinical suspicion exists (Bailey 1994). The measurement of IgM and IgG levels are often the most sensitive marker of EBV disease and can differentiate acute (IgM (+), IgG (+)) from previous (IgM (–), IgG (+)) disease (Fig. 12.2).

It is important to consider EBV as the cause of an upper respiratory infection, especially because of the risk for hepatosplenomegaly. It takes time for the body to produce antibodies to the EBV and thus an initial monospot will be negative despite infection, and thus follow up evaluations and repeat testing is often indicated. Splenic rupture most commonly occurs between days 4 and 21 of illness, and determining if an athlete's spleen is enlarged is often difficult on physical examination alone (Dommerby *et al.* 1986; Safran & Bloom 1990; Farley *et al.* 1992;

Grover *et al.* 1993). For this reason, in athletes that participate in contact sports, such as basketball, further assessment with either ultrasound or computed tomography (CT) is recommended. If there is concern for splenic leakage or rupture, CT is preferable.

Return to play after infectious mononucleosis

For the first three weeks of illness, the spleen can rupture even if it is not significantly enlarged, and for this reason participation should be prohibited once the diagnosis is confirmed or if clinical suspicion is high. After this point, participation should be limited if the spleen remains enlarged. Repeat measurement by ultrasound should be performed until resolution of splenomegaly is confirmed. In the basketball player, it is sometimes difficult to know if the spleen is enlarged, given that these athletes are often taller and larger than "normal". In general, the size of an athlete's spleen is unknown prior to the diagnosis of EBV disease. This makes it more difficult to discern when the spleen size is enlarged and at risk for rupture.

Other issues to consider in return to play after infectious mononucleosis include the energy level of the athlete, as well as other comorbidities. These return to play decisions must be individualized. Ensuring that the athlete's energy level is >90% may be helpful in allowing them to avoid prolongation of their illness. Though a flack jacket can provide some additional protection, it cannot protect an athlete completely. Knowing that an athlete has EBV disease, however, should help the medical team identify a problem if it does occur and respond quickly.

Cytomegolavirus (CMV) infection is similar to EBV, and should be considered in the differential of a viral illness with malaise, HSM and fatigue. Other infections to be considered in the differential include toxoplasmosis, rubella, hepatitis, HIV and adenovirus. These entities can be differentiated by proper diagnostic and laboratory testing.

Blood-borne pathogens

During basketball play, several injuries can occur, and exposure to blood is not uncommon. This is generally limited, and occurs as a result of abrasions or simple lacerations. Less common are nasal fractures or other traumatic injuries where more blood exposure is possible. The rules of play do not allow an athlete to participate if they are actively bleeding or if blood is evident on their body or uniform. The bleeding must be controlled, and all blood washed and removed from the players and court. There are guidelines developed by OSHA for the proper handling of blood exposed athletes and these are enforced to protect against blood borne pathogens. Universal precautions should be followed to protect the athlete as well as the medical care provider against transmission of blood borne pathogens, though these risks are small.

The popularity of Earvin "Magic" Johnson, a basketball player at Michigan State University and the LA Lakers, brought the issue of the HIV athlete and participation in sports to national attention. Though the risks of transmission of HIV is due to off court activities and not on court play, universal precautions should always be followed. The risk of transmission of HIV during professional football in the United States has been estimated as 1 in 85 million game contacts (Brown *et al.* 1995). There has never been a documented case of HIV transmission during sport. Whether an athlete with HIV can safely participate in basketball and not put their health, or the health of other participants, at risk, is also controversial. Whether an athlete can compete depends on their immune function as well as whether they have any other comorbid medical problems, and care must be individualized (McGrew, in press).

The blood-borne infections that an athlete is at risk for acquiring during basketball play include hepatitis B and C, although these risks remain minimal when universal precautions are utilized. There has been one report of transmission of hepatitis B during sumo wrestling in Japan (Kashiwagi *et al.* 1982), and hepatitis is more infective than HIV. Several recommendations have been made in regard to blood borne pathogens and their risk of transmission in sport (Calabrese & LaPerriere 1993; CASM 1993; AMSSM 1995; NCAA 2002). It is important to remember that off the court activities such as sexual activity, blood transfusions, and IV drug use are likely more important risk factors than basketball play. Evaluating these risk factors with the basketball player during the PPPE can be useful as a preventative measure for contracting these and other blood-borne and sexually transmitted diseases.

Environmental concerns

Potential hazards to consider in the basketball player when competing outdoors include thunderstorms, high winds, and either low or high temperatures. Sun protection is another environmental concern that should be considered for the outdoor basketball player, and using appropriate clothing, as well as a sunscreen with greater than 15 spf to protect the skin from ultraviolet light is recommended. In addition, taking breaks in the shade or going into an air conditioned building during half time can decrease the risk of sun exposure as well as heat-related illness.

Lightening can also be an environmental concern for the outdoor player, and medical staff should terminate play when lightening is present. Paying attention to weather reports, and using the National weather service Doppler reports on AM radio frequencies can help determine the risk for storms prior to an organized tournament or outdoor competition.

Hypothermia and hyperthermia can both be concerns, and how the athlete hydrates and their pre-existing level of hydration can become important. In addition, concomitant medical illness with fever or other physiologic demands can be exacerbated by or worsen hypo or hyperthermia. Hydration, nutrition, and prevention of both cold and heat related illness can become important considerations in the outdoor basketball player. Taking frequent water breaks, using electrolyte solutions, and appropriate clothing protection is imperative. These problems are considered in Chapters 2–4 and elsewhere in this book, and the reader is referred to these chapters for full discussion.

References

Abarbanel, J., Benet, A.E., Lask, D. & Kimche, D. (1990) Sports hematuria. *Journal of Urology* **143**, 887–890.

American Academy of Pediatrics Committee on Sports Medicine and Fitness (1997) Athletic participation by children and adolescents who have systemic hypertension. *Pediatrics* **99**, 637–638.

American Medical Society for Sports Medicine and American Orthopedic Society for Sports Medicine (1995) Position Statement on HIV and other bloodborne pathogens in sports. *Clinical Journal of Sports Medicine* **5**, 199–204.

Andiman, W.A., McCarthy, P., Markowitz, R.I. *et al.* (1981) Clinical, virologic, and serologic evidence of Epstein–Barr virus infection in association with childhood pneumonia. *Journal of Pediatrics* **99**, 880–886.

Appel, L.S., Moore, T.J., Obarnzanek, E. *et al.* (1997) A clinical trial of the effects of dietary patterns on blood pressure. *New England Journal of Medicine* **336**, 1117–1124.

Bailey, R. (1994) Diagnosis and treatment of infectious mononucleosis. *American Family Physician* **49**, 879–885.

Bartosh, S.M. & Aronson, A.J. (1999) Childhood hypertension: An update on etiology, diagnosis, and treatment. *Pediatrics Clinics of N America* **46** (22), 235–252.

Basler, R.S.W. (2002) Skin Problems in Athletes. In: *The Team Physician's Handbook*, 3rd edn. Mellion, M.B., Walsh, M.W., Madden, C., Putukian, M. & Shelton, G.L. (eds). Philadelphia: Hanley & Belfus, pp. 311–325.

Brown, L., Drotman, P., Chu, A. *et al.* (1995) Bleeding injuries in professional football; Estimates of the risk for HIV transmission. *Annals of Internal Medicine* **122**, 271–275.

Burroughs, K.E. & Hilts, M.J. (2002) Renal and Genitoruniary Problems. In: *The Team Physician's Handbook*, 3rd edn. Mellion, M.B., Walsh, M.W., Madden, C., Putukian, M. & Shelton, G.L. (eds). Philadelphia: Hanley & Belfus, pp. 254–261.

Butcher, J.D. (1999) Gastrointestinal Problems. In: *Handbook of Sports Medicine; a Symptom-Oriented Approach.* Lillegard, W.A., Butcher, J.D. & Rucker, K.S. (eds). Massachusetts: Butterworth-Heinemann, pp. 315–320.

Calabrese, L. & LaPerriere, A. (1993) Human immunodeficiency virus infection, exercise, and athletics. *Sports Medicine* **15**, 1–7.

Canadian Academy of Sports Medicine (1993) Position statement: HIV, as it relates to sport. *Clinical Journal of Sports Medicine* **3**, 63–68.

Carroll, M.F. & Tenite, J.L. (2000) Proteinuria in adults: a diagnostic approach. *American Family Physician* **62**, 1333–1340.

Dommerby, H., Stangerup, S., Stangerup, M. & Hancke, S. (1986) Hepatosplenomegaly in infectious mononucleosis assessed by ultrasonic scanning. *Journal of Laryngological Otology* **100**, 573–579.

Drazen, J.M., Israel, E. & O'Bryne, P.M. (1999) Treatment of asthma with drugs modifying the leukotriene pathway. *New England Journal of Medicine* **340**, 197–206.

Farley, D., Zietlow, S., Bannon, M. & Farnell, M. (1992) Spontaneous rupture of the spleen due to infectious mononucleosis. *Mayo Clinical Proceedings* **67**, 846–853.

Galeis, L.E. & Kass, E.J. (1999) Diagnosis and treatment of the acute scrotum. *American Family Physician* **59** (4), 817–824.

Glover, D. (in press) Hypertension. In: *Sports Medicine Secrets*, 3rd edn. Mellion, M., Putukian, M. & Madden, C. (eds). Philadelphia: Hanley & Belfus.

Green, G.A. (1992) Gastrointestinal disorders in the athlete. *Clinical Sports Medicine* **11**, 453–470.

Grover, S., Barkun, A. & Sackett, D. (1993) Does this patient have splenomegaly? *Journal of the American Medical Association* **270**, 2218–2221.

Helm, T.N. & Bergfeld, W.F. (2001) Sports Dermatology. In: *Principles and Practice of Primary Care Sports Medicine*. Garrett, W.E., Kirkendall, D.T. & Squire, D.L. (eds). Philadelphia: Lippincott Williams & Wilkins, pp. 231–246.

Kaplan, N.M. (2001) Systemic hypertension. Mechanisms and diagnosis. In: Braunwald, ed. *Heart Disease; A Textbook of Cardiovascular Medicine*, 6th edn. Philadelphia: WB Saunders, pp. 941–957.

Kaplan, N.M., Deveraux, R.B. & Miller, J.S. (1994) 26th Bethesda Conference: recommendations for determining eligibility for competition in athletes with cardiovascular abnormalities. Task Force 4: Systemic hypertension. *Journal of the American College of Cardiology* **24**, 885–887.

Kashiwagi, S. *et al.* (1982) Outbreak of hepatitis B in members of a high-school sumo wrestling club. *Journal of the American Medical Association* **248** (2), 213–214.

Kiselica, D. (1994) Group A beta-hemolytic streptococcal pharyngitis: current clinical concepts. *American Family Physician* **49**, 1147–1154.

Kobayashi, R.H. & Kobayashi, A.L. (2002) Exercise-Induced Bronchospasm, Anaphylaxis, and Urticaria. In: *The Team Physician's Handbook*, 3rd edn. Mellion, M.B., Walsh, M.W., Madden, C., Putukian, M. & Shelton, G.L. (eds). Philadelphia: Hanley & Belfus, pp. 287–293.

Martin, T. (2002) Infections in athletes. In: *The Team Physician's Handbook*, 3rd edn. Mellion, M.B., Walsh, M.W., Madden, C., Putukian, M. & Shelton, G.L. (eds). Philadelphia: Hanley & Belfus, pp. 225–244.

McGrew, C. (in press) HIV/AIDS in athletes. In: *Sports Medicine Secrets*, 3rd edn. Mellion, M., Putukian, M. & Madden, C. (eds). Philadelphia: Hanley & Belfus.

McIsaac, W.J., White, D., Tannenbaum, D. & Low, D.E. (1998) A clinical score to reduce unnecessary antibiotic use in patients with sore throat. *Canadian Medical Association Journal* **158**, 75–83.

Miser, W.F. (1999) Acute minor illnesses in the athlete. In: *Handbook of Sports Medicine*. Lillegard, W.A., Butcher, J.D. & Rucker, K.S. (eds). Boston: Butterworth-Heinemann, pp. 353–366.

Mitchell, J.H., Haskell, W.L. & Raven, P.B. (1994) 26th Bethesda Conference: Classification of Sports. *Journal of the American College of Cardiology* **24**, 864–866.

National Asthma Education Program (1991) Expert Panel Report: Guidelines for the diagnosis and management of asthma. National Heart, Lung, and Blood Institute, National Institutes of health, Bethesda, MD. *Journal of Allergy and Clinical Immunology* **88**, 425–534.

NCAA (2002) Sports Medicine Handbook (2001–2002): Guideline, 2-h: Blood Borne Pathogens and Intercollegiate Athletics. Indianapolis: National Collegiate Athletic Association, pp. 35–39.

Perkins, A. (1997) An approach to diagnosing the acute sore throat. *American Family Physician* **55**, 131–138.

Pichechero, M. (1995) Group A streptococcal pharyngitis: cost effective diagnosis and treatment. *Annals of Emergency Medicine* **25**, 390–403.

Putukian, M. (1997) Don't miss gastrointestinal disorders in athletes. *Physician and Sportsmedicine* **25**, 80–84.

Rupp, N.T., Brudno, D.S. & Guill, M.F. (1993) The value of screening for risk of exercise-induced asthma in high school athletes. *Annals of Allergy* **70**, 339–342.

Sachtleben, T.R. & Mellion, M.B. (2002) The Hypertensive Athlete. In: *The Team Physician's Handbook*, 3rd edn. Mellion, M.B., Walsh, M.W., Madden, C., Putukian, M. & Shelton, G.L. (eds). Philadelphia: Hanley & Belfus, pp. 277–287.

Sacks, F.M., Svetkey, L.P., Vollmer, W.M. *et al.* (2001) Effects on blood pressure of reduced dietary sodium and the dietary approaches to stop hypertension (DASH) diet. *New England Journal of Medicine* **344**, 3–10.

Safran, D. & Bloom, G. (1990) Spontaneous splenic rupture following infectious mononucleosis. *American Surgery* **56**, 601–605.

Schwartz, A.E., Vaagunas, A. & Kamel, P.L. (1990) Endoscopy to evaluate gastrointestinal bleeding in marathon runners. *Annals of Internal Medicine* **113**, 632–633.

Statement on Traveler's Diarrhea (1995) *Canadian Medical Association Journal* **152**, 205–208.

Steingard, S.A. (1993) Special Considerations in the Medical Management of Professional Basketball Players. *Clinics Sports Medicine* **12** (2), 239–246.

Swain, R. & Kaplan, B. (1997) Treating hypertension in active patients: which agents work best with exercise? *Physician and Sports Medicine* **25** (9), 47–65.

Vukmir, R. (1992) Adult and pediatric pharyngitis: a review. *Journal of Emergency Medicine* **10**, 607–616.

Wald, E.R., Green, M.D., Schwartz, B. & Barbadora, K. (1998) A streptococcal score care revisited. *Pediatric Emergency Care* **14**, 109–111.

Working Group Report (1996) Update on the 1987 Task Force Report on High Blood Pressure in Children and Adolescents: the National High Blood Pressure Education Program (1996). *Pediatrics* **98**, 648–658.

Chapter 13
Spine and pelvis

Jill Cook and Karim Khan

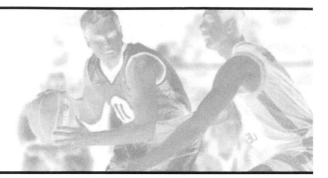

Back pain is a common complaint when basketball players attend for treatment. In a recent study of over 10 000 basketball participations, back injuries made up 5.3% of the total injuries (McKay *et al.* 2001). Furthermore, the therapist who travels with elite teams spends a great deal of time treating back pain and providing preventive mobilization for "stiff" backs, that might not be recorded in an injury surveillance study. The aim of this chapter is to provide an overview of common sports medicine problems that affect the back and pelvis in basketball players.

We first tackle problems arising in the axial skeleton by discussing the cervical spine, thoracic spine, and lumbar spine in turn. In each part we briefly review the anatomy, outline relevant biomechanics with a special emphasis on basketball, and then discuss management of the common conditions affecting that part of the spine. The remainder of the chapter concerns pelvic problems in basketball, and although these are not common, conditions such as stress fractures and osteitis pubis can severely limit a basketball player.

Axial skeleton—introduction

The vertebral column is comprised of 33 vertebrae, 24 of which are mobile and 9 in the sacrum and coccyx that are fixed. There are 7 cervical, 12 thoracic and 5 lumbar mobile vertebrae. The shape and function of these change from superior to inferior,

as mobility and diminutive size give way to stability and support. Both the vertebral bodies and the vertebral arch increase in size from cervical to lumbar spine. The vertebral bodies consist mainly of cancellous bone with strong lamellae making them light and strong while allowing them to store large amounts of energy.

A typical vertebra has a body with a pair of pedicles and lamina that form a vertebral arch. The pedicle has a notch on its inferior surface (the intervertebral foramen) for the spinal nerve. At the junction of the pedicle and lamina is the articular process that provides a single surface of a facet joint, which articulates with the vertebra above (Fig. 13.1). The

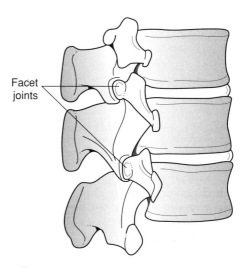

Fig. 13.1 Typical vertebral structure showing articulation between two vertebrae (the facet joint).

transverse process projects laterally from the pedicle/lamina junction and the spinous process projects posteriorly from the junction of the laminae.

The anterior part of the spinal column is comprised of the vertebral bodies and discs. The vertebrae are separated by intervertebral discs that make up more than a quarter of the length of the spine. The discs comprise an outer dense collagenous layer and a more gel-like interior portion. The outer layer, the annulus fibrosis, is a collagen-rich concentric ring of fibrocartilage the outer third of which is innervated and can be a source of pain without herniation or degeneration (Bogduk 1991). The nucleus pulposus, the central region of the disc is enclosed by the annulus and the vertebral cartilage endplates. It is a mesh of collagen fibers and large proteoglycans which absorb water into the disc (Melrose *et al.* 1998).

The posterior part of the spine comprises the vertebral arch and neural structures. The spinal cord is encased in the bony-ligamentous foramen formed by the vertebral body anteriorly and the lamina and pedicle laterally and posteriorly. The cord finishes at the first lumbar vertebra, below this is the cauda equina, the remaining segmental spinal nerves which run inferiorly and exit at the appropriate level. At each level, spinal nerves exit through the foramina, just below the pedicle of the vertebra above, and above the disc. Small nerves that supply the structures of the disc and facet joints also exit here.

The posterior spine, especially the joints, transmit 30% of the load through the spine. The joints are oriented more vertically in the thoracic region than in the cervical and lumbar regions and are loaded more in extension, a position common in basketball in rebounding. They are true synovial joints and the capsule is fully supported by ligaments.

The ligaments of the spine include those that run between the bodies (anterior and posterior longitudinal ligaments) and those between the posterior arch structures (interspinous ligament, supraspinous ligament and ligamentum flavum).

The spine stabilizes and supports the upper body and transmits body weight to the pelvis and legs, protects the neural structures and permits mobility of the head and arms. The curves of the spine provide resilience to weight bearing.

Table 13.1 "Red flags" alerting the clinician that back pain may have a serious cause.

Spinal cord symptoms (difficulty walking, tripping)
Corda equina signs (bowel and bladder dysfunction)
Vertebral artery signs (dizziness related to neck position)
Neural signs (motor and/or sensory loss)
Systemic symptoms (malaise, night pain)
Systemic disease and night pain

Clinical overview of spinal injury and pain

Pain in the spine is a diagnostic challenge, and an accurate assessment of the source of the pain is often difficult. In basketball, as in most sports, injury affects the soft tissue components of the spine more commonly than it does the osseous parts. In most cases, treatment aims to achieve symptom relief and functional recovery, rather than precise diagnosis and this is usually successful. However, all clinicians must be alert to "red flags" that reflect more serious manifestations of spinal pain (Table 13.1).

These symptoms and signs require rapid diagnosis that may include sophisticated imaging. Note that basketball players are not immune from general medical conditions, so persistent back pain must be assessed to exclude conditions such as malignancy, pelvic disease in women, renal disease and systemic arthropathies (Brukner & Khan 2001b). Nevertheless, in most cases of back pain in basketball players, imaging is not required. It is important to also note that abnormal imaging does not guarantee that the site is the source of the pain, as pathology can exist without pain and vice versa.

When using imaging, X-ray reveals spinal alignment and may indicate loss of disc height, significant pathology either of mechanical or other pathology. It is however, only useful as an exclusion examination for more serious pathology. A computed tomography (CT) scan can provide accurate morphological detail of both disc and facet joint pathology but does not provide the same quality of images as does magnetic resonance (MR) imaging. Furthermore, CT generates significant doses of radiation whereas MR uses none. In North American practice, MR is often the investigation of choice in the patient with persistent back pain, or suspicion of significant pathology. Where MR is not available, the combination of radionuclide bone scan and CT scan can provide information regarding bone, disc, and joint tissues.

Major spinal and pelvic injuries are rare in basketball and even simple fractures occur infrequently. One potentially dangerous setting occurs when a player is jumping high to dunk or rebound and an opponent runs underneath this player and knocks his or her legs away from underneath. This illegal move, called "tunneling", has the potential to cause a player to land head-first, which could cause axial loading injury to the cervical spine that can result in cervical fracture, although there is no suggestion that these occur in basketball. Assessment and management of any high force or velocity injury to the spine and pelvis should follow standard emergency procedure.

Cervical spine

The cervical spine requires great mobility but must also support the weight of the head. Hence, the cervical spine is prone to injury and degeneration and is a common source of pain both locally and regionally. Proximal pain referral to the head and distal pain referral to the arm, shoulder and thoracic spine are common. Basketball requires excellent cervical mobility, and similar to the lumbar spine, rebounding requires excellent extension.

Anatomy

The cervical spine is a complex anatomical region with two atypical and five typically shaped vetebrae. The first cervical vertebra has no body and the second has a large process that allows the first vertebra to rotate around. The remaining vertebrae have a typical vertebral shape, with small joints as well as discs between the vertebral bodies. The transverse processes have a foramen that permits passage of the vertebral artery.

Biomechanics

Functionally as well as anatomically the cervical spine is divided into two sections with the upper cervical segment (C1 and 2) considered separately from the lower segment. These two sections have different curves (upper neutral, lower lordotic) and can move independently of each other.

Flexion of the cervical spine occurs mainly in the lower segment, whereas extension occurs in the whole cervical spine. Flexion of the upper segment occurs when the chin is tucked in and the head is tipped forward and occurs more at the craniocervical joint than between C1 and 2. Rotation and lateral flexion occur as coupled movements, the relationship is complex and varies at different cervical levels.

Common pathology and presentation

Several syndromes are well known in the cervical spine, and can occur in basketball. Acceleration/deceleration injury (whiplash) can occur in a fall, when the head moves quickly without restraint or the head hits the ground or other object. The severity is usually less than that seen in higher velocity accidents. Lower velocity mechanisms as in sport result in a quicker recovery than high velocity injuries, but full recovery may take several weeks. The anterior structures are most commonly injured, but specific pathology may be hard to determine either clinically or with imaging.

Contact injury or falls on to the shoulder can lead to radiating pain, numbness, or tingling down one upper limb, usually lasting less than 1 min. This is commonly referred to as a "burner" or "stinger" in North American circles (Feinberg *et al.* 2000). Recurrences are common but have not been associated with permanent neurological deficit (Torg *et al.* 1997). Although much less common in basketball than in American football, the basketball physician must be aware of this phenomenon. Management includes restoration of neck motion and functional strengthening.

Acute loss of neck movement and pain (wry neck) is also seen, but most commonly occurs in a non-sporting environment. Wry neck can be due to apophyseal joint or disc injury. It responds well to symptomatic treatment of manual mobilization and exercise to restore range of movement.

Abnormal and sustained postural loads may result in pain, weakness and secondary pathology.

Muscle strain—acute, well localized muscle tenderness

Direct muscle injury is rare in all sports although pain from muscle spasm secondary to other pathology is common. Diagnosis and treatment should be directed at identifying the underlying cause of muscle pain and spasm, as well as directly treating the muscles.

A practical approach to treatment of basketball players

Whatever the suspected diagnosis of back pain, treatment in basketball players is usually symptomatic and is generally directed at more than one anatomical structure. Improving function requires increasing spinal joint mobility, strengthening spinal and abdominal muscles, and ensuring flexibility and appropriate function in the muscles of the pelvis and thigh. Finally sport-specific strength and function are required and in basketball this equates to normal spinal extension and lower limb function.

Hypomobility syndromes are easier to treat and respond more quickly than hypermobility syndromes. Irritable symptoms are difficult to treat. These athletes present with increasing pain after minimal treatment and may aggravate symptoms with small changes in functional levels. Treatment of disc disease is based on symptoms and an understanding of the underlying pathology. Treatment to improve musculoskeletal function in the surrounding structures will usually return the athlete to discal disease that is asymptomatic.

Range of movement

Treatment directed at recovering all range of movement of the spine is a crucial aspect of rehabilitation. In the basketball player, extension of the spine is essential, but recovery of all movements is desirable. Those unable to recover extension after disc prolapse may not respond conservatively and may require surgical intervention (Kopp et al. 1986).

Posture

Altering standing, sitting and sporting posture can be an important treatment. Sporting posture involves both the central stability and attention to techniques used in sport and the effect they have on the spine or the effect the spine has on the technique.

Muscular rehabilitation

There has been much interest in the role of the spinal muscles both anterior and posterior in the treatment of low back pain. It is apparent that muscle function is compromised in the acute and subacute phases of pain, and may not spontaneously recover with recovery from pain and function (Hides et al. 1995). Recruitment of both transverse abdominis and multifidus are abnormal in people with low back pain (Hodges & Richardson 1996). Research has also indicated that exercise can improve outcome in those patients with pain from anatomical instability (O'Sullivan et al. 1997). The local muscle systems that provide segmental stability require rehabilitation after back pain (Richardson & Jull 2000).

Close supervision of rehabilitation is paramount in all people with low back pain, but athletes that demand high levels of control and tall basketball players who have long levers and spines must be rehabilitated correctly and completely with close attention paid to muscular control and endurance.

Attention should be paid to the specific nature of this rehabilitation, as generic exercise prescription may not activate the appropriate muscles. Cocontraction of the deep abdominal and back muscles is another component of this rehabilitation; cocontraction supports the spinal segments. The muscles should be contracted at a low level of the maximal voluntary contraction as it is the tonic muscle fibers that provide the best joint stabilization. These fibers are most inhibited by pain and disuse. Similarly, the muscles should be worked with small regular repetitions during the day.

Initially, muscles should be worked isometrically, without movements of the limbs and then progressing to isometric contraction with limb movement.

The exercise should be performed with low load and in positions where the body weight is supported (4-point kneel).

Exercises should be progressed by increasing the time of contraction, increasing the load on the muscle by making body position more functional and by exercising with progressively greater range of motion. Ultimately, exercise should be completed in stressful positions with dynamic load.

Neural structures

Mobilization of neural tissue can be an important aspect of treatment of spinal pain (Butler 2000). In the lumbar spine, the nerves of the sacral and lumbar plexus course through large active muscle groups, leaving them vulnerable to irritation and intermittent compression. Adequate clinical examination of these structures and diagnosis of tightness and compression is essential in the complete examination and treatment of an athlete with low back pain.

Basketball-specific return to sport guidelines

Basketball allows graduated return to training and competition as it offers opportunity to increase the load on the spine in a progressive manner. Often players can return through shooting foul shots, jump shots, individual moves, offensive 1-on-1 moves, defensive 1-on-1 training, then quarter court, half court through to full training. Restriction of time on court and restriction of other fitness and weight work may also be necessary. Rehabilitation may require specific detailed limitation of basketball training. For example after a significant disc injury limitations on training and playing may exist until the back is capable of withstanding a charge and consequent fall onto the buttocks. Facet joint stiffness and pain may limit defensive training until full painfree extension has been regained. This requires a close working relationship between the clinician and the team coach.

Pelvis

Although not a common cause of many missed games in basketball players, the basketball team physician will come across players with both minor and moderately severe pelvic pain. One particularly challenging condition remains the chronic groin pain syndrome which may arise from a range of structures including the inguinal canal and herniae, the pubic symphysis, possible the abdominal or adductor tendons and rarely nerve entrapments. Several conditions are common in other sports and may occasionally be seen in the basketball player.

Anatomy

The pelvis is a bony ring comprised of the sacral and coccygeal vertebrae attached posteriorly through the sacroiliac joint to the pelvic ring which extends laterally and then anteriorly to join at the front at the pubic symphysis. The pelvic ring is made up of three bones the ilium, the ischium and the pubis.

Both the sacroiliac joint and the pubic symphysis are strong joints with little mobility, and the pubic symphysis has a fibrocartilaginous disc between the bone ends. There are also strong ligamentous connections between the sacrum and the spine.

Biomechanics of the pelvis

Movement of the pelvis occurs as a couple between the spine and legs. Movement of the anterior and posterior pelvic joints are related so abnormalities in the posterior pelvic joints may induce pain and pathology in the anterior joint (Major & Helms 1997).

The sacrum is a friction joint with bony and cartilaginous ridges which allow limited movement. The main movement of the sacrum on the ilium is a forward and backward tilting (Vleeming 1997). Forward tilting occurs in loaded positions such as standing, and tightens most SIJ ligaments and increases joint compression. Backward tilting occurs in unloaded position such as sitting and lying.

Common pelvic conditions

Stress fractures

Stress fractures are reported in running athletes, but appear rare in basketball players. Fractures of the pubic bones appear most common and only rare reports of sacral or other pelvic fractures appear in the literature. If these stress fractures occur, the physician should seek evidence of undernutrition as an underlying cause of poor bone health (Khan *et al*. 2002).

Sacroiliac joint dysfunction and pain

The role of the pelvic joints in producing low back and pelvic pain is well established. The relative emphasis afforded this structure in baskeball players' pain varies between authors. Diagnosis remains problematic as tests designed to evaluate sacroiliac joint movement overall have poor reliability. Palpation of the joint is also of doubtful clinical utility. Nevertheless, as the sacroiliac joint is a pain-producing structure, it is likely to be a cause of at least some pelvic pain.

Osteitis pubis

This is common in sports that have high load and change of direction such as football codes. Young, recently skeletally mature males seem most at risk, and many have had pain for a considerable period. Load through the pubic symphysis is considered to be the cause of the condition, but lack of hip joint rotation has been considered to be of significance (Verrall *et al*. 2001).

Typically, the athlete will have groin pain that may radiate to the adductors and the lower abdominal region with exquisite tenderness over the symphysis and adjacent pubic bone. Strength training has been shown to be critical to successful return to sport in soccer players (Holmich *et al*. 1999) and this approach should be incorporated into treatment of basketball players.

Apophysitis

There are several apophyses in the pelvis, all associated with large muscle groups, and vulnerable to injury in adolescence when under sporting loads. Basketball does not appear to be a sport associated with these injuries (Rossi & Dragoni 2001) as it does in the knee. Occasionally, however, the clinician may see acute or chronic apophysitis of the ischial tuberosity and the anterior iliac spines.

Muscular pain or trigger points

These have been well documented and the gluteal muscles may become an independent source of pain in the athlete with low back pain (Travell & Simons 1992). These can be assessed and treated with soft tissue techniques and stretches.

Conclusion

Back pain is a common problem in basketball and the team physician, therapists and coaches must understand the range of pathologies that exist. Various pathologies can have very different prognoses. Clinical assessment is the major guide to management as imaging findings do not correspond consistently with pain symptoms. Surgery is to be avoided unless there are signs of significant cord compression—muscle weakness or wasting, or there has been 6–12 months of failure of conservative management.

References

Bogduk, N. (1991) The lumbar disc and low back pain. *Neurosurgery Clinics of North America* **2** (4), 791–806.

Bogduk, N. (1997) *Clinical Anatomy of the Lumbar Spine and Sacrum*, 3rd edn. New York: Churchill Livingstone.

Brukner, P. & Khan, K. (2001a) Low back pain. In: *Clinical Sports Medicine*, 2nd edn. Sydney: McGraw-Hill, pp. 330–361.

Brukner, P. & Khan, K. (2001b) Pain: Where is it coming from? In: *Clinical Sports Medicine*, 2nd edn. Sydney: McGraw-Hill, pp. 30–35.

Butler, D. (2000) *The Sensitive Nervous System*. Adelaide: Noigroup Publications, pp. 91–106.

Feinberg, J. (2000) Burners and stingers. *Physical Medicine and Rehabilitation Clinics of North America* **11** (4), 771–784.

Frank, C.B. (1996) Ligament healing: current knowledge and clinical applications. *Journal of the American Academy of Orthopedic Surgeons* **4**, 74–83.

Hides, J.A., Richardson, C.A. & Jull, G.A. (1995) Magnetic resonance imaging and ultrasonography of the lumbar multifidus muscle. Comparison of two different modalities. *Spine* **20** (1), 54–58.

Hodges, P.W. & Richardson, C.A. (1996) Inefficient muscular stabilization of the lumbar spine associated with low back pain. A motor control evaluation of transversus abdominis. *Spine* **21** (22), 2640–2650.

Holmich, P., Uhrskou, P., Ulnits, L. *et al.* (1999) Effectiveness of active physical training as treatment for long-standing adductor-related groin pain in athletes: randomised trial. *Lancet* **353**, 439–453.

Janda, V. (1983) On the concept of postural muscles and posture in man. *Australian Journal of Physiotherapy* **29**, 83–84.

Khan, K.M., Liu-Ambrose, T., Sran, M.M., Ashe, M.C., Donaldson, M.G. & Wark, J.D. (2002) New critria for 'female athlete triad' syndrome? *British Journal of Sports Medicine* **36**, 10–13.

Kopp, J.R., Alexander, A.H., Turocy, R.H., Levrini, M.G. & Lichtman, D.M. (1986) The use of lumbar extension in the evaluation and treatment of patients with acute herniated nucleus pulposus. A preliminary report. *Clinical Orthopaedics* **202**, 211–218.

Major, N.M. & Helms, C.A. (1997) Pelvic stress injuries: the relationship between osteitis pubis (symphysis pubis stress injury) and sacroiliac abnormalities in athletes. *Skeletal Radiology* **26** (12), 711–717.

McKay, G.D., Goldie, P.A., Payne, W.R., Oakes, B.W. & Watson, L.F. (2001) A prospective study of injuries in basketball. A total profile and comparison by gender and standard of competition. *Journal of Science and Medicine in Sport* **4** (2), 196–211.

Melrose, J., Little, C.B. & Ghosh, P. (1998) Detection of aggregatable proteoglycan populations by affinity blotting using biotinylated hyaluronan. *Analytical Biochemistry* **256** (2), 149–157.

O'Sullivan, P.B., Phyty, G.D., Twomey, L.T. & Allison, G.T. (1997) Evaluation of specific stabilizing exercise in the treatment of chronic low back pain with radiologic diagnosis of spondylolysis or spondylolisthesis. *Spine* **22** (24), 2959–2967.

Richardson, C.A. & Jull, G.A. (2000) Muscle control–pain control. What exercises would you prescribe? *Manual Therapy* **1** (1), 2–10.

Rossi, F. & Dragoni, S. (2001) Acute avulsion fractures of the pelvis in adolescent competitive athletes: prevalence, location and sports distribution of 203 cases collected. *Skeletal Radiology* **30** (3), 127–131.

Schache, A.G., Blanch, P.D., Rath, D.A., Wrigley, T.V., Starr, R. & Bennell, K.L. (2002) Intra-subject repeatability of the three dimensional angular kinematics within the lumbo–pelvic–hip complex during running. *Gait & Posture* **15** (2), 136–145.

Torg, J., Corcoran, T., Thibault, L., Pavlov, H., Sennett, B. & Naranja, R. (1997) Cervical cord neurapraxia: classification, pathomechanics, morbidity, and management guidelines. *Journal of Neurosurgery* **87** (6), 843–850.

Travell, J. & Simons, D. (1992) *Myofascial Pain and Dysfunction: the Trigger Point Manual*. Baltimore: Williams & Wilkins.

Verrall, G.M., Slavotinek, J.P. & Fon, G.T. (2001) Incidence of pubic bone marrow oedema in Australian rules football players: relation to groin pain. *British Journal of Sports Medicine* **35** (1), 28–33.

Vleeming, A. (1997) *Movement, Stability, and Low Back Pain: the Essential Role of the Pelvis*. New York: Churchill Livingstone.

Weir, M.R. & Smith, D.S. (1989) Stress reaction of the pars interarticularis leading to spondylolysis. A cause of adolescent low back pain. *Journal of Adolescent Health Care* **10** (6), 573–577.

Chapter 14
Basketball injuries: upper extremity considerations

William F. Micheo and Eduardo Amy

Introduction

The game of basketball as we know it today requires nearly an equal amount of upper-extremity and lower-extremity coordination. The upper extremity

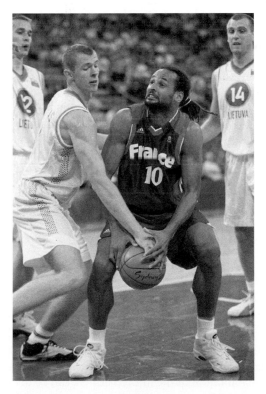

Fig. 14.1 The upper extremities are also vunerable in basketball. Photo © Getty Images/Darren McNamara.

used repeatedly in offense during the acts of dribbling and shooting may be exposed to overuse, and when used for defense or rebounding may be exposed to traumatic injury (Fig. 14.1). This fact alone sets it apart from many other highly skilled games. Over recent years, basketball has evolved into a contact collision sport in which athletes that participate have incredible quickness, stamina, conditioning, and muscle strength. In addition many athletes participate in practice and competition in a year round manner. This has lead to an increase in injuries associated to trauma and overuse.

Evaluation, management, and rehabilitation of basketball injury requires that the clinicians have an idea of the demands of the sport, the specific injuries associated to the sport, and keeping the goal of returning the athlete to competition in mind. Management of the injured athlete requires not only treatment of the symptoms but an accurate diagnosis, and specific management addressing not only the area of injury but the complete kinetic chain.

General concepts

Etiology of injury

Athletic injuries occur from an overload on the muscles, nerves, tendons, bones, or joints. The study of patterns of exercise and sports injuries is an important requisite in the development of preventive, therapeutic, and rehabilitative strategies. The distribution of injuries according to anatomical area and the frequency of specific diagnoses have been shown to vary with gender, age group, and type of athletic activity or sports (Frontera *et al.* 1994).

In our clinical experience basketball was the third most commonly seen sport with males injured more frequently than females. The shoulder was the second most common site of injury and tendonitis the most frequent diagnosis (Frontera *et al.* 1994). Other authors have reported that the vast majority of musculoskeletal injuries sustained by basketball players are to the lower extremity with ankle injuries being the most frequent (Sonzogni & Gross 1993; Kunkel *et al.* 1994). Injuries that result in the most time lost from play are knee injuries, followed by wrist, hand, and ankle injuries (Gomez *et al.* 1996).

In basketball each player has regular ball contact requiring fine hand function without protective gear such as splints or tape. The game is fast-paced with rapid, sudden changes in speed and direction. This combination of unprotected exposure with unpredictable changes in force sets the stage for upper extremity trauma. Hand injuries are common in basketball at all levels of play. Although upper extremity injuries are less common than lower extremity injuries, fractures of the hand and wrist are frequently seen in basketball. Although 3% to 9% of all sports injuries revolve around the wrist and the hand, in basketball injuries have been reported to be as high as 20%, most of these occurring during competition rather than practice (Wilson & McGinty 1993).

Classification of injury

For practical purposes an injury can be defined as a pathologic process that interrupts the athlete's training or competition and that leads the athlete to seek treatment. Athletic injury can be classified as acute, chronic or acute exacerbation of a chronic injury.

The method of presentation of injury is important to delineate. The athlete may present with an acute injury such as a shoulder dislocation which led to inability to continue sports participation, a chronic injury such as rotator cuff tendinopathy associated to gradual increase in symptoms, or acute presentation of a chronic injury such as lateral epicondylitis which was not appropriately treated and led to reduced performance.

Table 14.1 Framework for musculoskeletal injuries.

Clinical alterations
Symptoms

Anatomic alterations
Tissue injuries
Tissue overload

Functional alterations
Biomechanical deficits
Subclinical adaptations

Modified from Kibler (1994).

Patient evaluation

In evaluating an injured athlete the history and physical examination are very important and will give you the appropriate information needed to make a diagnosis and plan an appropriate treatment program. Pertinent information that should be obtained from the history includes: the mechanism of injury, the severity of the injury, and the previous treatment strategies. The physical exam should identify limitation of motion, lack of flexibility, muscle weakness, and imbalance, neurologic as well as propioceptive deficits, and ligamentous laxity.

Psychological issues that should be addressed include anxiety associated to competition, parental involvement in sports, and abnormal attitude towards eating.

Complete diagnosis of the athletic injury should be addressed using the musculoskeletal injury model described by Kibler (1994). This model identifies the anatomic site of injuries, the clinical symptoms and the functional deficits serving as a framework for initial diagnosis, appropriate management, and rehabilitation (Table 14.1).

Rehabilitation of injury

Athletic rehabilitation combines therapeutic modalities and exercise in order to return the competitor to unrestricted sports participation. It should start early in the postinjury period to reduce the deleterious effects of inactivity and immobilization. Rehabilitation of the injured athlete can be divided into acute, recovery, and functional phases (Table 14.2) (Micheo *et al.* 2001).

Table 14.2 Rehabilitation of musculoskeletal injuries goals.

Acute phase
Treat symptom complex
Protect anatomic injury site

Recovery phase
Correct biomechanical deficits
Improve muscle control and balance
Retrain propioception
Start sports specific activity

Functional phase
Increase power endurance
Improve neuromuscular control
Work on entire kinematic chain
Return to competition

The acute phase addresses the clinical symptoms complex and should focus on treating tissue injury. The goal at this stage should be to allow tissue healing while reducing pain and inflammation. Re-establishment of nonpainful range of motion, prevention of muscle atrophy and maintenance of general fitness should be addressed. This phase usually lasts 1–2 weeks.

Therapeutic strategies used in this phase include: ice, electrical stimulation, static exercise, and protected range of motion exercise. Symptom control should be accomplished prior to progressing to the next rehabilitation phase.

The recovery phase should focus on obtaining normal passive and active range of motion, improving muscle control, achieving normal muscle balance, and working on propioception. Biomechanical and functional deficits including inflexibilities, and inability to run or jump should begin to be addressed. This phase could last from 2 to 8 weeks after the injury occurs.

Therapeutic strategies used in this stage include: superficial heat, ultrasound, electrical stimulation, stretching and strengthening exercises. In addition, propioceptive retraining for the upper and lower extremities should be undertaken. Dynamic exercise for strengthening is the most important component of this stage. Open kinetic chain techniques in which the distal portion of the extremity is free to move in space can be combined with closed chain exercises in which the distal portion of the extremity is fixed.

Sports specific training should be initiated in this stage and progression without recurrence of symptoms is required prior to advancing to the next stage.

The functional phase should focus on increasing power and endurance while improving neuromuscular control. Rehabilitation at this stage should work on the entire kinematic chain addressing specific functional deficits. This program should be continuous with the ultimate goal of prevention of recurrent injury. The functional phase could last from 8 weeks to 4–6 months after the injury occurs.

Therapeutic strategies used in this stage include: plyometric exercises to gain power, sports specific training to improve technique, and maintenance strengthening as well as flexibility programs. The athlete should be pain free, exhibit full range of motion, normal strength, and muscle balance prior to returning to competition.

Shoulder injuries

The glenohumeral joint has a high degree of mobility at the expense of stability. Static and dynamic restraints maintain the shoulder in place with overhead activity. Muscle action, particularly of the rotator cuff and scapular stabilizers, is important in maintaining joint congruity in midranges of motion. Static stabilizers such as the glenohumeral ligaments, joint capsule, and glenoid labrum are important for stability in the extremes of motion. Injury can occur secondary to trauma or to overuse associated to repeated activity (Bahr *et al.* 1995; Cavallo & Speer 1998; Burkhart *et al.* 2000).

Glenohumeral dislocation

In the case of traumatic instability of the glenohumeral joint the individual usually falls on the outstretched externally rotated, and abducted arm with a resulting anterior dislocation. A blow to the posterior aspect of the externally rotated and abducted arm can also result in anterior dislocation. Posterior dislocation usually results from a fall on the forward flexed and adducted arm or by direct blow in the posterior direction when the arm is above the shoulder. An acutely dislocated shoulder can usually be recognized by the position of the arm. In anterior dislocation, the arm is held in external rotation while the humeral head can be palpated anterior to the glenoid. Posterior dislocations present with internal rotation and posterior fullness of the shoulder. Neurologic examination with special reference to the axillary nerve should be done before treatment is started.

The acute management of glenohumeral instability is nonoperative in the majority of cases. This includes relative rest, ice, and analgesic or anti-inflammatory medication. The goals at this stage include pain reduction, protection from further injury, and starting an early rehabilitation program.

In the case of acute anterior dislocation the injured individual presents with pain, decrease in active motion, and deformity. If the injury was observed and no evidence of neurologic or vascular damage is evident on clinical exam, reduction may be attemped with traction in forward flexion, slight abduction, and followed by gentle internal rotation (Bahr *et al.* 1995). If this fails, the patient should be transported away from the playing area and reduction may be attemped by placing the patient prone, sedating the individual, and allowing the injured arm to hang from the bed with a 5–10 pound weight attached to the wrist.

If there is a suspicion of fracture or posterior dislocation the patient should undergo radiologic evaluation prior to attemping a reduction. Following the reduction radiologic studies should be repeated. Controversy exists regarding treatment of first time anterior dislocations. Although some clinicians have recommended immobilization for as long as 6 weeks it is not clear that this will affect the long-term outcome. Many authors advocate functional rehabilitation following a shorter period of immobilization until the patient is pain free and able to progress in the treatment program. The young athlete returning to competition after a shoulder dislocation should be advised about the possibility of recurrence and the future need for surgical intervention (Nelson & Arciero 2000).

Acromioclavicular dislocation

Dislocations of the acromioclavicular joint are caused by a direct blow on the posterior aspect of the acromion and spine of the scapula such as when a player falls on the tip of his shoulder. They are classified from Type 1 to Type 6 based on the anatomic relationship between the acromion and the clavicle following the injury. Type 1 acromioclavicular dislocations represent complete tears of the joint capsule with no major break in continuity between the acromion and clavicle. Type 2 dislocations involve a complete tear of the joint capsule, but the coracoclavicular ligaments are intact. Point tenderness and compressibility are associated with this ligamentous disruption, and on visual examination the distal end of the clavicle appears to ride somewhat higher. Type 3 lesions involve a complete disruption of both the joint capsule and coracoclavicular ligaments. Type 4 injury results in posterior dislocation of the clavicle relative to the acromion; Type 5, in superior displacement of the clavicle through the trapezius tenting the skin with more than 100% of clavicle displacement; and Type 6, in inferior displacement of the clavicle (Wolin 1996).

Physical examination reveals an obvious depression of the scapula with what appears to be an elevation of the clavicle, localized tenderness to palpation and limited active shoulder motion. Radiographic examination should be performed with the patient upright, and a study holding on to weights is used by some clinicians in the diagnosis of type 1 or type 2 injuries.

Treatment of type 1 and type 2 injuries is nonoperative. A sling is used to support the arm, which should be kept at rest; heavy lifting or contact sports should be avoided until full range of motion is restored, with no pain on joint palpation. In type 1 injuries this process usually takes 2 weeks, whereas in type 2 injuries the period of protection may last up to 6 weeks. The treatment of type 3 acromioclavicular dislocation is somewhat controversial with some authors recommending surgical interventions while others recommend conservative treatment and rehabilitation after a period of immobilization. Type 4 to Type 6 injuries require surgical treatment (Wolin 1996).

Rotator cuff injury

With recurrent overhead activity such as shooting a basketball overload of the rotator cuff may occur, leading to symptoms of reduced motion, muscle weakness, and pain which interfere with activity. In the young patient this rotator cuff overload may be associated to shoulder instability. The repeated stresses of overhead activity place great demands on the dynamic and static stabilizers of the glenohumeral joint, including the rotator cuff, ligaments, capsule, and glenoid labrum (Cavallo & Speer 1998; Burkhart *et al.* 2000). These lead to increased translation of the humeral head and to pain associated with impingement of the rotator cuff. The individual may report that the shoulder slips out of the joint, the arm going "dead", or weakness associated to overhead activity. Continued symptoms of pain particularly at night in the older athlete may be secondary to a rotator cuff tear.

The shoulder should be inspected for the presence of deformity, atrophy of muscle, asymmetry, and scapular winging. The individual should be observed from the anterior, lateral, and posterior positions. Palpation of soft tissue and bone should be systematically addressed and include the rotator cuff, biceps tendon, subacromial region, and acromioclavicular as well as glenohumeral joints (Clarnette & Miniaci 1998).

Passive and active range of motion should be evaluated. Differences between passive and active motion may be secondary to pain, weakness, or neurologic damage. Repeated overhead activity may also lead to an increase in measured external rotation accompanied by a reduction in internal rotation. Strength testing should be performed to identify weakness of specific muscle of the rotator cuff and the scapular stabilizers. The supraspinatus muscle can be tested in the scapular plane with internal rotation or external rotation of the shoulder. The external rotators can be tested with the arm at the side of the body and the subscapularis muscle can be tested by using the "lift-off test" in which the palm of the hand is lifted away from the lower back. The scapular stabilizers such as the serratus anterior and the rhomboid muscles can be tested in isolation or by doing wall push-ups. Sensory and motor exam of the shoulder girdle should be performed to rule out nerve injuries (Micheo *et al.* 2001).

Rotator cuff impingement can be assesed by testing the shoulder in 90 degrees of forward flexion with internal rotation, or extreme forward flexion with the forearm supinated, looking for reproduction of symptoms. Glenohumeral translation testing looking for laxity or instability should be documented. Apprehension testing can be performed with the patient sitting, standing, or in the supine position. The shoulder joint is stressed in abduction and external rotation looking for reproduction of the feeling of instability in the patient. A relocation maneuver which reduces the symptoms also aids in the diagnosis. Other tests include the load and shift maneuver to document humeral head translation in anterior or posterior directions, the sulcus sign to document inferior humeral head laxity, and the Active Compression Test described by O'Brien in which a downward force is applied to the forward flexed, adducted, and internally rotated shoulder trying to reproduce pain associated to labral tears or acromioclavicular joint pathology. The across chest adduction maneuver may also be used to reproduce acromioclavicular symptomatology (O'Brien *et al.* 1998).

Management of rotator cuff injury should begin as soon as the injury occurs. The goals of nonsurgical management include reducing pain, restoring full motion, correction of muscle strength deficits, achieving muscle balance, and returning to full activity free of symptoms (Kibler 1994; Ellen & Smith 1999). Treatment can be divided into acute, recovery, and functional phases (Table 14.3).

The acute phase should focus on treating tissue injury, clinical signs and symptoms. The goal in this stage should be to allow tissue healing of the rotator cuff while reducing pain and inflammation. Reestablishment of nonpainful range of motion, prevention of muscle atrophy and maintenance of general fitness should be addressed.

Treatment strategies include the use of cryotherapy, high voltage galvanic stimulation, and static exercises to the rotator cuff and scapular muscles. In addition, pain free range of motion of the shoulder as well as strengthening of the trunk and lower extremities should be started.

The recovery phase should focus on obtaining normal passive and active glenohumeral range of motion, improve scapular muscle control, as well as achieving normal muscle strength, and balance. Biomechanical and functional deficits including abnormalities in the throwing motion should be addressed.

Table 14.3 Rotator cuff injury rehabilitation.

Acute phase	Recovery phase	Functional phase
Therapeutic intervention	*Therapeutic intervention*	*Therapeutic intervention*
Active rest	Modalities: superficial heat, ultrasound, electrical stimulation	Power and endurance in upper extremities: diagonal and multiplanar motions with tubings, light weight medicine balls
Cryotherapy		
Electrical stimulation	Range of motion exercises, flexibility exercises for posterior capsule	Plyometrics, increase multiple-plane neuromuscular control
Protected motion		
Isometric exercise to shoulder and scapular muscles	Scapular control: closed chain exercises, propioceptive neuro-muscular facilitation, patterns	Maintenance: general flexibility training, strengthening, power and endurance exercise program
General conditioning		
NSAIDs	Dynamic upper extremity strengthening exercise: isolated rotator cuff exercises	Sports-specific progression
	Sports-specific exercises, surgical tubing, multiplanar joint exercises, trunk and lower extremity	
	General conditioning	
	Gradual return to training	

Treatment strategies include superficial heat, ultrasound, shoulder girdle mobilization, posterior capsule stretching, and strengthening exercises. The strengthening program should include closed kinetic chain exercises for the rotator cuff and scapular stabilizers including wall pushups. In addition, pain free strengthening of the rotator cuff muscles and scapular stabilizers could be undertaken with the use of light weights or surgical tubing in an open kinetic chain mode of exercise. Functional activities to improve trunk and lower extremities strength as well as sports specific training should be incorporated into the treatment program as muscle strength and scapular control improve. A supervised return to sport program in which the patient progresses without symptoms is required prior to progressing to the next rehabilitation phase.

The functional phase should focus on increasing power and endurance of the upper extremities while improving neuromuscular control. Rehabilitation at this stage should work on the entire kinematic chain addressing specific functional deficits. This program should be continuous with the ultimate goal of prevention of recurrent injury.

In this phase treatment should include strengthening in a sports specific range of motion, plyometric training, return to sports participation with supervision, and a muscle balance as well as propioceptive training program.

Recurrent shoulder instability

The spectrum of shoulder instability ranges from acute traumatic dislocation which is usually unidirectional to recurrent subluxation which is usually not related to trauma and multidirectional. Patients with recurrent instability may have history of recurrent dislocations, but more commonly that of subluxation or pain associated to repeated overhead activity. In addition, the patient may complain or weakness, locking, transient giving way of the shoulder or the feeling of a "dead arm". Some patients may present with impingement symptoms of the rotator cuff secondary to failure of the capsuloligamentous structures which stabilize the shoulder at the extremes of range of motion (Laurencin *et al*. 1998; Meister 2000a).

A complete physical examination should be performed similar to the one described for the patient with rotator cuff pathology. The key to diagnosing recurrent shoulder instability is the demonstration of asymmetry of glenohumeral translation from side to side. This is particularly important in the patient with evidence of generalized ligamentous laxity such as elbow and knee hyperextension. Apprehension testing can be performed with the patient sitting, standing, or in the supine position. The shoulder joint is stressed in abduction and external rotation looking for reproduction of the feeling of instability in the patient. A relocation maneuver with reduces the symptoms also aids in the diagnosis. Other tests include the load and shift maneuver to document humeral head translation in anterior or posterior directions, the sulcus sign to document inferior humeral head laxity, and the Active Compression Test described by O'Brien in which a downward force is applied to the forward flexed, adducted, and internally rotated shoulder trying to reproduce pain associated to labral tears or acromioclavicular joint pathology.

Initial treatment of patients with multidirectional or microtraumatic instability is nonoperative (Meister 2000b). Reduction of acute symptoms followed by appropriate rehabilitation addressing weakness of the scapular stabilizers, rotator cuff, and appropriate sports specific mechanics should be undertaken before surgery is considered. In this situation, emphasis should be placed on working the scapular and rotator cuff muscles in a "closed chain" cocontraction method. This method emphasizes joint stabilization activities in the muscles (Kibler 1994; Ellen & Smith 1999; Micheo *et al.* 2001). If despite conservative treatment the patient persists with recurrent episodes of instability surgical reconstructive surgery should be considered (Speer 1995; Nelson & Arciero 2000).

Elbow injuries

Elbow injuries result from acute trauma and repetitive overuse as seen primarily in throwing sports, such as baseball. In basketball, elbow injuries are less common, however, repeated activity as well as trauma such as that associated to a fall on the outstretched arm may lead to injury. Forces that may damage the elbow include valgus tension of the medial structures, compression of the lateral structures, and extension overload of the posterior structures. Because of a stable joint structure single traumatic events require substantial forces which may result in fracture or dislocation (Plancher & Lucas 2001).

Elbow dislocation—fracture

Single-event injuries are most often a result of collision of an outstretched hand with the ground. If the elbow is somewhat flexed, postero-lateral dislocation may occur. If the elbow is fully extended, transmission of force up the radius may result in a fracture of the radial head or capitellum. Varus/valgus shear forces at the time of impact may result in fracture of the condylar and supracondylar structures. Direct impact of the elbow is another mechanism of injury that may result in fractures about the elbow, most likely the olecranon (Plancher & Lucas 2001).

Early reduction, management of associated fractures, ongoing assessment of the neurovascular status, and early protected range of motion to minimize the risk of flexion ankylosis are the basics of proper treatment (Wiesner 1994). In most cases complete immobilization should not exceed 2 weeks, as prolonged positioning leads to increased flexion contractures with associated pain. Use of a removable splint that permits active elbow range of motion including flexion–extension and supination–pronation may be considered after 3–4 days. By 10 days to 2 weeks, if the fracture or dislocation are stable the splint should be discontinued and a full elbow flexibility and strengthening program pursued. On return to play, the elbow may be braced or taped to limit elbow hyperextension and provide for protection from valgus forces.

Soft tissue injuries

Injuries to the soft tissue include lateral epicondylitis, medial epicondylitis, ulnar collateral ligament injury, and ulnar neuropathy. Although these are more common in throwing and racquet sports they may occur in the basketball player during training or competition.

The patient with lateral epicondylitis presents with pain anterior and distal to the lateral elbow involving the proximal extensor musculature and lateral epicondyle. The pain is commonly increased on resisted wrist extension with the elbow extended and the forearm pronated. In addition, the athlete may complain of pain with gripping activities. The examination reveals localized tenderness anterior to the lateral epicondyle over the forearm extensors origin, wrist extension weakness, and loss of passive wrist flexion in chronic cases.

Management includes control of acute symptoms with relative rest, icing, and therapeutic modalities as well as anti-inflammatory medications. Stretching and eccentric strengthening of the wrist extensor muscles should be combined with generalized conditioning (Wiesner 1994). In some cases, a local corticosteroid injection may allow a more rapid progression in the rehabilitation program. The use of a counterforce brace to reduce the force load of the extensor muscles has been advocated when athletes return to practice or competition.

The athletes with medial epicondylitis usually present with injury to the flexor pronator muscles group associated to eccentric overload. Pain occurs distal to the medial epicondyle at the origin of the flexor pronator group and increases with resisted forearm pronation or wrist flexion.

Management includes symptomatic treatment combined with stretching and strengthening of the flexor pronator group, proximal shoulder girdle muscles and generalized conditioning. In severe cases, a local injection and counterforce bracing may be used as previously described for lateral epicondylitis.

Some patients with chronic medial symptoms may have injury to the capsule ligamentous structures or the ulnar nerve. Symptoms are related to repeated activity in which valgus and extension forces are applied to the elbow. Stability testing with the elbow in 20–30 degrees of flexion may reproduce pain symptoms in ulnar collateral ligament injury. Patients with ulnar neuropathy may present with pain or paresthesias in the distribution of the nerve. In many instances sensory symptoms may not be present at rest and are only reproduced following activity.

Management of medial injury to the ulnar collateral ligament includes avoidance of activity with valgus stress, strengthening of the whole upper extremity kinetic chain, improvement of sports specific technique and in some cases surgical repair. This injury is uncommon in basketball players.

Ulnar neuropathy at the level of the elbow cubital tunnel can be treated with protection by the use of an elbow pad, to avoid direct pressure over the nerve, or in severe cases with an elbow orthosis made of rigid thermoplastic material in 45 degrees of flexion. In the early stages of recovery the orthosis should be worn during most of the day and as the patient's symptoms improve it should be used only at night. Appropriate stretching, strengthening of the whole kinetic chain, and sports biomechanics should also be addressed.

Wrist and hand injuries

Hand and upper extremity injuries are among the most common injuries sustained by athletes. Unfortunately, there is a tendency to minimize their severity as the hand does not bear weight and the injuries rarely render the athlete unable to compete. Wrist and hand injuries are fairly common and described to occur in 3% to 9% of all athletic injuries (Wilson & McGinty 1993).

Although soft tissue injuries are more common, fractures are also seen quite frequently. Hand and wrist injuries are more common in adolescents than in adults due to the fact that they suffer a high incidence of epiphyseal trauma. The most common hand and wrist injuries in basketball include metacarpal fractures, phalangeal fractures, scaphoid fractures, proximal interphalangeal (PIP) dislocations and mallet finger (Speer 1995).

Mechanisms of injuries

Hand and wrist injuries may occur secondary to throwing, repeated overhead activity, weight bearing or direct impact. Throwing typically causes overuse injuries from repetition. Examples of these are De Quervain's tendinitis, carpal tunnel syndrome, extensor carpi ulnaris (ECU) subluxation and tendonitis. All of these injuries are more common in adolescents than in the adult population. Weight bearing on the dorsiflexed wrist and hand causes dorsal carpal impingement, distal radial physis stress fractures, scaphoid stress fractures as well as triangular fibrocartilage (TFCC) injuries. Impact stresses on the hand and wrist can cause scaphoid fracture of the wrist, scapholunate dissociation, metacarpal fractures as well as the more common PIP joint, dorsal dislocation and mallet finger.

Wrist injuries

Soft tissue injuries

De Quervain's disease

In basketball De Quervain's results from an overuse syndrome of the hand and the wrist. De Quervain's is a tenosynovitis of the abductor pollicis longus and the extensor pollicis brevis, which occurs in activities that require forceful grasp coupled with radial and ulnar deviation as well as the repetitive use of the thumb. Pain is the most common presenting symptom.

The physical examination reveals tenderness of the first dorsal compartment of the wrist and reproduction of symptoms with the Finkelstein's test in which the thumb is placed inside the palm of the hand and the wrist is ulnarly deviated. The treatment for this condition is initially rest, immobilization and anti-inflammatory medications. Physical therapy modalities such as ultrasound and electrical stimulation may also be used. If the patient does not improve a steroid injection in the first dorsal compartment of the wrist is indicated. If these conservative measures fail to help the athlete referral for a surgical release of the first dorsal compartment is indicated.

ECU tendinitis

The ECU is the second most common site for upper extremity tenosynovitis. ECU tendinitis clinically presents as pain and swelling along the dorsal ulnar aspect of the wrist, and it is seen in basketball due to repetitive twisting and dorsiflexion of the wrist. The treatment for this condition is initially nonsteroidal anti-inflammatory medication with splinting, but if this fails an injection at the area of the tendon sheath usually takes care of the problem. In some recalcitrant cases the pain continues, and surgical release of the tendon sheath along with repair may have to be performed.

Trigger finger

A trigger finger is another one of the overuse syndromes of soft tissues of the hand that may be seen associated with basketball, although it is more common in racket sports which require repeated grasping. It is associated with thickening of the A-1 pulley at the level of the metacarpophalangeal joint due to repetitive impact, causing pressure and swelling over the flexor tendon sheath. This condition usually responds to steroid injections of the flexor tendon sheath under the A-1 pulley. If the patient does not respond to conservative treatment referral for surgical release of the A-1 pulley is indicated.

Closed tendon injuries

These injuries result from trauma to either the flexor or the extensor tendons of the hand, and are commonly seen associated to basketball. They are often believed to be minor injuries and may go untreated. If these injuries are not diagnosed early and treatment not initiated promptly permanent deformity could result.

Mallet finger

The mallet finger, the most common of the closed tendon injuries of the hand, is also referred to as baseball finger or drop finger. It is caused by direct impact of the basketball against an extended distal interphalangeal (DIP) joint of any of the fingers of the hand. The patient presents with pain, swelling on the dorsum of the DIP joint and inability to extend the joint. This injury usually occurs at the substance of the extensor tendon, however, it can also be associated with an avulsion fracture of the dorsal aspect of the distal phalanx at the DIP joint. The treatment of the mallet finger when it occurs at the substance of the extensor tendon consists of applying a dorsal splint in extension of the DIP joint for approximately 6 weeks. The splint is to be used continuously for 6 weeks followed by an additional 4 weeks of dorsal night splinting to prevent the occurrence of the deformity. It is important that after treatment with the splint the athlete should wear a protective splint maintaining the DIP in extension during the next 2 months following the completion of the treatment to protect the joint from further reinjury during the game.

It is to be noted that even if treatment is delayed

in this condition by as much as 3–4 months after the injury, good results can be obtained with late treatment. This however, is not an excuse to delay treatment in the acute phase, which will provide the best results. Failure to heal the extensor tendon may result in a permanent deformity with the development of a swan neck.

In the event of an avulsion fracture at the dorsal aspect of the DIP joint, if the fracture does not involve the articular surface it can still be treated with dorsal splinting. However, if the avulsion fracture involves the articular surface, especially greater than one third of the articular surface, with palmar subluxation at the DIP joint, the treatment of choice is open reduction and internal fixation.

Boutonnière deformity

The boutonnière deformity (boutonnière is French for button hole), occurs as a result of an injury to the central slip of the extensor tendon at or near its insertion into the base of middle phalanx. There are two mechanisms by which this injury occurs. The first one is a blow to the dorsal aspect of the middle phalanx forcing the PIP joint into flexion while the athlete is actively extending the PIP joint. The second mechanism occurs as an unrecognized palmar dislocation of the PIP joint either spontaneously reduced or reduced on the field by the athlete or the medical personnel, and this is the most commonly seen mechanism causing the boutonnière deformity.

Clinically the classic deformity, which consists of flexion of the PIP joint and hyperextension of the DIP joint, is rarely seen acutely. Acutely the clinical presentation is that of weakness of PIP extension or an extensor lag at the PIP joint with swelling, pain and tenderness at the dorsal aspect of the joint. If the acute injury goes untreated, the central slip retracts, the triangular ligament becomes stretched, and the lateral bands fall palmar to the axis of rotation. In this case the lateral bands actually become flexors of the PIP joint and retract proximately hyperextending the DIP joint creating the classic deformity.

The history of the injury is very important in this condition, and it is important to be suspicious of the risk of developing a boutonnière deformity every time we encounter a PIP injury, especially a palmar dislocation. The treatment of choice of an acute boutonnière deformity consists of a volar or palmar splint as early as possible after the injury. This palmar splint holds the metacarpophalangeal (MCP) and PIP joint in extension while allowing active and passive flexion at the DIP joint. This DIP flexion is important to allow the lateral bands to assume and maintain the anatomic position at the PIP joint. The splint should be worn continuously for 5 weeks and then for two more weeks as a night splint. After 5 weeks of splinting gentle active and passive range of motion exercises are begun at the PIP joint. In the event that the injury has been overlooked and the classic boutonnière deformity develops, surgical referral for surgical release with reconstruction will be necessary.

Pseudoboutonnière deformity

This condition must be differentiated from boutonnière deformity, although the appearance is similar the mechanism of injury is different. It is caused by hyperextension injury to the PIP joint, causing an injury to the volar plate and one of the collateral ligaments. In this condition the central slip in the dorsal aspect is not injured. In the pseudoboutonnière deformity the treatment consists of dorsal splinting in slight flexion.

Avulsion of the flexor digitorum profundus tendon

Avulsion of the flexor digitorum profundus (FDP) tendon is also known as the "Jersey" finger. It is a relatively common injury seen in many sports, football being the most common. It occurs in the ring finger more than 75% of the time with a mechanism of injury of a forceful extension of the finger during a maximum contraction of the profundus muscle (Wilson & McGinty 1993). Acutely the athlete presents with swelling and pain of the palmar aspect of the hand and inability to actively flex the DIP joint of the involved finger. This injury is classified into three types.

In type 1 injury the profundus tendon retracts to the palm of the hand. The patient presents with pain and swelling at the palm of the hand at the level of the lumbrical muscles. Due to the fact that the blood supply of the tendon is at risk this injury should be recognized early and treated within the first week of the injury for the tendon to survive. The treatment consists of surgical rethreading of the tendon and attachment of the tendon to the distal phalanx of the finger. Dorsal splinting and passive flexion is allowed post operatively for the first 3 weeks followed by protective splinting for the next 6 weeks after the repair.

In type 2 injury the profundus tendon retracts back to the level of the PIP joint and it is held there by the intact long vinculum, therefore the blood supply to the tendon is preserved. Clinically the patient presents with pain and swelling at the level of the PIP joint as well as loss of active flexion at the level of the DIP joint and at the level of the PIP joint. The treatment for this type of avulsion is similar to type 1 avulsion of the profundus tendon.

In type 3 injury the avulsion of the profundus tendon is associated with a large boney fragment that gets held in place by the A-4 pulley. As with a type 2 injury since the tendon is not retracted to the palm of the hand the nutrition is preserved. Clinically the patient presents with pain and swelling over the distal aspect of the middle phalanx. X-rays of the hand usually show a boney fragment just proximal to the DIP joint. The treatment for a type 3 injury is open reduction and internal fixation followed by splinting for 4–6 weeks which is then followed by active and passive range of motion.

Ligament injuries

Thumb ulnar collateral ligament

The most common soft-tissue injury of the thumb is rupture of the ulnar collateral ligaments (game-keeper's thumb) (Kunkel *et al.* 1994). Injury may occur from a fall on the hand or from trauma associated to thumb abduction and hyperextension. The ligaments may be partially or completely torn and failure to diagnose this injury may lead to chronic instability.

First and second degree tears may be treated with immobilization in 30 degrees of flexion with a short-arm thumb spica cast for 4 weeks. After 2 weeks the cast may be changed and if the patient is pain free a removable splint may be used and range motion exercises started (Wilson & McGinty 1993).

When the UCL is completely torn stress radiographs may help in the diagnosis. The radiographs are also helpful in detecting an avulsion fracture. Nondisplaced avulsion fracture may be treated with the cast for 4–6 weeks. If the avulsion fracture is greater than 10–15% of the articular surface, displacement is more than 2–3 mm, then angulater operative treatment should be considered (Kunkel *et al.* 1994).

Scapholunate dissociations

Ligamentous injuries of the wrist usually result from falls on the outstretched hand. The ligaments provide alignment and stability and coordinate the complex motion patterns between the bony articulations during normal wrist function. Difficulties in diagnosis arise because the ligaments are not easily visualized. Instead, we must look for altered bony relationships that occur secondarily. The commonest wrist ligament injury is scapholunate dissociation. In the static form, a separation between these two bones is seen on posteroanterior radiographs. The scaphoid rotates from a longitudinal to a horizontal position, while the lunate simply angulates. This situation results in carpal collapse and is described as a dorsal intercalary segmental instability. Dynamic and partial scapholunate dissociations may sometimes be demonstrated on a clenched fist or radial–ulnar deviation views (Lewis & Osterman 2001).

Treatment of acute static or dynamic scapholunate ligament dissociations is by closed reduction and pinning, or open reduction and repair of the ligament. Acute partial ligament injuries without any of the collapse deformities are best treated in a short-arm thumb spica cast for at least 6 weeks (Wilson & McGinty 1993; Kunkel *et al.* 1994).

Fractures of the wrist

Carpal fractures

Scaphoid fractures

The scaphoid is the most commonly fractured carpal bone, and the injury occurs in sports in which the individuals are subjected to violent forces. The mechanism of injury is a fall on the outstretched hand causing hyperextension of the wrist.

The patient will present with complaints of wrist pain localized to the anatomic snuffbox area. X-rays should be obtained in any athlete who presents with this symptom complex in order to diagnose a fracture of the scaphoid. If the X-rays are negative, and there is a strong clinical suspicion of fracture a thumb spica splint should be applied for 2 weeks, followed by a re-examination to confirm that the pain has disappeared. If the patient is still symptomatic repeat X-rays, and a bone scan or MRI should be performed.

The treatment for a nondisplaced scaphoid fracture consists of a thumb spica cast for approximately 6–8 weeks until the fracture clinically and radiographically heals. The more proximal the fracture of the scaphoid the longer it will take to heal due to its blood supply. If the fracture is very proximal in the scaphoid an early open reduction and internal fixation may be recommended to improve the healing time of the fracture. For displaced fracture of the scaphoid an open reduction and internal fixation is recommended as the treatment of choice. Usually the athlete returns to sports within 3–4 months after an open reduction of a scaphoid fracture.

Capitate fractures

These fractures, similar to the scaphoid fractures, should be considered inherently unstable. Like the proximal scaphoid fracture the head and neck of the capitate is subjected to major vascular disruption when fractured. Healing is commonly prolonged and nonunion as well as avascular necrosis (AVN) are commonly seen at the usual site of fracture which is the junction of the body and the neck of the capitate. Usually the optimal treatment for this fracture is open reduction and internal fixation.

Pisiform fractures

Pisiform fractures can occur when the basketball player sustains a fall landing on an outstretched hand on its ulnar aspect receiving direct trauma to the bone. These fractures can be diagnosed using oblique radiographs of the wrist to isolate the pisiform bone. The treatment consists of cast immobilization for 3–6 weeks for undisplaced fractures or removal of the pisiform bone for fractures which are comminuted or displaced.

Hand fractures and dislocations

In basketball hand fractures are very common particularly in young athletes. Usually these occur as a result of torque, angular forces, compressive forces or direct trauma.

Distal phalanx fractures

These fractures constitute more than half of all hand fractures, with the distal phalanx of the middle finger the most commonly involved in basketball. Usually this fracture is caused by a crush injury or a direct blow to the area. This fractures in general are stabilized by the nail plate dorsally and the pulp septa volarly. The treatment for proximal nondisplaced fractures is with a DIP extension splint for 3 weeks. For a displaced distal phalanx fracture treatment consists of closed reduction and K-wire pin fixation of the fracture for 3 weeks.

Middle phalanx fractures

Middle phalanx fractures usually occur as a result of a direct blow to the finger producing a short oblique or transverse fracture line. It is important to determine the stability of the fracture. If the fracture has less than 10 degrees of angulation in either plane, no malrotation, and minimal motion at the fracture site, treatment is with splinting or buddy taping to the next finger and the athletes are allowed to return to sports as soon as they don't have tenderness over the fracture site. If the alignment is unacceptable or the fracture displaced, then closed reduction and percutaneous pin fixation is recommended.

Proximal phalanx fractures

These fractures although less common than the distal fractures in basketball in our experience are the source of significant time loss from the sport and if not treated properly significant functional deficit may result. These fractures can be spiral, oblique or transverse depending on the stresses applied to the bone. In adolescents this is commonly seen at the physeal plate at the base of the phalanx.

If these fractures are stable with no rotational deformity they can be treated with splinting and buddy taping. Return to sports can be done as soon as the patient tolerates the pain. If the fracture is unstable or if there is rotational deformity present then closed or open reduction with internal fixation is necessary. In fractures where the articular surface is involved, if less than 1 mm of displacement is noted, the fracture can be treated with splinting for 3–4 weeks, however, if the fracture has greater than 1 mm of displacement then open reduction and internal fixation will be needed.

Metacarpal fractures

Metacarpal fractures are very common fractures associated to basketball. In some series up to 36% of all hand injuries are metacarpal fractures. Metacarpal fractures which involve the middle and ring fingers, are usually more stable than the index and small finger, due to the support provided by the transverse metacarpal ligament. Treatment is closed reduction and splinting or 3–4 weeks followed by active range of motion. Fractures through the diaphysis of the metacarpals tend to shorten or rotate as well as angulate, and percutaneous pinning may be necessary.

Metacarpal neck fractures

Metacarpal neck fractures are most frequently seen involving the ring and little finger. They usually angulate volarly and in more distal fractures more angulation can be accepted during treatment. Some angulation is acceptable in the ring and small finger because of greater carpometacarpal (CMC) motion

of these fingers. Up to 40–50 degrees of angulation can be accepted for the ring and little fingers, while only 15 degrees of angulation is accepted in the middle and index fingers. The treatment for metacarpal neck fractures involves closed reduction and splinting for 3–4 weeks followed by active range of motion and physical therapy.

Metacarpal shaft fractures

In the treatment of these fractures if there is full flexion and extension, no malrotation, and the fracture is stable it can be treated with splinting. Unacceptable findings includes shortening greater than 4–5 mm, angulation greater than 50 or 60 degrees in the ring and the small finger, or 15–20 degrees in the middle and index fingers, and any malrotation. In these unacceptable cases closed reduction or open reduction with internal fixation are recommended as the treatment of choice.

Metacarpal fractures of the thumb

The thumb is frequently traumatized because of its unprotected position. Thumb fractures are usually caused by impact to the radial side of the thumb and usually occur at the proximal one third of the thumb metacarpal. Fracture angulation is usually in adduction and volar flexion, approximately 35 degrees of angulation is acceptable and closed treatment can be used for this fracture. However, for any greater degree of angulation or malrotation open reduction and internal fixation is recommended.

Another fracture, which is commonly seen at the thumb metacarpal, is Bennett's fracture which is a fracture of the base of the thumb metacarpal at its articular surface with the trapezium. This fracture at times can be associated with dislocation or subluxation of the base of the thumb metacarpal. For undisplaced fractures closed treatment with a splint can be used, however, for any displacement of these fractures open reduction and internal fixation is recommended.

Dorsal dislocations of the PIP joint

Dorsal dislocation is the most common type of dislocation of the PIP joint and probably the most common dislocation associated to basketball injuries. For a dorsal dislocation to occur the volar plate must be torn and this leads to a dorsal displacement of the middle phalanx of the finger.

The treatment of this dislocation is immediate reduction on the field, followed by buddy taping for 3–6 weeks. Usually the player can return to the sport immediately after reduction using the buddy tape technique, however, it is recommended that the athlete is a immobilized with a dorsal splint in 30 degrees of flexion when not playing to promote the healing of the volar plate. Inadequately treated dorsal dislocations can develop into a pseudobouton-nière deformity.

References

Bahr, R., Craig, E. & Engerbretsen, L. (1995) The Clinical Presentation of Shoulder Instability Including On-Field Management. *Clin Sports Med* **14**, 761–776.

Burkhart, S.S., Morgan, C.D. & Kibler, W.B. (2000) Shoulder Injuries in Overhead Athletes: The "Dead Arm" Revisited. *Clin Sports Med* **19**, 125–158.

Cavallo, R.J. & Speer, K.P. (1998) Shoulder: Instability and Impingement in Throwing Athletes. *Med Sci Sports Exerc* **30** (S), 18–25.

Clarnette, R.C. & Miniaci, A. (1998) Clinical Exam of the Shoulder. *Med Sci Sports Exerc* **30** (S), 1–6.

Ellen, M. & Smith, J. (1999) Musculosketeletal Rehabilitation and Sports Medicine: Shoulder and Upper Extremity Injuries. *Arch Phys Med Rehabil* **80** (S), 50–58.

Frontera, W.R., Micheo, W.F., Amy, E. *et al.* (1994) Patterns of Injuries in Athletes Evaluated in An Interdisciplinary Clinic. *PR Health Sci J* **13**, 165–170.

Gomez, E., DeLee, J.C. & Farney, W.C. (1996) Incidence of Injury in Texas Girl's High School Basketball. *Am J Sports Med* **24** (5), 684–687.

Kibler, W.B. (1994) A Framework for Sports Medicine. *PM and R Clin N Am* **5** (1), 1–8.

Kibler, W.B., Livingston, B. & Bruce, R. (1995) Current Concepts in Shoulder Rehabilitation. *Adv Oper Orthop* **3**, 249–300.

Kunkel, S.S. (1994) Basketball Injuries and Rehabilitation. In: R.M. Bushbacher & R.L. Braddom (eds) *Sports Medicine and Rehabilitation: a Sport Specific Approach*, pp. 95–109. Philadelphia: Hanley & Belfus.

Laurencin, C.T. & O'Brien, S.J. (1998) Anterior Shoulder Instability: Anatomy, Pathophysiology, and Conservative Management. In: J.R. Andrews, B. Zarims & K. Wilk (eds) *Injuries in Baseball*, pp. 189–197. Philadelphia: Lippincott-Raven.

Lewis, D.M. & Osterman, A.L. (2001) Scapholunate Instability in Athletes. *Clin Sports Med* **20**, 131–140.

Meister, K. (2000a) Current Concepts. Injuries to the Throwing Athlete. Part One: Biomechanics/ Pathophysiology/Classification of Injury. *Am J Sports Med* **28**, 265–275.

Meister, K. (2000b) Current Concepts. Injuries to the Throwing Athlete. Part Two: Evaluation/Treatment. *Am J Sports Med* **28**, 587–601.

Micheo, W.F. & Ramos, E. (2001) Glenohumeral Instability. In: W.R. Frontera, J.K. Silver (eds) *Essentials of Physical Medicine and Rehabilitation*, pp. 76–89. Philadelphia: Hanley & Belfus.

Nelson, B.J. & Arciero, R.A. (2000) Arthroscopic Management of Glenohumeral Instability. *Am J Sports Med* **28**, 602–614.

O'Brien, S.J., Pagnani, M.J., Fealy, S. *et al.* (1998) The Active Compression Test: a New and Effective Test for Diagnosing Labral Tear and Acromioclavicular Joint Abnormality. *Am J Sports Med* **26**, 610–613.

Plancher, K.D. & Lucas, T.S. (2001) Fracture Dislocations of the Elbow in Athletes. *Clin Sports Med* **20**, 59–76.

Sonzogni, J.J. & Gross, M.L. (1993) Assessment and Treatment of Basketball Injuries. *Clin Sports Med* **12**, 221–237.

Speer, K.P. (1995) Anatomy and Pathomechanics of Shoulder Instability. *Clin Sports Med* **14**, 751–760.

Ticker, J.B. & Warner, J.J.P. (2000) Selective Capsular Shift Technique for Anterior and Anterior-Inferior Glenohumeral Instability. *Clin Sports Med* **19**, 1–17.

Wiesner, S.T. (1994) Rehabilitation of Elbow Injuries in Sports. *PM and R Clin N Am* **5**, 81–113.

Wilson, R.L. & McGinty, L.D. (1993) Common Hand and Wrist Injuries in Basketball Players. *Clin Sports Med* **12**, 265–291.

Wolin, P.M. (1996) Soulders Injuries. In: W.B. Kibler (ed.) *ACSM's Handbook for the Team Physician*, pp. 253–271. Baltimore: Williams & Wilkins.

Chapter 15
Lower extremity considerations

Karim Khan and Jill Cook

Anterior thigh pain

The anterior thigh is the site of common basketball injuries such as quadriceps muscle contusion and strain of the quadriceps muscle. Referred pain from the hip, sacroiliac joint or lumbar spine may also cause anterior thigh pain. A list of causes of anterior thigh pain is shown in Table 15.1. In this section, we illustrate the functional anatomy of the anterior thigh (Fig. 15.1) and outline clinical assessment (history and physical examination). For those conditions that are common in basketball we share our approach to investigation, as well as detailing treatment and rehabilitation. Finally we highlight rare, but important causes of thigh pain the basketball physician must keep in mind when treating players with this presentation.

The main muscle of the anterior thigh is the rectus femoris muscle that spans the anterior inferior iliac crest and the patella, on its way to the tibial tuberosity as the patellar tendon. Sartorius runs

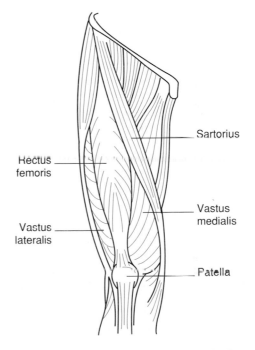

Fig. 15.1 Functional anatomy of the anterior thigh.

Table 15.1 Causes of anterior thigh pain in basketball players.

Common	Less common	Not to be missed
Quadriceps muscle	Referred pain	Slipped capital femoral epiphysis
Contusion	Upper lumbar	(in a young player)
Strain (rectus femoris)	Sacroiliac joint	Tumor (e.g., osteosarcoma
Myositis ossificans	Hip joint	of the femur)
	Sartorius muscle strain	
	Gracilis strain	

more medially, arising from the anterior superior iliac crest and attaching at the medial aspect of the proximal tibia. It is important to remember that hip pathologies can refer to the anterior thigh and knee, so proximal pathologies must be considered when the patient presents with thigh (or knee) pain.

Clinical approach—history and physical examination

The two most important aspects of the history of a basketball player with anterior thigh pain are the exact site of the pain and the mechanism of injury. The site of the pain is usually well localized in cases of contusion or muscle strain. Muscle strains occur in the mid belly, although a contusion can occur anywhere in the quadriceps muscle, most commonly anterolaterally or in the vastus medialis obliquus.

The mechanism of injury may help differentiate between the two conditions. A contusion is likely to be the result of a direct blow, usually by an opponent's knee during running. A muscle strain usually occurs when the player is striving for extra speed while sprinting or extra elevation in rebounding.

In anterior thigh pain of acute onset, the diagnosis is usually straightforward and examination is confined primarily to local structures. In more complicated cases, examination should include sites that refer pain to the thigh, such as the lumbar spine, sacroiliac joint (SIJ) and hip. The aim of the examination is to determine the exact site of the pathology and to assess range of motion and muscle strength.

Quadriceps contusion

If the history suggests a direct blow to the anterior thigh and examination confirms an area of tenderness and swelling with worsening pain on active contraction and passive stretch, thigh contusion with resultant hematoma is the most likely diagnosis. This is known colloquially as a "charley horse". In severe cases with marked swelling, the patient may complain of being unable to sleep because of the severity of pain.

It is important to assess the severity of the contusion in order to give the patient an idea of the prognosis (which can vary from several days to a number of weeks off sport) and plan an appropriate treatment program. It is also necessary to identify the exact muscle involved to optimize treatment and accurately monitor progress. Contusions that occur in the lower third of the thigh are of particular concern as the bleeding may track down to the knee and result in irritation of the patellofemoral joint.

Investigations

Investigations are usually not required in athletes with anterior thigh pain. In cases of quadriceps contusion that fail to respond to treatment and have persistent pain, tenderness and swelling, an X-ray may demonstrate the development of myositis ossificans. This is usually not evident until at least 3 weeks after the injury. Ultrasound examination will confirm the presence of a hematoma and may demonstrate early evidence of calcification.

Treatment

The treatment of a thigh contusion can be divided into four stages:
1 Control of hemorrhage
2 Restoration of pain-free range of motion
3 Functional rehabilitation
4 Graduated return to activity.
Progression within each stage, and from one stage to the next, will depend on the severity of the contusion and the rate of recovery.

The most important period in the treatment of a thigh contusion is in the first 24 h following the injury. Once a thigh contusion occurs, the player should be removed from the field of play and the RICE regimen instituted immediately. The importance of rest and elevation of the affected leg must be emphasized. The use of crutches ensures adequate rest if full weight bearing is painful and encourages the athlete to recognize the serious nature of the condition. Ice should be applied in a position of pain-free muscle stretch. The patient must be careful not to aggravate the bleeding by excessive activity, alcohol ingestion or the application of heat.

Loss of range of motion is the most significant finding after thigh contusion and emphasis needs to be placed on regaining this range of movement in a gradual, pain-free progression.

After a moderate to severe contusion there is a considerable risk of rebleed in the first 7 to 10 days. Therefore, care must be taken with stretching, electrotherapy, heat and massage. During this period the patient must be careful not to overstretch. Stretching should be pain-free.

Emphasis should be placed on the prevention of quadriceps contusion. In those who are recovering from a previous contusion, protection may help prevent a recurrence.

Complication of thigh hematoma—myositis ossificans

Occasionally after a thigh contusion, the hematoma calcifies. This condition is known as myositis ossificans and can usually be seen on a plain X-ray approximately 3 weeks after the injury. The more severe the contusion the more likely is the development of myositis ossificans.

Symptoms of developing myositis ossificans include an increase in morning pain and pain with activity. Patients often complain of night pain. On palpation, the developing myositis ossificans has a characteristic "woody" feel. Initial improvement in range of motion ceases with subsequent deterioration.

Once myositis ossificans is established, there is very little that can be done to accelerate the resorptive process. Treatment may include local electrotherapy to reduce muscle spasm and gentle, painless range of motion exercises. Corticosteroid injection is absolutely contraindicated in this condition.

Quadriceps muscle strain

Basketball-related strains of the quadriceps muscle, most commonly the rectus femoris, usually occur during sprinting or jumping. Like all muscle strains, they may be graded into mild (grade I), moderate (grade II) or severe, complete tears (grade III). The athlete feels the injury as a sudden pain in the anterior thigh during an activity requiring explosive muscle contraction. There is local pain and tenderness and, if the strain is severe, swelling and bruising.

Grade I strain is a minor injury with pain on resisted active contraction and on passive stretching. An area of local spasm is palpable at the site of pain. An athlete with such a strain may not cease activity at the time of the pain but will usually notice the injury after cooling down or the following day.

Moderate or grade II strains cause significant pain on passive stretching as well as on unopposed active contraction. There is usually a moderate area of inflammation surrounding a tender palpable lesion. The athlete with a grade II strain is generally unable to continue the activity.

Complete tears of the rectus femoris are uncommon. They occur with sudden onset of pain and disability during intense activity. A muscle fiber defect is usually palpable when the muscle is contracted. In the long term, they resolve with conservative management, often with surprisingly little disability.

Treatment

Although loss of range of motion may be less obvious than with a contusion, it is important to regain pain-free range of movement as soon as possible. Loss of strength may be more marked than with a thigh contusion and particular emphasis needs to be placed on regaining strength in the rehabilitation program. As with the general principles of muscle rehabilitation, the program should commence with low resistance, high repetition exercise. Concentric and eccentric exercises should begin with very low weights. General fitness needs to be maintained by activities such as swimming (initially with a pool buoy) and upper body training. Functional retraining should be incorporated as soon as possible. Full training must be completed prior to return to sport.

Occasionally, it may be difficult to distinguish between a minor contusion and a minor muscle strain. However, clinically, this difference is important as an athlete with a thigh strain should progress more slowly through a rehabilitation program than should the athlete with quadriceps contusion. The athlete with thigh strain should avoid sharp acceleration and deceleration movements in the early stages of injury.

Less common causes of thigh pain

Referred pain may arise from the hip joint, the sacroiliac joint, the lumbar spine (especially upper lumbar) and neuromeningeal structures. Patients with referred pain may not have a history of injury and have few signs suggesting local pathology. If the history and clinical examination point to hip joint pathology a plain X-ray is indicated. This may show degenerative change in older players and rarely, but importantly, a slipped capital femoral epiphysis in an adolescent.

Acute knee injuries

Acute knee injuries are, unfortunately, a relatively common problem in basketball players. The demands of basketball—especially stopping suddenly to change direction—mean that the sport is rife with major ligament and cartilage injuries. Entire textbooks are devoted to acute knee injuries so this section focuses on specific concerns for basketball players, therapists, and physicians. The reader is directed elsewhere for definitive resources about managing acute knee injuries in general (Ellenbecker 2000; Cooper *et al.* 2001).

Functional anatomy

The knee contains two joints: the tibiofemoral joint with its associated collateral ligaments, cruciate ligaments and menisci; and the patellofemoral joint, which obtains stability from the medial retinaculum and the large patellar tendon passing anteriorly over the patella. In this section we refer to the tibiofemoral joint as the knee joint. The anatomy of the knee joint is shown in Fig. 15.2.

The anterior cruciate ligament (ACL) prevents forward movement of the tibia in relation to the femur, and controls rotational movement. The ACL is essential for controlling the pivoting movements that are fundamental to patterns of play in basketball. Without an intact ACL, a player can suffer an episode of giving way while landing from a rebound, or trying to fake a change of direction. The posterior cruciate ligament (PCL) prevents the femur from sliding forwards off the tibial plateau.

The two collateral ligaments, the medial and lateral, provide medial and lateral stability to the knee joint. The two menisci, medial and lateral, are intra-articular and attach to the tibial plateau and absorb some of the forces placed through the knee joint, thus protecting the otherwise exposed articular surfaces from damage. By increasing the concavity of the tibia, they play a role in stabilizing the knee. In

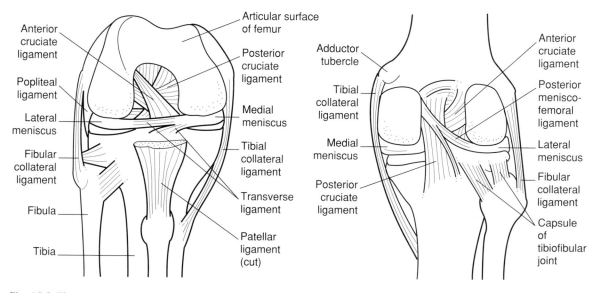

Fig. 15.2 The anatomy of the knee joint.

Table 15.2 Common and less common causes of acute knee pain in a basketball player. All these conditions may occur in isolation or, commonly, in association with other conditions.

Common	Less common
Medial meniscus tear	Fracture of the tibial plateau
MCL sprain	Acute patellofemoral joint injury
ACL rupture	Avulsion fracture
Lateral meniscus tear	Acute fat pad impingement
Articular cartilage injury	Low quadriceps hematoma
PCL sprain	Avulsion of biceps femoris tendon
Patellar dislocation	Dislocated superior tibiofibular joint

ACL, anterior cruciate ligament; MCL, medial collateral ligament; PCL, posterior cruciate ligament.

addition, the menisci contribute to joint lubrication and nutrition. As a result, it is important to preserve as much of the menisci as possible after injury.

Clinical perspective and diagnosis

The acute knee injury of greatest concern to the basketball player is the tear of the ACL. Meniscal injuries are also common. With the advent of arthroscopy and more sophisticated imaging techniques, it has become evident that the articular cartilage of the knee is often damaged in association with ligamentous or meniscal injuries. A list of acute knee injuries occurring in basketball is shown in Table 15.2.

Clinical assessment

Important components of the history include the description of the precise mechanism of injury and the subsequent symptoms, for example, pain and giving way. If the player reports pain without contact—such as while changing direction or while landing from a rebound, an ACL tear must be suspected. If the player reports twisiting the knee while the foot remained planted on the floor, then a meniscal injury is more likely.

The key feature of the knee examination is that each structure that may be injured must be examined. Clues to diagnosis are gleaned from the presence or absence of effusion, assessment of the state of the ligaments and menisci, and range of motion testing. The most important test is the Lachmann's test for anterior cruciate ligament stability.

Investigations

It is necessary to perform an X-ray in cases of moderately severe acute knee injuries in order to detect an avulsion fracture associated with an ACL injury or a tibial plateau fracture following a high-speed injury. An osteochondral fracture may be evident after patellar dislocation. MRI is an excellent adjunct to clinical assessment in cases of uncertain diagnosis, especially if a meniscal abnormality is suspected. MRI is also a useful investigation in determining the extent of ACL injury, articular cartilage damage and patellar tendon injury.

Meniscal injuries

Medial meniscal injuries occur more frequently than lateral meniscal injuries and generally have less morbidity.

The most common mechanism of meniscal injury is a twisting injury with the foot anchored on the ground, often by another player's body. The twisting component may be of comparatively slow speed. The degree of pain associated with an acute meniscal injury varies considerably. Some patients may describe a tearing sensation at the time of injury. Meniscal injuries often occur in association with ACL tears. In these patients a history of locking may be due to either the ACL or the meniscal injury.

On examination, the most important signs of a meniscal tear are joint line tenderness and the presence of a joint effusion. The flexion/rotation (McMurray's) test is positive when pain is produced by the test and a clunk is heard or felt that corresponds to the torn flap being impinged in the joint. MRI examination will usually demonstrate a torn meniscus and is often performed as a preoperative assessment.

The management of meniscal tears varies depending on the severity of the condition. A small tear or a degenerative meniscus should initially be treated conservatively. On the other hand, a large painful "bucket handle" tear, causing a locked knee, requires immediate arthroscopic surgery. The majority of meniscal injuries fall somewhere between these two extremes and the decision on whether to proceed immediately to arthroscopy must be made on the basis of the severity of the symptoms and signs, as well as the demands of the player.

The aim of surgery is to preserve as much of the meniscus as possible. Some peripheral meniscal lesions are suitable for repair by meniscal suture, which can be performed arthroscopically. Partial tears may require removal of the damaged flap of the meniscus. Following meniscal suture, the knee may need full or partial immobilization in a cast or brace for 6 weeks to allow the meniscus to heal.

Arthroscopic partial meniscectomy is usually a straightforward procedure followed by a fairly rapid return to activity. The length of the rehabilitation process depends on the degree of knee injury, especially if the lateral meniscus is injured. The presence of associated abnormalities, such as articular cartilage damage or ligament (MCL, ACL) tears, slows down rehabilitation.

Medial collateral ligament injury

Injury to the medial collateral ligament (MCL) usually occurs when an opponent falls across the knee from lateral to medial. MCL tears are classified on the basis of their severity into grade I (mild, first degree), grade II (moderate, second degree) or grade III (complete, third degree).

In patients with a grade I MCL tear, there is local tenderness over the MCL on the medial femoral condyle but usually no swelling. When a valgus stress is applied at 30° flexion, there is pain but no laxity. A grade II MCL tear is produced by a more severe valgus stress. Examination shows marked tenderness, sometimes with localized swelling. A valgus stress applied at 30° knee flexion causes pain. Some laxity is present but there is a distinct endpoint.

A grade III tear of the MCL results from a severe valgus stress that causes a complete tear of the ligament fibers. The patient often complains of a feeling of instability and a "wobbly knee". The amount of pain is variable and frequently not as severe as one would expect given the nature of the injury.

The treatment of MCL injuries involves a conservative rehabilitation program. Patients with grade III MCL injuries that have been treated conservatively have been shown to return to sport as well as those treated surgically. The rehabilitation program following MCL injury varies depending on the severity.

The more severe MCL injury (the severe grade II or grade III tear) requires a longer period of rehabilitation.

Anterior cruciate ligament tears

Anterior cruciate ligament tears are the most common cause of prolonged absence from basketball. Most ACL tears occur when the athlete is landing from a jump, pivoting or decelerating suddenly. Occasionally, a tear will occur as the result of another player falling across the knee. It is often surprising to patients how a relatively simple movement can result in a torn ACL. At the time of the injury the patient often describes an audible "pop", "crack" or feeling of "something going out and then going back". Most complete tears of the ACL are extremely painful, especially in the first few minutes after injury. Athletes are initially unable to continue their activity, although occasionally they may attempt to resume later when the intense initial pain has settled.

Tear of the ACL is usually accompanied by the development of a hemarthrosis. This may be visible as a large, tense swelling of the knee joint within a few hours of the injury. Occasionally, swelling is minimal or delayed.

The examination findings, although difficult to elicit at times, are also very typical. Athletes with an ACL tear often have restriction of movement, especially loss of extension. They may have widespread mild tenderness. Medial joint line tenderness may be present if there is an associated medial meniscus injury. Lateral joint tenderness is often present, as the knee stretches the lateral joint capsule while subluxating. The Lachman's test is positive in ACL disruption and is the most useful test for this condition.

X-ray of the knee should be performed when an ACL tear is suspected. It may reveal an avulsion of the ligament from the tibia or a "Segond" fracture at the lateral margin of the tibial plateau, pathognomonic of ACL rupture. MRI may be useful in demonstrating an ACL tear when the diagnosis is uncertain clinically. A bone bruise is usually present in conjunction with an ACL injury. The most common site is over the lateral femoral condyle. At present it is not clear whether the presence of a bone bruise is significant in the long term. It may be that those patients with a bone bruise are more prone to the development of osteoarthritis.

Surgical treatment

There are numerous surgical techniques used in the treatment of ACL injuries including using the patellar tendon, iliotibial band, semitendinosus and gracilis tendons. ACL reconstructions are now performed through a small incision with the aid of the arthroscope.

The aim of an ACL reconstruction is to replace the torn ACL with a graft that reproduces the normal kinetic functions of the ligament. In most cases, an autogenous graft, taken from around the knee joint, is used. The most common grafts used are the bone–patellar tendon–bone (BTB) autograft involving the central third of the patellar tendon, or the hamstring (semitendinosus +/– gracilis tendons) graft. The decision on whether to perform a patellar tendon or hamstring reconstruction is dependent on a number of factors. Other graft options include the iliotibial band and allografts.

Management principles have changed dramatically in recent years, resulting in greatly accelerated rehabilitation after ACL reconstruction (Shelbourne & Trumper 1997; Shelbourne et al. 1997). The principle of complete immobilization has been replaced with protected mobilization, with a resultant dramatic decrease in stiffness and increase in range of motion of the knee joint. This has allowed earlier commencement of a strengthening program and rapid progression to functional exercises. The average time for rehabilitation after ACL reconstruction to return to sport has been reduced from around 12 months to 6–9 months.

The timing of return to basketball depends on several different factors, including the surgeon's assessment, the nature of the sport, the therapist and coach's opinion and the confidence of the patient. Functional testing should be used to help assess readiness to return to sport. Functional tests include agility tests, the standing vertical jump and the "Heiden hop". The patient performs the "Heiden

hop" by jumping as far as possible using the uninjured leg, landing on the injured leg. In the light of all these factors and the varying progress of different athletes, the time for return to sport after ACL reconstruction may vary from 4 to 12 months. There are some quantitative measures of function after ACL reconstruction (Mohtadi 1998).

The use of a brace on return to sport is not necessary but may help the athlete's confidence. There is some evidence that wearing a neoprene compression sleeve improves proprioception after ACL reconstruction (Kuster et al. 1999). Some sporting codes have restrictions on the type of brace and material used.

Conservative management

When the clinical diagnosis of an ACL tear is made and the patient selects initial conservative management, an arthroscopy should probably be performed. The aim of this arthroscopy is to assess stability of the knee under anesthesia, to wash out the hemarthrosis, and to assess and treat other injuries such as meniscal tears and articular cartilage damage. Articular cartilage damage indicates a poor prognosis as patients tend to have persistent problems with pain and swelling even after surgery. This is aggravated if a full or partial meniscectomy is required, as the stresses placed on the articular cartilage are increased.

Derotation knee braces may be used as part of the conservative management of ACL tears to provide additional stability when returning to basketball. The effectiveness of these braces varies depending on the degree of instability and the type of brace.

The rehabilitation program for the conservatively managed ACL injury is similar to management after reconstruction. The principles of initial reduction of swelling and pain, restoration of full range of motion, increase of muscle strength and power, functional rehabilitation and, finally, return to sport all apply. Depending on the degree of instability and other associated abnormalities (e.g., articular cartilage damage), the rate of progress may be slower or faster than after a reconstruction. The final stages of the rehabilitation program, the agility work and sport specific drills may not be possible in the patient with ACL deficiency.

Other ligament tears and less common knee injuries

Tears of the PCL do not appear to be as common as of the ACL, due partly to the greater strength of the PCL. However, the condition is probably under-diagnosed (Harner & Hoher 1998). The mechanism of PCL injury is either a hyperextension injury or, more commonly, a direct blow to the anterior tibia with the knee in a flexed position. Lateral collateral ligament tears are much less common than MCL tears and rare in basketball.

Articular cartilage damage varies from gross, macroscopically evident defects in which the under-lying bone is exposed, to microscopic damage that appears normal on arthroscopy but is soft when probed. Articular cartilage damage in the knee has both short-term and long-term effects. Various methods have been used to encourage healing of articular cartilage defects.

Patellar dislocation can occur in basketball when the patella moves out of its groove laterally onto the lateral femoral condyle. Patients who suffer patellar dislocation usually complain that, on twist-ing or jumping, the knee suddenly gave way with the development of severe pain. Often the patient will describe a feeling of something "popping out". Swelling develops almost immediately. The dis-location usually reduces spontaneously with knee extension; however, in some cases this may require some assistance or regional anesthesia (e.g., femoral nerve block).

Treatment of traumatic patellar dislocation may be conservative, although arthroscopic surgery per-mits inspection of the articular surfaces, removal of any osteochondral fragments, joint lavage and perhaps early repair of the medial patellofemoral ligament.

The most important aim of rehabilitation after patellofemoral dislocation is to reduce the chances of a recurrence of the injury. As a result, the rehabil-itation program is lengthy and emphasizes vastus medialis obliquus strength and stretching of the lateral structures. Recurrent patellar dislocation requires surgery.

The patellar tendon occasionally ruptures spon-taneously. This is usually in association with a sud-den severe eccentric contraction of the quadriceps muscle, which may occur when a player jumps or stumbles. The patient may have had a previous his-tory of patellar tendinopathy but this is usually not the case. There may have been a history of previous corticosteroid injection into the tendon.

Patients complain of a sudden acute onset of pain over the patellar tendon accompanied by a tearing sensation and are unable to stand. There is a visible loss of fullness at the front of the knee as the patella is retracted proximally. The athlete finds knee extension impossible. Surgical repair of the tendon is mandatory and must be followed by 6–9 months of intensive rehabilitation.

Anterior knee pain

Anterior knee pain is a common presentation in basketball and one that is feared by many players because the condition "jumper's knee" may be career threatening. This, together with the much more benign condition, the patellofemoral joint syndrome, are the most common causes of anterior knee pain and garner most of the attention in this section (Fig. 15.3). A list of causes of anterior knee pain in basketball players is shown in Table 15.3. Acute knee injuries such as the anterior cruciate ligament rupture are discussed in the previous sec-tion (see Acute knee injuries, p. 194).

After briefly discussing functional anatomy of the patellar and its tendon, we outline clinical assess-ment (history and physical examination) of the bas-ketball player with anterior knee pain. For each of these conditions we discuss the approach to invest-igation, as well as detailing treatment and rehabil-itation. We also alert the reader to a common cause of anterior knee pain in growing children, many of whom play basketball enthusiastically. Finally we highlight rare, but important causes of anterior knee pain which may need to be considered if a player is not responding to treatment.

Functional anatomy

The patellar tendon and the patellofemoral joint, two intimately related structures, are most commonly the culprits when basketball players present with

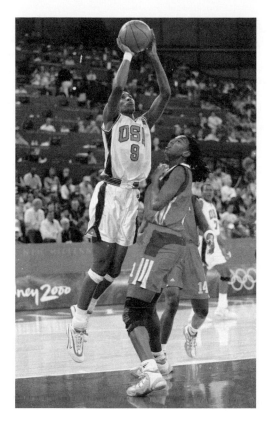

Fig. 15.3 Basketball players can be painfully aware of patellofemoral joint problems. Photo © Getty Images/ Andy Lyons.

anterior knee pain (Fig. 15.4). The patellar tendon pathology generally lies proximally, at the attachment to the patella, on the deep surface. One of the key structures implicated in patellofemoral pain is the large vastus medialis muscle. If its distal fibers contract effectively, it serves to maintain patellar alignment in the femoral trochlea. If basketball players with patellofemoral pain are unable to contract the vastus medialis effectively, they are taught to palpate the region and feel it contract with knee flexion. Also, biofeedback units can be used, with electrodes on the appropriate muscles to train the athlete to contract the muscle appropriately.

Clinical approach—history and physical examination

Distinguishing between patellofemoral syndrome and jumper's knee as a cause of anterior knee pain can be difficult and it is not uncommon for basketball players to have both conditions. The conditions may appear simultaneously as a result of the same biomechanical abnormality or because of overuse, or one may occur first and predispose to the other (see below) (Table 15.4).

Although it is difficult for the patient with anterior knee pain to be very specific in pinpointing the pain, the area of pain often gives an important clue as to which structure is causing pain. For example, medial patellar pain suggests the patellofemoral joint is a likely culprit, predominantly lateral patellofemoral pain indicates excessive lateral pressure syndrome or iliotibial friction syndrome, and inferior patellar pain indicates patellar tendon or infrapatellar fat pad involvement.

The type of activity producing pain also aids diagnosis. Precipitating activities that involve repetitive eccentric loading of the patellar tendon, such as rebounding and plyometrics training suggest the diagnosis of patellar tendinopathy. On the other hand, a player developing anterior knee pain after

Table 15.3 Causes of anterior knee pain in basketball players.

Common	Less common	Not to be missed
Patellofemoral syndrome	Fat pad impingement	Referred pain from the hip
Jumper's knee—patellar tendinopathy	Patellofemoral instability	Osteochondritis dissecans
	Synovial plica	Slipped capital femoral epiphysis
	Quadriceps tendinopathy	Tumor (especially in the young)
	Infrapatellar bursitis	
	Tenoperiostitis of upper tibia	
	Stress fracture of the patella	
	Osgood–Schlatter disease	
	Sinding–Larsen–Johansson syndrome	

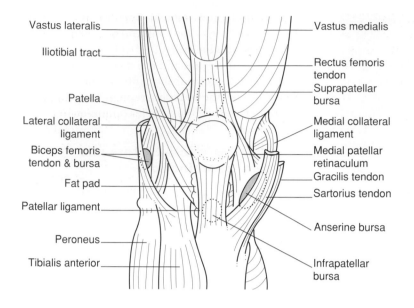

Vastus lateralis

Iliotibial tract

Patella

Lateral collateral
ligament

Biceps femoris
tendon & bursa

Fat pad

Patellar ligament

Peroneus

Tibialis anterior

Vastus medialis

Rectus femoris
tendon

Suprapatellar
bursa

Medial collateral
ligament

Medial patellar
retinaculum

Gracilis tendon

Sartorius tendon

Anserine bursa

Infrapatellar
bursa

Fig. 15.4 The anatomy of the anterior knee.

Table 15.4 Comparison of clinical features of two common causes of anterior knee pain in basketball players.

Signs	Patellofemoral syndrome	Patellar tendinopathy
Onset	Running (especially downhill), steps/stairs training, hill running	Activities involving jumping and landing (e.g., rebounding, repeated jump shot practice, plyometrics)
Pain	Vague/nonspecific, may be medial, lateral or infrapatellar	Usually around inferior pole of patella, aggravated by jumping and mid to full squat
Inspection	Generally normal or vastus medialis muscle wasting	Generally normal or vastus medialis muscle wasting
Tenderness	Usually medial or lateral facets of patella but may be tender in infrapatellar region. May have no pain on palpation due to areas of patella being inaccessible	Most commonly inferior pole of patellar tendon attachment. Occasionally in midtendon, rarely at distal attachment to tibial tuberosity
Patellofemoral joint movement	May be restricted in any direction. Commonly restricted medial glide due to tight lateral structures	May have normal PFJ biomechanics. In combined problem will have PFJ signs
Vastus medialis obliquus	May have obvious wasting, weakness or more subtle deficits in tone and timing	May have generalized quadriceps or vastus medialis obliquus weakness
Functional testing	Squats, stairs may aggravate. PFJ taping should decrease pain	Squats (especially fast) may aggravate. PFJ taping should have no effect

PFJ, patellofemoral joint.

doing a great deal of long distance running in preparation for training camp may be more likely to have patellofemoral syndrome.

During clinical assessment, it is critical to reproduce the patient's anterior knee pain. This is usually done with either a double or single leg squat. This is important both for diagnostic purposes and to provide a baseline measure from which to determine the effectiveness of treatment. The clinician should palpate the anterior knee carefully to determine the site of maximal tenderness. Biomechanical examination is important in determining any predisposing factors.

Jumper's knee or patellar tendinopathy

Jumper's knee is also known as patellar tendinopathy, patellar tendinosis, and, in the past, patellar tendinitis. We use the term "jumper's knee" because it is well entrenched in basketball circles and is apt in this sport. Clinicians generally use the term "patellar tendinopathy" to refer to this condition, as athletes in sports that don't primarily involve jumping can also suffer the condition (e.g., soccer players, sprinters, skiers). The prevalence of jumper's knee is 40–50% among high-level basketball players. Extrinsic factors that predispose to it are total training load, hardness of the floor surface and amount of weight training. Information on intrinsic etiological factors is sparse, but these may be important as almost one in two players have symptoms of jumper's knee in spite of identical extrinsic etiological factors. Studies of the dynamic performance of the leg extensor apparatus suggest that volleyball players with jumper's knee perform generally better than controls. The right knee was affected more often than the left knee among basketball players.

Clinical scenario: jumper's knee

A typical presentation is an Olympic basketball player reporting to the team physician or therapist with infrapatellar pain that is aggravated by jumping. Pain may arise after particularly arduous on-court training, or after activities such as weight training or plyometrics. The player may have previously had problems like this, or, in the younger player, this may be the first episode of such pain. Usually, the player localizes the pain to the inferior pole of the patella.

In this scenario, jumper's knee is suspected and X-ray is generally not required. However, ultrasound (US) or magnetic resonance (MR) imaging both display the patellar tendon well. The presence of hypoechogenicity (US) or high signal abnormality (MR) increases the likelihood that jumper's knee is the diagnosis. However, asymptomatic athletes may have patellar tendons that reveal regions of "abnormal" imaging.

Treatment of jumper's knee

Studies of the outcome of jumper's knee indicate that some players have prolonged symptoms and require more than 6 months treatment before they can return to sport. To tackle this challenging problem, practitioners usually combine treatments that include self-care, medical management and exercise

prescription. If these fail, then surgical intervention is indicated. Each of these components of treatment is discussed below.

Immediate self-care

Basketball players must recognize that jumper's knee is potentially a very serious injury requiring a long period of rehabilitation. Thus, players should present early to their practitioner and report this condition—there is some evidence that early diagnosis and treatment helps minimize the need for time off from basketball.

Ice is one of the most effective therapies that a player can begin. Ice should be applied for no more than 15 min at least once a day. Whether or not a player should begin on nonsteroidal anti-inflammatory medication (which is available without prescription in many countries) is discussed under medical management below.

Medical management

The main pharmaceutical agents used to treat jumper's knee have traditionally been nonsteroidal anti-inflammatory drugs (NSAIDs) and to a lesser extent, corticosteroids. This is unfortunate as jumper's knee is now known to be due to collagen disruption—either due to degeneration or failed healing. Thus, it appears that these medications are playing a decreasing role in management of tendinopathy, particularly in chronic cases.

For the same reason that oral anti-inflammatory medication would appear inappropriate in treatment of tendinopathy, the role of corticosteroids also remains controversial. Jozsa and Kannus (1997) provide guidelines for use of corticosteroid injections (Table 15.5) and these should be adhered to. Note that after injection a tendon is at increased risk of rupture until appropriate strengthening has been undertaken.

Relative tendon unloading

This is critical for treatment success and means the patient may be able to continue playing or training if it is possible to reduce the amount of jumping or sprinting, or the total weekly training hours. Tendon unloading can be achieved by activity modification and by biomechanical correction. Biomechanical abnormalities may be anatomical (static and

Table 15.5 Guidelines for the use of corticosteriod injections.

No repeated injections. Injections should be limited to 2 or 3 spaced a minimum of 2 weeks apart. The 2nd and 3rd injection should only be given if the first injection produced clear improvement

No intratendinous injection

No injection before a competition to make participation possible

No injection for chronic tendon problems that are likely to be due to degeneration

Dilute the corticosteroid with local anesthetic before injection as this reduces the incidence of adverse effects and permits evaluation of any diagnostic pain-relief

Order rest from 1–6 weeks after the injection combined with a gradual tendon strengthening program before allowing return to full activity

dynamic) or functional (resulting from regional dysfunction).

Correcting biomechanics improves the energy-absorbing capacity of the limb both at the affected musculoskeletal junction and at the hip and ankle. The ankle and calf are critical in absorbing the initial landing load transmitted to the knee as about 40% of landing energy is transmitted proximally. Compared with flat-foot landing, forefoot landing generates lower ground reaction forces and if this technique is combined with a large range of hip or knee flexion, vertical ground reaction forces can be reduced by a further 25%.

Common functional biomechanical abnormalities include inflexibility of the hamstrings, iliotibial band, and calf muscles that can lead to functionally restricted knee and ankle range of motion and thus, increase the load on the patellar tendon. Hamstring tightness (decreased sit and reach test) is associated with increased prevalence of jumper's knee. Weakness of the gluteal, lower abdominal, quadriceps and calf muscles lead to fatigue and aberrant movement patterns that may alter forces acting on the knee and restrict range of motion during activity. Therefore, proximal and distal muscles also need assessment in patients with patellar tendinopathy.

Eccentric strengthening

Eccentric strength training refers to the performing of "drop squats" among other exercises with the theoretical goal of stimulating tendon healing and the clinical goal of reducing pain. The drop squat is performed in different ways by different practitioners but one description suggests beginning by standing and then dropping to about 100–120° of knee flexion. In published studies patients perform 3 sets of 10 repetitions per session (one session daily). An effective strength program embraces the principles outlined in Table 15.6.

Because basketball players with jumper's knee tend to "unload" the affected limb to avoid pain, progression should also include single leg exercises. As an additional training stimulus to the tendon, squats performed on a 30° decline board appear to be more effective than those done on flat ground with the heels fixed. The therapist can help the patient progress by adding load and speed to the exercises, and then endurance can be introduced once the patient can do these exercises well. After that, combinations such as load (weight) and speed, or height (e.g., jumping exercises) and load can be added. These end-stage eccentric exercises can provoke tendon pain, and are only recommended after a sufficiently long rehabilitation period and when the sport demands intense loading. Nevertheless, in sports such as basketball, it is essential to add jump training to the rehabilitation program. Ice is used to cool the tendon after the eccentric training.

Table 15.6 Strengthening program for treatment of patellar tendinopathy.

Timing	Type of overload	Activity
0–3 months	Load endurance	Hypertrophy and strengthen the affected muscles, focus attention on the calf as well as the quadriceps and gluteal muscles
3–6 months	Speed endurance	Weight-bearing speed-specific loads
6+ months	Combinations dependent on sport (e.g., load, speed)	Sports-specific rehabilitation

Under close clinician supervision to adjust the program as needed, this type of eccentric training regimen brought complete relief to 30% of patients and marked decrease in symptoms to a further 64%. The remaining 6% had worsening symptoms. A randomized pilot study found eccentric strengthening to provide about 75% success in treating in jumper's knee. The condition often took 12 weeks to resolve. Given the natural history of jumper's knee, these results are encouraging.

Causes of failure in rehabilitation strength programs include: too rapid a progression of rehabilitation; inappropriate loads (not enough strength or speed work, eccentric work too early or aggressively, insufficient single leg work); too many electrotherapeutic modalities, and lack of monitoring patients' symptoms during and after therapy.

Surgery
Patellar tendon surgery is generally reserved for basketball players with jumper's knee who have not improved after at least 6 months of conservative management. A variety of surgical techniques have been used but the outcome of surgery remains rather unpredictable. A review of 23 papers found that authors reported surgical success rates of between 46 and 100%. In the three studies that had more than 40 patients, authors reported combined excellent and good results of 91%, 82%, and 80% in series of 78, 80, and 138 subjects, respectively. The mean time for return to preinjury level of sport varied from 4 months to greater than 9 months. A long-term study of outcome in patients who underwent open patellar tenotomy for patellar tendinosis showed that only 54% were able to return to previous levels of sport activity.

Patellofemoral syndrome

Patellofemoral syndrome is the term used to describe pain in and around the patella. From the 1930s until the 1970s, the term "chondromalacia patellae" was synonymous with patellofemoral pain, because softening was noted on the undersurface of the patella. This term is now out of vogue and has been replaced by nonspecific terms such as patellofemoral syndrome (which we advocate), patellofemoral pain syndrome, patellofemoral joint

Table 15.7 Factors that predispose to patellofemoral syndrome.

Factors	Cause
Abnormal biomechanics	Excessive pronation
	Femoral anteversion (internal femoral torsion)
	High small patella (patella alta)
	Increased Q angle*
Soft tissue tightness	*Muscles*
	Gastrocnemius
	Hamstrings
	Rectus femoris
	Iliotibial band
	Lateral structures
	Lateral retinaculum
	Iliotibial band
	Vastus lateralis
Muscle dysfunction	Vastus medialis obliquus
Training	Hip abductors/external rotators (gluteus medius)
	Distance running
	Hills, stairs

* Angle between line of pull of quadriceps muscle and line of patellar tendon.

syndrome, anterior knee pain, extensor mechanism disorder.

A number of factors predispose to patellofemoral syndrome (Table 15.7) and their role must be assessed as some of them can be corrected (e.g., pronation, soft tissue hip joint stiffness).

Traditionally, one of the major causes of patellofemoral pain was thought to be dysplasia/insufficiency of the vastus medialis obliquus muscle. However, this notion is slowly falling out of favor. It may be that appropriate timing of contraction, rather than muscle bulk may be a key to normal patellofemoral joint biomechanics. Taping the patella of patellofemoral pain sufferers causes an earlier activation of the vastus medialis obliquus and a delayed activation of the vastus lateralis particularly on stair descent. This suggests that the vastus medialis obliquus of the patellofemoral pain sufferers needs to fire earlier to overcome the abnormal tracking forces.

Another predisposing factor for patellofemoral pain is the type and amount of training. Increased training (e.g., increased volume and intensity, hills, steps or squats) increases the load on the patello-femoral joint and this often contributes to the knee pain along with other predisposing factors.

Assessment of patellar position and muscle function

A major component of the treatment of the patellofemoral syndrome is correction of patellofemoral biomechanics, so it is essential to assess the relationships between the patella and the femur and the patella and its surrounding soft tissues. The aim of patellar taping is to site the bone in an ideal position—approximately midway between the two femoral condyles. The most common abnormality is a laterally sited patella which is described as having restricted medial glide. The medial and the lateral patellar borders should be of equal height. A common abnormality is a lower lateral border, a reflection of tight deep retinacular fibers. This is called a lateral tilt. The long axis of the patella should be parallel with the long axis of the femur and deviation is described as a rotational abnormality. The superior and inferior poles of the patella should lie in the same plane. The abnormality seen most commonly in this axis is called posterior tilt and clinically results in the inferior pole being difficult to palpate as it is embedded in the infrapatellar fat pad.

Assessment of muscle function

The clinician must assess the state of the vastus medialis obliquus in weight bearing. In severe cases, there may be frank muscle wasting but for reasons outlined above, it is important also to assess the timing of the vastus medialis obliquus contractions to ensure it is synchronous with the rest of the quadriceps mechanism. Even if the vastus medialis obliquus is strong and bulky it may be rendered ineffective due to its incoordinate action.

Treatment

The management of a patient with patellofemoral syndrome requires an integrated approach which may involve:

- reduction of pain and inflammation;
- taping to correct abnormal patellar position;
- vastus medialis obliquus strengthening;
- stretching;
- massage therapy;
- bracing; and
- correction of abnormal biomechanics.

Reduction of pain and inflammation
This is achieved with a combination of rest from aggravating activities, ice, NSAIDs and electrotherapeutic modalities. Taping should also provide immediate pain relief.

Taping
The aim of taping is to correct the abnormal position of the patella in relation to the femur. Taping the patella relieves pain but the mechanism of the effect is still being investigated. Taping that caused an earlier activation of the vastus medialis obliquus relative to the vastus lateralis was associated with significant pain reduction. Patellar taping has been associated with increases in loading response knee flexion, as well as increases in quadriceps muscle torque. Taping is an effective interim measure to relieve patellofemoral pain while other biomechanical abnormalities (e.g., vastus medialis obliquus weakness, excessive pronation) are being corrected. Taping can cause adverse skin reactions. Therefore, the area to be taped should be shaved and a protective barrier applied beneath the rigid strapping tape to reduce both the reaction to the zinc oxide in the tape adhesive and the reaction to shearing stresses on the skin.

Muscle training
To spread forces more evenly through the patellofemoral joint the basketball player usually needs to train the vastus medialis obliquus and the gluteus medius muscles. This can be done by palpating the vastus medialis. A dual channel biofeedback machine may also be used. The patient needs to be free of patellofemoral pain before these exercises can become effective, otherwise muscle action may be inhibited. Therefore, taping may be required to facilitate the exercise program. The patient should attempt to recruit the vastus medialis obliquus to contract before the rest of the quadriceps. Closed

chain exercise, i.e., when the foot is on the ground, is the preferred method of training, as this improves patellar alignment.

Stretching
Treatment should include stretching of tight lateral structures (e.g., lateral retinaculum).

Braces
Some commercially available braces are available to maintain medial glide. Although braces are less specific than taping and are unable to affect tilt or rotation, they may play a role in those patients who suffer recurrent patellar subluxation or dislocation and in those who are unable to wear tape.

Orthotics
Orthotics can correct excessive subtalar pronation that increases internal rotation of the lower limb and compromises patellar alignment in the femoral groove.

Surgery
The need for surgery in patellofemoral syndrome has been almost eliminated due to the improved understanding of its etiology and the introduction of the vastus medialis obliquus strengthening and taping program. The only indication for surgery in this condition is failure of an appropriate conservative management program.

Osgood–Schlatter disease

Osgood–Schlatter disease is an osteochondrosis that occurs at the tibial tuberosity and is a very common presenting complaint among young basketball players who attend a sports medicine clinic. It arises in girls of around 10–12 and boys of around 13–15 years (but these ages vary) and results from excessive traction on the soft apophysis of the tibial tuberosity by the powerful patellar tendon. It occurs in association with high levels of activity during a period of rapid growth.

Treatment consists of reassurance that the condition is self-limiting and correcting underlying biomechanical abnormalities. Whether or not to play sport depends on the severity of symptoms. Children with mild symptoms may wish to continue

to play some or all sport—others may choose some modification of their programs. If the child prefers to cease sport because of pain he/she should be supported. However, the amount of sport played does not seem to affect the time the condition takes to heal.

Rare conditions not to be missed

If the clinician only focuses on the common conditions, she or he will miss conditions such as hip problems that cause knee pain (e.g., slipped upper femoral epiphysis in 12–14-year-old boys, early osteoarthritis in older athletes). Also in younger people, osteochondritis dissecans can present as knee pain and/or joint effusion, without history of trauma. If the young basketball player has constant tibial tuberosity pain, suggestive of Osgood–Schlatter disease, but it is not alleviated with relative rest, the possibility of benign (osteoid osteoma) or malignant (e.g., osteosarcoma) tumor must be entertained. Although tumors are rare, bone tumors occur in childhood, and the proximal tibia is one of the more commonly affected sites.

Shin pain

Shin pain is commonly a problem for basketball players, particulary those that are attempting to increase their amount of training. This often happens when a player is a freshman joining a college team, or a player making a national or professional training program for the first time. The term "shin splints" has been used in the past to describe the pain along the medial border of the shin but we recommend physicians make a more precise pathological diagnosis and eschew the term "shin splints". A list of the causes of shin pain is shown in Table 15.8. In this section, we illustrate the functional anatomy of the shin (Fig. 15.5) and outline clinical assessment (history and physical examination). We share our approach to management of the three major conditions that cause shin pain in basketball players. Finally we highlight rare, but important causes of shin pain that have caused diagnostic challenges for us on occasions.

Table 15.8 Causes of shin pain in basketball players.

Common	Less common	Not to be missed
Bone (tibia/fibula)	Referred pain	Tumors
Stress fracture	Lumbar spine	Osteosarcoma
Tenoperiostitis	Neuromeningeal structures	Vascular insufficiency
Medial border of the tibia	Superior tibiofibular joint	Acute anterior compartment syndrome
Chronic compartment syndrome	Chronic compartment syndrome	
Deep posterior	Peroneal	
Anterior	Entrapment syndrome	
	Popliteal artery	
	Anterior tibial artery	
	Superficial peroneal nerve	

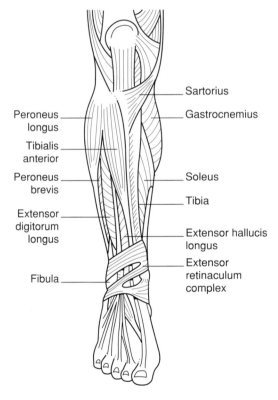

Fig. 15.5 The anatomy of the shin.

Labels: Sartorius; Gastrocnemius; Peroneus longus; Tibialis anterior; Peroneus brevis; Soleus; Tibia; Extensor digitorum longus; Extensor hallucis longus; Extensor retinaculum complex; Fibula

Functional anatomy

Shin pain generally occurs in one or more of three anatomical structures.

• *Bone.* A continuum of increased bone damage exists from bone strain to stress reaction and stress fracture.

• *Tenoperiosteum.* Inflammation develops at the aponeurotic insertion of muscles, particularly tibialis posterior and soleus to the medial border of the tibia.

• *Muscle compartment.* The lower leg has a number of muscle compartments each enveloped by a thick inelastic fascia. The muscle compartments of the lower leg are shown in Fig. 15.6. As a result of overuse, these muscle compartments may become swollen and painful, particularly if there is excessive scarring of the fascia. There are two common compartment syndromes. The deep posterior compartment containing flexor hallucis longus, flexor digitorum longus and tibialis posterior is usually associated with posteromedial tibial pain. The other common compartment syndrome is the anterior compartment syndrome.

Clinical perspective

When a basketball player present with shin pain, the three major pathologies, bone, tenoperiosteum and muscle compartment can usually be distinguished on the basis of history, examination and investigations. It is important to remember that two or all three of these conditions exist together. For instance, it is not uncommon to have a stress fracture develop in a patient with chronic tenoperiostitis.

One of the major causes of all three injuries is abnormal biomechanics. Basketball players who have a rigid, cavus foot have limited shock attenuation which increases the strain placed on bone. Players with excessively pronated feet, must use the muscles of the superficial and deep compartments excessively

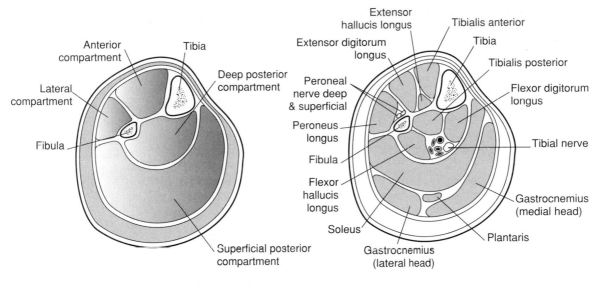

Fig. 15.6 The muscle compartments of the lower leg.

and eccentrically to resist pronation after heel strike. On toe-off, these same muscles then contract concentrically to accelerate supination. With fatigue, these muscles fail to provide the normal degree of shock absorption. This mechanism may lead to the development of a stress fracture or tenoperiostitis and will exacerbate a tendency to develop compartment syndromes.

The most important aspect of the history is the relationship of pain to exercise. If pain improves after warming up and with continued exercise, then tenoperiosteal problems are most likely. If the pain worsens with exercise and is accompanied by a feeling of tightness, then compartment syndrome may be present. If the pain is increased by jumping activities or if there is pain at rest or a night ache, a stress fracture must be considered. A pain that disappears relatively quickly with rest is indicative of compartment syndrome. The presence of associated features, such as numbness, a "dead" feeling in the leg or pins and needles in the foot, is suggestive of compartment syndrome. In the examination of the patient with shin pain, it is important to palpate the site of maximal tenderness and assess the consistency of soft tissue. Determine whether bony tenderness is diffuse, along a stretch of bone (more likely to represent tenoperiostitis) or focal (which may represent a stress fracture). If bony pathology is

suspected, assess whether this is on the anterior cortex of the tibia, or the posteromedial border, as these stress fractures require very different management and have different prognoses (see below).

Stress fracture of the tibia

The athlete with stress fracture of the tibia presents with gradual onset of shin pain, aggravated by exercise. Pain may occur with walking, at rest or even at night. There is localized tenderness over the tibia. Investigation with plain X-ray may reveal a stress fracture of the tibia or fibula but in most cases it is not helpful in the diagnosis of shin pain. Radioisotopic bone scan or MRI are the two best tests for stress fracture. They show a discrete, focal area of increased uptake (bone scan) or high signal abnormality (MRI) on either the tibia or fibula.

Treatment

The treatment of stress fracture of the tibia requires an initial period of rest (sometimes requiring a period of nonweight-bearing on crutches for pain relief) before the pain settles. The patient should continue to rest from basketball and other sporting activities until she/he is able to perform activities of daily living without pain for 2 weeks, and until bony tenderness disappears (4–8 weeks). Then the player can gradually return to training and increase the quality and quantity of play over the following month. Alternative exercises such as swimming, cycling and water running should be prescribed during the enforced lay-off. It is important to determine which factors have precipitated the stress fracture. The most common causes are excessive training and biomechanical abnormalities. If a female player is suffering amenorrhea, it strongly suggests insufficient energy availability, which compromises bone formation.

Tenoperiostitis

The patient with tenoperiostitis complains of pain along the medial border of the tibia which usually decreases with warming up. The athlete can often complete the training session but pain gradually recurs after exercise and is worse the following morning. On examination, there is commonly an area of maximal tenderness along the medial border of the tibia which may extend along the entire tibia or may be as little as 2 cm in length. This usually occurs at the junction of the lower third and upper two-thirds of the tibia.

Investigation with isotopic bone scan or MRI may show a linear increased uptake along the medial border of the tibia (bone scan) or increased abnormal signal at that site (MRI). In the early stages, however, imaging may be normal.

Treatment

Initial treatment is to reduce inflammation by the use of rest, NSAIDs, ice and electrotherapeutic modalities. The most effective definitive treatment involves deep soft tissue massage. The massage therapist should treat the thickened muscle fibers of the soleus, flexor digitorum longus and tibialis posterior adjacent to their bony attachment, avoiding the site of periosteal attachment which may prove too painful. The entire calf muscle should be assessed for areas of tightness or focal thickening that can be treated with appropiate soft tissue techniques. Significant biomechanical abnormalities should be corrected with orthotics. Training should recommence on alternate days only, wearing appropriate footwear and trying to be on a basketball floor that is relatively shock-absorbent.

Chronic compartment syndrome

There are two common chronic compartment syndromes that cause shin pain in basketball players. Deep posterior compartment syndrome typically presents as an ache in the region of the medial border of the tibia or as chronic calf pain. In chronic anterior compartment syndrome, exertional pain is felt lateral to the anterior border of the shin. There may be reduced sensation in the first web space. This condition affects the anterior compartment containing the tibialis anterior, extensor digitorum longus, extensor hallucis longus and peroneus tertius muscles.

In both cases, the patient describes a feeling of tightness or a bursting sensation. Pain increases with exercise. There may be associated distal symptoms (e.g., weakness, pins and needles), which may be indicative of nerve compression. Small muscle hernias occasionally occur along the medial or anterior borders of the tibia after exercise.

In chronic compartment syndromes, imaging may be normal or it may show a linear uptake similar to that of tenoperiostitis. The definitive test for this condition is a compartment pressure test.

Treatment

Treatment consists initially of a conservative regimen of reduced exercise and deep soft tissue therapy. Longitudinal release work with passive and active dorsiflexion is performed to reduce fascial thickening. Transverse frictions are used to treat chronic muscular thickening. Assessment and correction of any biomechanical abnormalities, especially excessive pronation, must be included. If this conservative treatment fails, then surgery is indicated. Fasciotomy (release of the fascial sheath around the compartment) alone is insufficient as the sheath re-forms. It is necessary to perform a fasciectomy (removal of the fascial sheath) in addition to the fasciotomy.

Acute compartment syndrome—a medical emergency

Occasionally, acute compartment syndrome may develop following a direct blow. This is a medical emergency and has a very different treatment pathway to chronic, or exertional, compartment syndrome.

Ankle injuries in basketball

It has been estimated that there are 25 000 ankle sprains each day in the USA (Kannus & Renstrom 1991). Although the term "sprained ankle", is sometimes thought to be synonymous with "lateral ligament injury" and thus, implies a rather benign injury, this is not always the case. If the ankle injury is indeed a lateral ligament sprain, inadequate rehabilitation can lead to prolonged symptoms, decreased sporting performance and high risk of recurrence. Thus, the first half of this section focuses on clinical assessment and management of lateral ligament injuries after ankle sprain in basketball.

The seemingly benign presentation of "sprained ankle" can also mask damage to other structures in addition to the ankle ligaments, such as subtle fractures around the ankle joint, osteochondral fractures of the dome of the talus and dislocation of the peroneal tendons (Brukner & Khan 2001). Such injuries are frequently not diagnosed and, thus, cause ankle pain that persists much longer than would be expected with a straightforward ankle sprain. This is often referred to as "the difficult ankle" and this presentation is discussed in the second half of this section (pp. 212–213).

Clinical scenario: ankle sprain

A typical presentation is a basketball player reporting to the team physician or therapist after having sprained his or her ankle. Sprains usually occur when landing on a teammate or opposition player's foot after a rebound. They can also occur when a player is driving to the basket in traffic (i.e., moving among many players in the crowded key area toward the basket). Players experience immediate pain on the lateral aspect of the ankle, and swelling begins after only a few minutes in the same region unless adequate first aid is given on site. Players are often unable to bear any weight on the leg, or they can partially weight bear. Players have often suffered several previous sprains to the same ankle.

Clinical approach

Although lateral ligament sprain is by far the most common result of an ankle injury, other possible outcomes have to be considered as listed in Table 15.9. The most important issue is to distinguish between ligament injuries and fractures. Fractures are rare among adolescent and young adult players, but fractures of the lateral malleolus and 5th metatarsal occur more often in the older recreational athlete. Since they may require early surgery, it is also important not to miss growth plate injuries in children or injuries to the syndesmosis. History should be taken carefully, since the mechanism of injury is an important clue to diagnosis after ankle sprain. A precise examination will reveal whether it is necessary to submit the patient to an X-ray examination to rule out fractures. If a fracture is suspected, an X-ray examination should be completed

Table 15.9 Common, less common, and important but rare conditions resulting from ankle sprain.

Common	Less common	Not to be missed
Ligament sprain	Osteochondral lesion of the talus	Reflex sympathetic dystrophy (postinjury)
Lateral ligaments	Ligament sprain	Greenstick fractures (children)
	Medial ligament	Ruptured syndesmosis
	AITFL	
	Fractures	
	Lateral/medial/posterior	
	Malleolus (Pott's)	
	Tibial plafond	
	Base of the fifth metatarsal	
	Other fractures	
	Dislocated ankle (fracture/dislocation)	
	Tendon rupture/dislocation	

AITFL, anteroinferior tibiofibular ligament.

without delay. Acute fracture surgery—if necessary—should be performed within six hours before the swelling is excessive.

The goal of the initial examination therefore, is to decide whether the patient has a lateral ligament injury, and not a different injury which may require surgery or immobilization.

History

The typical injury mechanism is stepping on an opponent's foot while stepping or landing from a jump with the foot in an inverted position, i.e., plantarflexed, internally rotated and supinated. The ligaments rupture from an anterior to a posterior direction. The forces involved determine the number of partially or completely injured ligaments. In about half the cases, there is an isolated tear of the anterior talofibular ligament only, in about 25% there is a combined rupture of the anterior talofibular and calcaneofibular ligaments, whereas additional rupture of the posterior talofibular ligament is rare (1%). If there is an eversion injury (pronation and external rotation), a medial ligament injury must be suspected, but this is rare. The practitioner needs to be aware that if the injury mechanism is atypical, it may cause injuries other than the routine lateral ligament injury.

Clinical examination

The main objective of the clinical examination is to rule out ankle fractures and syndesmosis injury. Ankle X-rays are only required if there is bone tenderness to palpation according to the Ottawa ankle rules or the patient is unable to bear weight both immediately and at the clinical assessment. The sensitivity of this procedure to detect clinically significant fractures is 100%.

Injury to the syndesmosis can be revealed by a number of specific tests. The squeeze test is performed by compressing the fibula against the tibia about halfway between the knee and ankle. If the syndesmosis is injured, this test will cause pain at the site. Another test is the external rotation test, which is done by externally rotating the foot with the ankle in 90 degree flexion. Again, the test is positive if it elicits pain in the syndesmosis region.

These tests usually do not cause significant pain if only the lateral ligaments are injured. Further X-ray investigations are necessary if these tests raise suspicion that the syndesmosis may be injured.

Traditional dogma posits that the anterior drawer and talar tilt tests can be used to evaluate whether the ankle is mechanically unstable after a significant lateral ligament injury. The anterior drawer test should be positive if the anterior talofibular ligament is torn. If the talar tilt test is positive, this may be taken as a sign that the calcaneofibular ligament is ruptured as well. However, clinical studies have shown that these tests have very limited value in the acute phase and that it is not possible to distinguish between total and partial ruptures, or between isolated or combined lateral ligament based on these tests. Therefore, the anterior drawer and talar tilt tests are not helpful in the management of the acutely injured ankle.

Imaging

If there are signs indicating that a fracture may be present according to the Ottawa ankle rules, a routine X-ray investigation including anteroposterior (AP), lateral and mortise views are indicated. Also, the same investigations are indicated if the physical examination has raised suspicion of a syndesmosis injury. Other imaging studies are usually not indicated in the acute phase.

Treatment of ankle injuries

The management of lateral ligament injuries is conservative, even if there is a combined injury to the anterior talofibular and calcaneofibular ligament. Functional treatment has been shown to give at least equal results to surgical repair and/or casting regardless of degree of lateral ligament injury. Functional treatment provides the quickest recovery of full range of motion and return to physical activity, does not compromise mechanical stability more than other treatments, and is safer and cheaper.

The goals of a functional treatment program is to minimize initial injury, swelling and pain, to restore range of motion, muscle strength and proprioception, and then graduate to a sport-specific exercise program.

Immediate self-care

Initial management

Lateral ligament injuries require RICE treatment. This essential treatment limits hemorrhage and subsequent edema that would otherwise cause an irritating synovial reaction and restrict joint range of motion. The injured athlete must avoid factors that will promote blood flow and swelling, such as hot showers, heat rubs, alcohol or excessive weight bearing.

Reduction of pain and swelling

Pain and swelling can be reduced with the use of electrotherapeutic modalities (e.g., TENS, interferential stimulation, magnetic field therapy). Analgesics may be required. After 48 h, gentle soft tissue therapy and mobilization may reduce pain. By reducing pain and swelling, muscle inhibition around the joint is minimized, permitting the patient to begin range of motion exercises.

The indications for the use of NSAIDs in ankle injuries are unclear. The majority of practitioners tend to prescribe these drugs after lateral ligament sprains although their efficacy has not been proven. The rationale for commencing NSAIDs 2–3 days after injury is to reduce the risk of joint synovitis with return to weight bearing.

Restoration of full range of motion

If necessary, the patient may be nonweight-bearing on crutches for the first 24 h but then should commence partial weight bearing in normal heel–toe gait. This can be achieved while still using crutches or, in less severe cases, by protecting the damaged joint with strapping or bracing. Thus, partial and, ultimately, full weight bearing can take place without injury. Lunge stretches, accessory and physiological mobilization of the ankle, subtalar, and midtarsal joints should begin early in rehabilitation. As soon as pain allows, the practitioner should prescribe active range of motion exercises (e.g., stationary cycling).

Muscle conditioning

Active strengthening exercises including plantarflexion, dorsiflexion, inversion and eversion should begin as soon as pain allows. They should be progressed by increasing resistance (a common method is to use rubber tubing). Strengthening eversion with the ankle fully plantarflexed is particularly important in prevention of future lateral ligament injuries. Weight-bearing exercises (e.g., shuttle, wobble board exercises) are encouraged as soon as pain permits.

Proprioceptive training

An important factor in the rehabilitation after an ankle sprain is to train neuromuscular control during balance exercises. Proprioceptive function is impaired in patients with residual functional instability after previous sprains, can be improved by balance board exercise, and the risk of reinjury can be reduced to the level of a previously uninjured ankle. Proprioceptive training should be carried out for 6–10 weeks after an acute injury.

Functional exercises

Functional exercises (e.g., jumping, hopping, twisting, figure-of-eight running) can be prescribed when the athlete is pain-free, has full range of motion and adequate muscle strength and proprioception. Specific technical training not only accelerates a player's return to sport, but it can also substantially reduce the risk of reinjury (Bahr *et al*. 1997).

Return to sport

Return to sport is permitted when functional exercises can be performed without pain during or after activity. While performing rehabilitation activities and upon return to sport, added ankle protection should be provided with either taping or bracing. The relative advantages of taping and bracing have been discussed in Chapter 6. As both seem equally effective, the choice of taping or bracing depends on patient preference, cost, availability and expertise in applying tape.

Any athlete who has had a significant lateral ligament injury should use protective taping or bracing while playing sport for a minimum of 6–12 months postinjury (Bahr *et al*. 1994). There are a number of methods to protect against inversion injuries. The three main methods of tape application are stirrups, heel lock, and the figure of six. Usually at least two of these methods are used simultaneously.

Braces have the advantage of ease of fitting and adjustment, lack of skin irritation and reduced cost compared with taping over a lengthy period. There are a number of different ankle braces available. The lace-up brace is popular and effective.

Treatment of grade III injuries

A review of 12 prospective randomized trials concluded that rehabilitation was the treatment of choice for acute complete tears of the lateral ligaments of the ankle (Kannus & Renstrom 1991). Also, Finnish researchers compared surgical treatment (primary repair plus early controlled mobilization) with early controlled mobilization alone in a prospective study of 60 patients with grade III lateral ankle ligament injuries (Kaikkonen *et al*. 1996). Of the patients treated with rehabilitation alone, 87% had excellent or good outcomes compared with 60% of patients treated surgically. Thus, early mobilization alone provided a better outcome than surgery plus mobilization in complete tears of the lateral ankle ligaments.

Thus, all grade III ankle injuries warrant a trial of initial conservative management over a 6-week period, irrespective of the caliber of the athlete. If, despite appropriate rehabilitation and protection, the patient complains of recurrent episodes of instability or persistent pain, then surgical reconstruction of the lateral ligament is indicated. Suitable grafts include one of the peroneal tendons or a fibular periosteal flap. Following surgery, it is extremely important to undertake a comprehensive rehabilitation program to restore full joint range of motion, strength and proprioception. The principles of rehabilitation outlined under "treatment and rehabilitation of lateral ligament injuries" above, are appropriate.

"The difficult ankle"—persistent pain or instability

While most patients with a lateral ligament injury do well after functional treatment, some have resid-

ual complaints. The prevalence of problems ranges from 18% to 78% in different studies. In the acute phase it is therefore important to inform patients to return for follow-up if they have persisting problems after the completion of functional rehabilitation. It is useful to classify patients with residual complaints into separate categories—those complaining of pain, stiffness, and swelling, and patients with recurrent sprains and instability episodes.

The cause of pain, stiffness and residual swelling is often chondral or osteochondral injury in the ankle joint. Such lesions are more common after high energy injuries, such as when landing after a maximal jump—and may therefore be expected to occur more often in basketball players than in some other sports. Focal uptake on a bone scan may indicate that there is an osteochondral injury. A CT or MRI scan can be used to differentiate between subchondral fractures and chondral fractures with or without separation and/or displacement. Patients with persistent symptoms and chondral injuries should be referred to an orthopedic surgeon. Pain may also result from impingement of scar tissue, in particular in the anterolateral corner of the ankle joint.

Instability may result from mechanical or functional instability. Mechanical instability can occur after complete ligament tears if the scar tissue is lengthened and provides inadequate mechanical support, while functional instability results from inadequate sensorimotor control. Some patients can suffer from both mechanical instability and loss of sensorimotor control. Subtalar instability may also result from ankle sprains, and the sinus tarsi pain syndrome may occur as a sequel to an ankle sprain.

The anterior drawer and talar tilt tests may be used to check the mechanical stability of the ankle joint in chronic cases. Stress X-rays are generally unhelpful and falling out of favor. A simple functional balance test may be used to estimate sensorimotor control, although the predictive value of the test has not been properly documented. The patient is instructed to stand on one leg for one minute with arms held across the chest, eyes fixed forward and the opposite leg straight down. The test is said to be normal if the patient can complete one minute on one leg and stand for more than 45 s without balance adjustments other than in the ankle. The test result is above normal if the patient can complete an additional 15 s with eyes closed.

Patients with persistent instability symptoms should complete at least 10 weeks of intensive proprioceptive training during which time they should wear tape or a brace to prevent reinjuries. If instability episodes persist even after an adequate proprioceptive training program has been completed, the patient should be referred to an orthopedic surgeon for evaluation.

Foot problems in basketball

Foot problems in basketball players range from common inconveniences such as calluses, ingrown toenails, and blisters to potentially career threatening conditions such as the Jones' fracture and navicular stress fractures. In this section we focus on these two particularly challenging basketball fractures. It is widely known that Michael Jordan suffered a navicular stress fracture early in his professional career, but he was fortunate to receive expert medical advice, undergo appropriate nonweight-bearing cast treatment, and make the full recovery that the basketball world witnessed with such great pleasure.

Rear foot pain—plantar fasciitis

The most common cause of rear foot (inferior heel) pain in basketball players is plantar fasciitis. Players often refer to this as "heel spur(s)". Plantar fasciitis is an overuse condition of the plantar fascia at its attachment to the calcaneus. The player may report that pain in the heel is worse in the morning and improves during the day. There may be a history of other leg or foot problems in patients with abnormal biomechanics.

There is point tenderness at the medial process of the calcaneal tuberosity that may extend some centimeters along the medial border of the plantar fascia. Stretching the plantar fascia may reproduce pain.

Excessive pronation is frequently associated with plantar fasciitis (Cornwall & McPoil 1999). An abducted gait or calf tightness may reduce the athlete's ability to supinate, increasing the strain on the plantar fascia. X-ray may show a calcaneal spur

even though these spurs are not causally related to pain (Lu *et al.* 1996).

Treatment includes avoidance of aggravating activity, cryotherapy after activity, stretching of the plantar fascia, gastrocnemius and soleus, the insertion of a heel cup or wedge, the use of shoes with adequate support and flexibility, NSAIDs, electrotherapy and taping. A night splint may be helpful in some individuals (Batt *et al.* 1996; Probe *et al.* 1999). Corticosteroid injection may be very effective when combined with biomechanical correction. Surgery is sometimes required in players with a rigid, cavus foot who do not respond to conservative management.

Stress fractures of the navicular

Stress fractures of the navicular are among the most common stress fractures seen in the jumping athlete, which is why they are not uncommonly seen in basketball players (Khan *et al.* 1994). The history is usually one of a poorly localized midfoot ache associated with activity. Unlike most stress fractures, pain settles quickly with rest. If, however, palpation confirms tenderness over the "N spot" the athlete should be considered to have a navicular stress fracture until proven otherwise.

Sensitivity of X-ray in navicular stress fracture is poor (Khan *et al.* 1992). Thus, either MR imaging or isotopic bone scan (with CT scan if positive) is required.

Treatment of navicular stress fracture is *strict* nonweight-bearing immobilization in a cast for 6 weeks (Khan *et al.* 1992). At the end of this period the cast should be removed and the "N spot" palpated for tenderness. Generally, the "N spot" will be nontender but, if tenderness is present, the patient should have the cast reapplied for a further 2 weeks of nonweight-bearing immobilization. Management must be based on the clinical assessment as the radiological defect persists on CT scan well after clinical union of the stress fracture has occurred (Khan *et al.* 1992).

Often, patients with these fractures will present after a long period of pain or after a period of weight-bearing rest. All patients, even if they have been unsuccessfully treated with prolonged weight-bearing rest or short-term cast immobilization, should undergo cast immobilization for a 6-week period. This method of treatment produces excellent results and may be successful even in long-standing cases.

Following removal of the cast, it is essential to mobilize the stiff ankle, subtalar and midtarsal joints. The calf muscles require soft tissue therapy and exercise to regain strength. This must be done before resuming running. Activity must be resumed gradually, building up to full training over a period of 6 weeks. Predisposing factors to navicular stress fractures may include tarsal coalition, excessive pronation and restricted dorsiflexion of the ankle. These factors need to be corrected before resuming activity.

Midtarsal joint sprains

The midtarsal joints are occasionally sprained and most commonly result in sprain of the calcaneo-navicular ligament. Local tenderness and limitation of midtarsal movement are usually present. Electrotherapeutic modalities may be helpful and taping may provide additional support. Orthotics may be required. Following a joint sprain, joint inflammation occasionally develops. This generally responds well to NSAIDs but if it persists the patient may benefit from a corticosteroid injection into one of the midtarsal joints.

Lisfranc's fracture-dislocation

Lisfranc's fracture-dislocation is rare in sport but because of its disastrous consequences if untreated, must be considered in all cases of "midfoot sprain" in a basketball player. The eponym Lisfranc's joint refers to the tarsometatarsal joints—the bases of the five metatarsals with their corresponding three cuneiforms and cuboid. The most common mechanism of injury is via an axial load applied to a plantarflexed foot, rupturing the weak dorsal tarsometatarsal ligaments. As the injury progresses the plantar aspect of the metatarsal base fractures, or the plantar capsule ruptures and the metatarsal may displace dorsally. Thus, a fracture at the plantar base of a metatarsal can be a clue to a subtle Lisfranc's injury.

A patient with this injury may complain of midfoot pain and difficulty weight bearing (Mantas & Burks 1994). Bony deformity may range from none to the most obvious. The dorsum of the foot is diffusely swollen. The injured joints will be tender. Gentle stressing of the forefoot into plantarflexion, particularly with rotation, reproduces pain. Neurovascular examination is mandatory as the dorsalis pedis artery can be compromised in the initial injury, or by subsequent swelling of the foot.

Investigation requires weight-bearing plain X-ray (Faciszewski et al. 1990) but even with this technique the diagnosis is often missed (Preidler et al. 1999). Also, spontaneous reduction may follow severe injury so subtle radiologic signs must be noted. These include the fracture of the dorsal base of the 2nd metatarsal ("fleck sign") and compression fracture of the cuboid. If there is clinical suspicion of a Lisfranc's injury and X-ray is normal, CT should be ordered as this has greater sensitivity. Bone scan may also be used to rule out occult fracture.

Treatment depends on the severity of injury. Precise anatomic reduction is required. If that is present and there is no gross instability on testing, then 6 weeks below-knee cast immobilization is indicated (Faciszewski et al. 1990). Close neurovascular observation is indicated, especially during early stages. In cases of joint displacement, closed reduction with traction is indicated. It can be difficult to maintain anatomic reduction in plaster because of the swelling and the inherent instability of the injury, so percutaneous wires are often used to stabilize the joint. Some difficult cases require open reduction with internal fixation (Anderson 1993). This is a significant injury that has a much better prognosis if managed correctly initially, rather than being salvaged once there is prolonged joint malalignment and nonunion (Curtis et al. 1993).

Fractures of the fifth metatarsal

Two different fractures affect the base of the fifth metatarsal (Yu & Shapiro 1998). The fracture of the tuberosity at the base of the fifth metatarsal is usually an avulsion injury that results from an acute ankle sprain. This uncomplicated fracture heals well with a short period of immobilization for pain relief.

A serious fracture of the fifth metatarsal is the fracture of the diaphysis known as a Jones' fracture.

This may be the result of an inversion plantarflexion injury or, more commonly, as a result of overuse. A Jones' fracture requires 6–8 weeks of nonweight-bearing cast immobilization (DeLee *et al.* 1983). Non-union may be treated by bone grafting or screw fixation. Because of the prolonged healing time, immediate screw fixation may be considered in certain clinical situations.

Sesamoid injuries

The medial and lateral sesamoid bones act as pulleys for the flexor hallucis brevis tendons. They stabilize the first MTP joint. The sesamoid bones may be injured by traumatic fracture, stress fracture, sprain of a bipartite sesamoid and sprain of the sesamoid-metatarsal articulation. Sesamoid pathology involves inflammatory changes and osteonecrosis around the sesamoid. The medial sesamoid is usually affected. The patient complains of pain with forefoot weight bearing and will often walk with weight laterally to compensate. There is marked local tenderness and swelling.

Inflammation may be caused by landing heavily after a jump, increased forefoot weight-bearing activities (e.g., preseason training with much full court sprinting) or after traumatic dorsiflexion of the hallux. Pronation may cause lateral displacement or subluxation of the sesamoids within the plantar grooves of the first metatarsal. This subluxation of the sesamoids may lead to erosion of the plantar aspect of the first metatarsal resulting in pain underneath the first metatarsal head, arthritic changes and ultimately decreased dorsiflexion. Sprain of a bipartite sesamoid also occurs. A bipartite sesamoid is present in approximately 30% of individuals.

Treatment of sesamoid pain is with ice and electrotherapeutic modalities to reduce inflammation. Padding is used to distribute the weight away from the sesamoid bones and technique correction is mandatory in activities such as dance. In ballet, this injury arises because of excessive rolling in of the foot, which is commonly due to "forcing turnout". Corticosteroid injection into the joint space between the sesamoid and metatarsal may prove effective if underlying abnormalities have been corrected. Orthotics are required if foot mechanics are abnormal.

Surgery should be avoided if possible as the removal of a sesamoid bone causes significant muscle imbalances and may contribute to a hallux abducto-valgus deformity (Leventen 1991). However, excision is required in cases of significant osteonecrosis. Partial sesamoidectomy has been used without success and there are now reports of an arthroscopic approach to this joint (Perez Carro *et al.* 1999).

Stress fractures of the sesamoid bones are not uncommon in basketball players (Brukner *et al.* 1999). Radioisotopic bone scan confirms the presence of a stress fracture. These stress fractures are prone to nonunion and sometimes require nonweight-bearing for a period of 6 weeks.

Corns and callus

Basketball players are prone to excessive pressure on skin which may cause hypertrophy of the squamous cell layer of the epidermis and manifest as corns and calluses. Treatment involves the removal of circumscribed corns and diffuse areas of callus with a scalpel, the wearing of well-fitting footwear and, if abnormal foot mechanics are present, orthotic therapy. Petroleum jelly over the corn or callus and on the outside of the sock can also help.

References

Anderson, R.B. (1993) In: Pfeffer, G.B. & Frey, C.C. (eds) *Current Practice in Foot and Ankle Surgery*. New York: McGraw-Hill, pp. 129–159.

Bahr, R., Karlsen, R., Lian, O. & Ovrebo, R.V. (1994) Incidence and mechanisms of acute ankle inversion injuries in volleyball. A retrospective cohort study. *American Journal of Sports Medicine* **22**, 595–600.

Bahr, R., Lian, O. & Bahr, I.A. (1997) A twofold reduction in the incidence of acute ankle sprains in volleyball after the introduction of an injury prevention program: a prospective cohort study. *Scandinavian Journal of Medicine and Science in Sports* **7**, 172–177.

Batt, M.E., Tanji, J.L. & Skattum, N. (1996) Plantar fasciitis: a prospective randomized clinical trial of the tension night splint. *Clinical Journal of Sport Medicine* **6**, 158–162.

Brukner, P., Bennell, K. & Matheson, G. (1999) *Stress Fractures*. Melbourne: Blackwell Science.

Brukner, P. & Khan, K. (2001) *Clinical Sports Medicine*, 2nd edn, pp. 553–573. Sydney: McGraw-Hill.

Cooper, R., Crossley, K. & Morris, H. (2001) Low back pain. In: Brukner, P. & Khan, K. (eds) *Clinical Sports Medicine,* 2nd edn, pp. 426–463. Sydney: McGraw-Hill.

Cornwell, M. & McPoil, T. (1999) Plantar fasciitis: etiology and treatment. *Journal of Orthopedic Sports Physical Therapy* **29**, 756–760.

Curtis, M.J., Myerson, M. & Szura, B. (1993) Tarsometatarsal joint injuries in the athlete. *American Journal of Sports Medicine* **21**, 497–502.

DeLee, J.C., Evans, P. & Julian, J. (1983) Stress fractures of the fifth metatarsal. *American Journal of Sports Medicine* **11**, 349–353.

Ellenbecker, T.S. (2000) *Knee Ligament Rehabilitation.* New York: Churchill Livingstone.

Faciszewski, T., Burks, R.T. & Manaster, B.J. (1990) Subtle injuries of the Lisfranc joint. *Journal of Bone and Joint Surgery* **72**, 1519–1522.

Harner, C.D. & Hoher, J. (1998) Evaluation and treatment of posterior cruciate ligament injuries. *American Journal of Sports Medicine* **26**, 471–482.

Jozsa, L. & Kannus, P. (1997) *Human Tendons.* Champaign, IL: Human Kinetics.

Kaikkonen, A., Kannus, P. & Jarvinen, M. (1996) Surgery versus functional treatment in ankle ligament tears. A prospective study. *Clinical Orthopaedics* **326**, 194–202.

Kannus, P. & Renstrom, P. (1991) Treatment of acute tears of the lateral ligament of the ankle. *Journal of Bone and Joint Surgery* **73**, 305–312.

Khan, K.M., Fuller, P.J., Brukner, P.D., Kearney, C. & Burry, H.C. (1992) Outcome of conservative and surgical management of navicular stress fracture in athletes. Eighty-six cases proven with computerized tomography. *American Journal of Sports Medicine* **20**, 657–666.

Khan, K.M., Brukner, P.D., Kearney, C., Fuller, P.J., Bradshaw, C.J. & Kiss, Z.S. (1994) Tarsal navicular stress fracture in athletes. *Sports Medicine* **17**, 65–76.

Kuster, M.S., Grob, K., Kuster, M., Wood, G.A. & Gachter, A. (1999) The benefits of wearing a compression sleeve after ACL reconstruction. *Medicine and Science in Sports and Exercise* **31**, 368–371.

Leventen, E.O. (1991) Sesamoid disorders and treatment. An update. *Clinical Orthopaedics* **269**, 236–240.

Lu, H., Gu, G. & Zhu, S. (1996) Heel pain and calcaneal spurs. *Chung Hua Wai Ko Tsa Chih* **34**, 294–296.

Mantas, J.P. & Burks, R.T. (1994) Lisfranc injuries in the athlete. *Clinics in Sports Medicine* **13**, 719–730.

Mohtadi, N. (1998) Development and validation of the quality of life outcome measure (questionnaire) for chronic anterior cruciate ligament deficiency. *American Journal of Sports Medicine* **26**, 350–359.

Perez Carro, L., Echevarria Llata, J.I. & Martinez Agueros, J.A. (1999) Arthroscopic medial bipartite sesamoidectomy of the great toe. *Arthroscopy* **15**, 321–323.

Preidler, K.W., Peicha, G., Lajtai, G. *et al.* (1999) Conventional radiography, CT, and MR imaging in patients with hyperflexion injuries of the foot: diagnostic accuracy in the detection of bony ligamentous changes. *American Journal of Roentgenology* **173**, 1673–1677.

Probe, R.A., Baca, M., Adams, R. & Preece, C. (1999) Night splint treatment for plantar fasciitis. A prospective randomized study. *Clinical Orthopaedics* **368**, 190–195.

Shelbourne, K.D. & Trumper, R.V. (1997) Preventing anterior knee pain after anterior cruciate ligament reconstruction. *American Journal of Sports Medicine* **25**, 41–47.

Shelbourne, K., Klootwyk, T. & DeCarlo, M. (1997) Rehabilitation program for anterior cruciate ligament reconstruction. *Sports Medicine Arthritis Review* **5**, 77–82.

Yu, W.D. & Shapiro, M.S. (1998) Fractures of the fifth metatarsal. Careful identification for optimum treatment. *The Physician and Sportsmedicine* **26**, 47–64.

Index

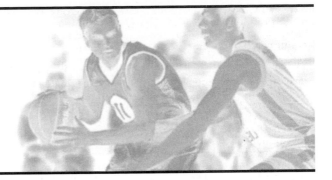